The Self in Emotional Distress

The Self in Emotional Distress

Cognitive and Psychodynamic Perspectives

Edited by
ZINDEL V. SEGAL
Clarke Institute of Psychiatry,
University of Toronto

SIDNEY J. BLATT
Yale University

THE GUILFORD PRESS
New York London

A Division of Guilford Publications, Inc.
72 Spring Street, New York, NY 10012

Printed in the United States of America

This book is printed on acid-free paper.

Last digit is print number: 9 8 7 6 5 4 3 2 1

Library of Congress Cataloging-in-Publication Data

The Self in emotional distress : cognitive and psychodynamic perspectives / edited by Zindel V. Segal, Sidney J. Blatt.
p. cm.
Includes bibliographical references and index.
ISBN 0-89862-256-5
1. Self-perception. 2. Psychology, Pathological. 3. Self psychology. I. Segal, Zindel V., 1956– . II. Blatt, Sidney J. (Sidney Jules)
[DNLM: 1. Behaviorism. 2. Mental Disorders—etiology. 3. Psychoanalytic Theory. 4. Self Concept. WM 100 S465]
RC455.4.S42S445 1993
616.89071—dc20
DNLM/DLC
for Library of Congress 92-49988
CIP

For Lisa Ann
—Z. V. S.

For the Grandchildren:
Lesley, William, Ruth, Sarah, and Madeline . . .
—S. J. B.

Contributors

SUSAN A. BERS, Ph.D., Department of Psychiatry, Yale University, New Haven, Connecticut

SIDNEY J. BLATT, Ph.D., Departments of Psychiatry and Psychology, Yale University, New Haven, Connecticut

ROBERT P. COHEN, Ph.D., Detroit Psychiatric Institute, Detroit, Michigan; Michigan Psychoanalytic Institute, Southfield, Michigan

STEVEN H. COOPER, Ph.D., Harvard Medical School, Boston, Massachusetts; Boston Psychoanalytic Society and Institute, Boston, Massachusetts

TRACY D. EELLS, Ph.D., Department of Psychiatry and Behavioral Sciences, University of Louisville, Louisville, Kentucky

LINDA S. EWALD, M.A., Department of Psychology, University of Hawaii, Honolulu, Hawaii

BRAM FRIDHANDLER, Ph.D., Department of Psychiatry, University of California, San Francisco, San Francisco, California

HEIDI L. HEARD M.A., Department of Psychology, University of Washington, Seattle, Washington

E. TORY HIGGINS, Ph.D., Department of Psychology, Columbia University, New York, New York

MARDI J. HOROWITZ, M.D., Department of Psychiatry, University of California, San Francisco, San Francisco, California

HOWARD D. LERNER, Ph.D., Department of Psychology, University of Michigan, Ann Arbor, Michigan

MARSHA M. LINEHAN, Ph.D., Department of Psychology, University of Washington, Seattle, Washington

RICHARD J. MCNALLY, Ph.D., Department of Psychology, Harvard University, Cambridge, Massachusetts

J. CHRISTOPHER MURAN, Ph.D., Beth Israel Medical Center, Mount Sinai School of Medicine, New York, New York

ZINDEL V. SEGAL, Ph.D., Cognitive Behavioral Therapy Unit, Clarke Institute of Psychiatry, Departments of Psychiatry and Psychology, University of Toronto, Toronto, Ontario, Canada

TIMOTHY J. STRAUMAN, Ph.D., Departments of Psychology and Psychiatry, University of Wisconsin, Madison, Wisconsin

CHARLES H. STINSON, M.D., Department of Psychiatry, University of California, San Francisco, San Francisco, California

KELLY BEMIS VITOUSEK, Ph.D., Department of Psychology, University of Hawaii, Honolulu, Hawaii

DREW WESTEN, Ph.D., Department of Psychiatry, Harvard University, Cambridge, Massachusetts; Cambridge Hospital, Cambridge, Massachusetts

Preface

How do people with emotional disorders view themselves? Is there a relationship between a sense of self (self-perception and representation) and psychological difficulties? This book seeks to address these two questions of enduring importance to the study of mental disorder. Much has been written on this subject, and if there is a prevailing consensus, views of the self play an important role in personality development, many forms of psychopathology, and the regulation of feelings of well-being or inadequacy and unworthiness. Furthermore, a sense of self is often a central building block of more global strivings for emotional satisfaction and the capacity for adaptive coping in the face of adversity.

What is unique about this book is that it seeks to address the role of the self in different forms of psychological difficulties from within the cognitive–behavioral and psychodynamic traditions and allows authors to comment on each other's work. In our view, this is an especially auspicious time for such an ecumenical undertaking, since strong trends in both traditions have pointed to a greater role of the self in psychopathogenesis (e.g., depressive self-schemas in cognitive therapy or Kohut's contributions to self psychology). The intent behind structuring the book in this way was to provide a survey of new developments in theorizing about the self within both theoretical models, and to facilitate a dialogue between these perspectives that would serve to articulate points of convergence and divergence as well as to identify points of neglect or underemphasis. The inclusion of commentaries on chapters written from a differing theoretical framework was meant to generate a sense of exchange within the volume itself rather than, as is often the case, leaving readers wondering how an author would evaluate work of a complementary nature. In reading through these contributions, we are struck by the compelling manner in which the commentaries illustrate both the limits and potentialities of dialogue between these perspectives.

In order to help ensure that contributors addressed the core issues in this area, we circulated a series of common questions with which we hoped each author would grapple: (1) Provide a definition of the self; (2) What elements of the self are represented and how might they develop? (3) Are there different consequences associated with representation at different levels? (4) How can we best assess self constructs? and (5) What is the relationship between change in these constructs and response to treatment?

The first two chapters are meant to orient readers to current thinking about self constructs in both cognitive–behavioral and psychodynamic theory. Following this is an examination of self-representation in four clinical disorders (anxiety, depression, eating disorders, and borderline personality disorder) along with a final integrative section.

In many ways this book is actually telling two stories: on the one hand, it presents the role of the self in emotional distress; and on the other hand, it speaks to the possibility of integrating the two perspectives portrayed in its chapters. In working together on this project, we have experienced these two aspects personally, whether in the form of having to put aside misconceptions, considering new ways of looking at phenomena, or challenging views that seemed incomplete. We believe it has been a mutually enriching process.

We wish to thank each of the contributors for their participation in the present volume. We would also like to acknowledge the support of the John D. and Catherine T. MacArthur Foundation, both through the Program for Conscious and Unconscious Mental Processes and for a research grant to Sidney J. Blatt for the study of therapeutic change. Finally, we owe a particularly warm note of thanks to Seymour Weingarten of The Guilford Press for his consistent encouragement and ongoing support of this work.

Contents

PART III. DEPRESSION

PART IV. EATING DISORDERS

PART V. BORDERLINE PERSONALITY DISORDER

PART VI. EPILOGUE

I

Clinical Theories

1

The Self Construct in Social Cognition: Past, Present, and Future

TIMOTHY J. STRAUMAN
University of Wisconsin—Madison

E. TORY HIGGINS
Columbia University

Understanding the Self in this widest sense, we may begin by dividing the history of it into three parts, relating respectively to:

1. *Its constituents;*
2. *The feelings and emotions they arouse;*
3. *The actions to which they prompt.*

—*William James,* The Principles of Psychology

WHEN JAMES FIRST wrote those now-famous words about an ephemeral yet intriguing psychological construct called the *self*, he was well aware of the long, muddled history that the self as a concept possessed. Indeed, his seminal analysis of the self construct provided both an astute summarization of the construct's philosophical underpinnings and a remarkably prescient glimpse of how it would develop and mature over a century of psychological enterprise. Currently, the self and its implications for behavior are central topics of investigation for the field of social cognition. Nonetheless, despite the enormous literature on the self that has emerged over the last decades, it remains in some respects as nebulous and complex a concept as it appeared to James.

While it is beyond the scope of this chapter to provide a comprehensive summary of the self literature, we believe it is useful to consider the major trends in theory and research that have characterized the study of the self among social (and, more recently, social-cognitive) investigators. In doing so, it will be advantageous to examine the various approaches to studying the self by means of a general thematic structure. James (1890/1948) himself suggested several possibilities. As described in the quotation, the self can be delineated according to the major psychological domains for which it is relevant (i.e., cognition, emotion, and action). James also examined the self in terms of its function as a template for constructing the individual's past, present, and future. Our survey of the self construct in social-cognitive theory considers both this template and the relevant psychological domains. Our organizational theme, however, will be in terms of the psychological investigation of the self construct, which itself has a past, present, and future.

THE SELF IN THE PAST: THE HISTORY OF THE SELF CONSTRUCT

Origins of the Social Perspective on the Self

James's famous chapter in his *Principles of Psychology* (1890/1948) examined several aspects of the normal self, including what he called the "empirical self," or the "me." This empirical self is the self as an object of perception or knowledge, analogous to what is called "self-concept" by many contemporary theorists (e.g., Greenwald & Pratkanis, 1984; Wylie, 1979). He divided the "me" into three categories: *material* (body, family, material possessions), *social* (recognition from others), and *spiritual* (inner experiences, values, ideals). James postulated that the experience of selfhood is essentially a social experience, in that the self is largely dependent on relationships with others; in fact, he alluded to the threatening consequences for the self if all one's relationships were lost. In addition to the empirical self, or "me," James also described the self as knower, or "I," and discussed what aspects of the self correspond to the presence of an experiencing agent.

Central to James's ideas about the empirical self is the proposition that individuals possess not one, but many, selves: "A man has as many social selves as there are individuals who recognize him and carry an image of him in their mind. . . . But as the individuals who carry the images form naturally into classes, we may practically say that he has as many different social selves as there are distinct *groups* of persons about whose opinions he cares" (1948, Vol. 1, p. 924). This proposition remains an important theme in contemporary social psychology (e.g., Stryker & Statham, 1985), suggesting that although people assume that they are fairly consistent and stable beings, some individuals may be strikingly inconsistent in the selves that they present and experience under different circumstances. This inconsistency would be particularly likely to arise when the opinions of significant others toward them (either actual or anticipated) are at stake and when the significant others have different standards for their behavior or personal attributes.

Other emerging viewpoints on the self also adopted a social, role-taking approach. Cooley (1902/1964) and Mead (1934), who originated the perspective known as *symbolic interactionism*, stressed that participants in social interactions attempt to take the perspective of the other and learn to see themselves as they believe others see them. These two theorists were among the first to be concerned with the importance of relationships as they predispose the individual to role-appropriate identity and behavior. In terms of the self construct, both Cooley and Mead noted that the self-concept is essentially a social phenomenon, since it develops from the variety of roles the individual embraces in social interaction and reflects the anticipated responses of others. According to Mead, the person internalizes the attitude of the "generalized other" toward her/himself. Cooley referred to the self-concept as a "looking-glass self" because it consists of the individual's beliefs about how she/he appears to others and expectations of how others judge her/his behavior and appearance.

This emphasis on the social origins of self-knowledge has been highly influential throughout the century. Anticipating later developments in cognitive social psychology, Sarbin (1952) argued that social behavior is organized around the individual's collection of knowledge structures, including the self (which consists of two substructures, the somatic and social selves). As with the theories of James, Cooley, and Mead, each person is said to possess a number of "empirical selves" that correspond to the different social roles that she/he is called upon to play. This role-taking framework is based in part upon qualitative research techniques in which individuals describe themselves (e.g., Bugental, 1964; Gordon, 1968; McGuire & McGuire, 1982). Interestingly, studies using this approach have demonstrated that people tend to describe themselves in ways that are distinctive or that set them apart from their actual social background, even though their actual behavior usually emphasizes role-determined, common response patterns.

The work of Kelly (1955) exemplifies a particularly significant extension of the classic literature on the social self that again prefigured the current emphasis on the self as a cognitive structure. In Kelly's theory, the self, or personality, comprises what individuals represent themselves to be (e.g., "I am an outgoing person"), as determined by their hypotheses and interpretations regarding social events and interactions. The individual acquires *personal constructs* out of a fundamental need to understand the world, through a continuous process of testing hypotheses about the events occurring in her/his life. The construct system that she/he accrues as she/he interacts with the social world forms the basis for self-evaluation and social behavior. Kelly emphasized a number of features of this self-as-scientist framework: (1) personal constructs permit individuals to anticipate as well as interpret events; (2) individuals differ from one another in their constructions of events; (3) constructs are organized into hierarchical systems, within which a "self" can be located; and (4) the construct system is modified and extended by continuing social interaction.

Origins of Theories Relating Self and Affect

Although the origin of the self in social interaction was a primary focus of a number of classic theories, a separate emphasis on the self construct emerged focusing on the relation between self and affect. The thrust of this literature has almost uniformly involved notions of conflict, inconsistency, or discrepancy. In social psychology, for example, various early theories proposed a relation between "inconsistency" in a person's attitudes or beliefs and discomfort. The notion that people who hold conflicting or incompatible beliefs about themselves are likely to experience discomfort or distress is quite prevalent in self theory. Among a wide array of possible inconsistencies in various aspects of the self, three basic types of incompatibilities can be identified (Higgins, 1987): (1) inconsistencies between one's self-perceived attributes and external, behavioral feedback related to one's self-perceptions; (2) contradictions among one's self-perceived attributes that impede a coherent and unified self-concept; and (3) discrepancies between one's self-perceived attributes and some self-standard or self-guide. While several theories contain aspects of more than one type, all these theories share three basic assumptions: that holding conflicting beliefs is intolerable or uncomfortable, that people are cognitive creatures who think about their beliefs and make choices (conscious or otherwise) based on them, and that people will be motivated to change either their beliefs or their behavior in order to maintain consistency. This section reviews the theories relating self and affect, grouped according to the type of self-belief incompatibility.

Inconsistencies between the Self and External Feedback

The first type of self-inconsistency, that involving external feedback, can occur either from one's own behavior or the responses of others. The well-known theory of cognitive dissonance (Festinger, 1957) proposed that when two cognitions (opinions, beliefs, or feelings about oneself or one's environment) are inconsistent, the individual experiences psychological distress and is motivated to reduce the inconsistency (and thus the discomfort). For example, an individual who believed that he was an honest person but knew that he had cheated on an exam would be holding two inconsistent cognitions, which would induce distress and motivation to reduce or eliminate the inconsistency. Dissonance theory has had great influence on social psychological theories of the self, generating a succession of useful and insightful models. For example, Aronson (1969) refined the theory by emphasizing the role of self-expectancies in dissonance. He proposed that dissonance involves the relation between cognitions and the self-concept: when people behave in a manner that is inconsistent with their self-concept, they experience discomfort and a resultant motivation to reduce the dissonance. Secord and Backman (1964) applied a dissonance perspective to the domain of social roles and the impact of role expectations on affect and behavior. They described the origins and effects of role conflict, that is, incompatible expectations associated with different roles that an individual might hold. More recently, Swann (1983) proposed a model of self-verification that focused on people's attempts to obtain responses from others confirming their self-conceptions. According to this model, people experience distress when they receive social feedback that is inconsistent with their self-concept, even when the feedback disconfirms a negative self-conception. Wicklund and Gollwitzer's (1982) theory of symbolic self-completion postulates that people who are committed to a particular self-definition but have been unable to sufficiently achieve it experience a psychological tension that motivates the emergence of self-completion strategies and behaviors. Steele (e.g., Steele & Liu, 1983) offered a self-affirmation interpretation of dissonance phenomena. This approach posits a need to affirm the self as an important factor in determining both when dissonance-generating conflict and discomfort will arise and how such discomfort can be reduced.

Inconsistencies among Self-beliefs

A number of theories have proposed that people need to maintain consistency among their self-perceived attributes in order to form a coherent and unified self-concept. Allport (1937, 1943) suggested that the mature personality is distinguished by three attributes exemplifying an underlying process of self-unification: (1) *self-extension*, the capacity to deter momentary gratification or pain in favor of pursuing long-term goals; (2) *self-objectification*, in which the individual "surveys his own pretensions in relation to possible objectives for himself, his own equipment in comparison with the equipment of others, and his opinion of himself in relation to the opinions others hold of him" (1937, p. 214); and (3) a *unifying philosophy of life*, in which mature individuals attempt to live their lives by overarching guiding principles. Similarly, Lecky (1961) offered a theory of self-consistency in which the formation and maintenance of consistency among self-attributes is considered a primary task of psychological development.

More recent additions to the self literature manifest this central focus on consistency among elements of the self. Epstein (1973, 1980) postulated that the self-concept represents the individual's theory about her/himself used in an active, information-gathering interchange with the social environment. Epstein also proposed that the self-concept is responsible for the considerable degree of unity and consistency in one's identity. Individuals' unique self-theories involve postulates that guide their behavior but may not be directly accessible to awareness (and so must be inferred from observation of the individual's behavior and affect across situations). Among developmental theorists, Harter (1986) has traced the emergence of the self-system and the corresponding development of self-consistency. She observed that adolescents are able to distinguish between self-perceived opposite traits that are in conflict or inconsistent with one another (e.g., "smart" vs. "fun-loving" in school) and those that are not in conflict because they occur in different contexts (e.g., "outgoing" with friends vs. "shy" with a potential romantic partner). As theories proposing the need for self-consistency would suggest, the adolescents in Harter's research were distressed by their self-perceived conflicting traits unless the traits were viewed as pertaining to different social contexts.

Discrepancies between Self-concept and Self-standard

The first two categories of self-inconsistency theories emphasize the interrelation among self-perceived attributes, behaviors, and experiences—that is, the interrelation among different pieces of information about the self as actually perceived or construed (the "actual" self). The third type of theory emphasizes the relation between the actual self and some self-standard or self-guide. Theories in this category propose that discrepancies between self-perceived attributes and contextually salient standards, personal aspirations, or values produce discomfort. In his writings, James (1890/1948) highlighted the motivational role of the self in prompting and regulating action (e.g., self-seeking, self-preservation) and in influencing the processes of self-evaluation. Specifically, James distinguished between the "spiritual" self, which includes one's own moral sensibility and conscience, and the "social" self, which includes the self that is worthy of being approved by the highest social judge. Freud's (1923/1961) structural model of the psyche posited continual conflict and struggle between the id and the superego, respectively, and the ego. Interestingly, two of the three primary psychic structures (ego and superego) embody internalized "identifications" with significant others, demonstrating the importance of socializing forces even within classic psychodynamic models of personality. Sullivan (1953) distinguished among behavioral standards incorporated within the self-system according to the types of self–other contingencies with which they were typically associated (i.e., "good me," "bad me," and "not me"). Other neo-Freudians such as Erikson (1950/1963) and Horney (1950) also emphasized the role of socialization-based internal standards in the genesis and maintenance of neurotic symptomatology. Rogers (1961) generated a theory of the healthy personality in which discrepancies between an individual's self-concept and her/his ideals were said to be minimized. Rogers distinguished between what others believe a person should or ought to be (the normative standard) and a person's own beliefs about what he/she would "ideally" like to be. He also pioneered a method for idiographic assessment of the self-concept, the Q-sort technique, that has been widely used in social, personality, and clinical investigations of self-beliefs.

More recent contributions to the self literature also focus on actual self/self-standard inconsistency. Duval and Wicklund's (1972) theory of objective self-awareness described a process whereby behavior was contrasted with salient internal standards, with resultant positive or negative consequences. Carver and Scheier (1981) proposed a cybernetic model of self-regulation in which behavior is continually compared with standards for desirable and/or undesirable outcomes. Cantor and Kihlstrom (1986) and Markus (Markus & Nurius, 1986) have also made important contributions, focusing on self-regulatory processes that involve actual self/self-standard comparison processes. These models will be described in greater detail in the next section.

The History of the Social Self: A Summary

Even as James was drafting his authoritative treatise on the nature and origins of the self, a diverse literature already existed describing the self and its psychological characteristics. The above section traces the evolution of important research and theoretical traditions in the social-psychological study of the self. Despite the diversity of these theories, they share many features: (1) the tendency to view the self as comprising multiple elements or aspects, in terms of self-belief content (behavior-specific, situation-specific, standard-specific), time frame (past, present, future), and standpoint (one's own, a significant other's, a generalized other); (2) recognizing the importance of the psychological origins of the self for understanding its structure and function; and (3) addressing the intimate and complex links between self and affect. Each of the major theories cited emphasized at least two of these themes. A number of recent reviews have concluded (e.g., Gergen, 1984; Greenwald & Pratkanis, 1984; Kihlstrom, Cantor, Albright, Chew, Klein, & Niedenthal, 1988), as James himself did, that none of the theories represents a truly comprehensive and integrative theory of the self. Given the present state of psychological theory and technology, however, it is unrealistic to expect models of the self to deal adequately with all of the issues raised by contemporary reviewers—or even those raised by James and the other classic self theorists.

THE SELF IN THE PRESENT: CURRENT MODELS OF THE SELF CONSTRUCT

The diversity of classic self theories is equalled by the heterogeneity of current models of the self in social-cognitive psychology. Nonetheless, recent reviews of social-cognitive research on the self (Higgins & Bargh, 1987; Kihlstrom & Cantor, 1984; Markus & Wurf, 1987; Strauman, 1989a) have identified two key premises shared by most investigators in the field. First, it is typically accepted that the self mediates between the environment and behavior and is not simply a reflection or epiphenomenon of how the individual behaves. The self system is viewed as actively organizing behavior, as interpreting and responding to contextual cues, and as involved in complex regulatory processes. Second, most social-cognitive self researchers have appropriated information-processing principles into their models. These principles offer useful concepts for such self functions as environment monitoring ("reality testing"), allocation of attentional resources, response selection, and behavior-standard discrepancy reduction. Although it has been argued that exclusive reliance on a "cold" computer metaphor may result in a less-than-optimal understanding of the "hot," affective/motivational aspects of the self (Sorrentino & Higgins, 1986), the utility of the information-processing perspective for self research is rarely disputed. This section will examine salient issues in the application of cognitive principles to the study of the self, describe representative social-cognitive theories of the self, and briefly review cognitive theories of psychopathology with implications for the self.

Information Processing and the Self: Current Theories

The increasing prevalence of an information-processing perspective may be the most significant development within the self literature over the last 20 years. Since the quantity of information available at any moment is far greater than an individual could ever comprehend or attend to, she/he must select subsets of information to process. The nonrandom manner in which individuals selectively notice, assimilate, and respond to self-relevant stimuli implies the existence of knowledge structures that function as "templates" for construing and interpreting events. Although not everyone has concluded that the self is a unique cognitive structure (e.g, Bower & Gilligan, 1979; Fiske & Taylor, 1984) or even that it is necessarily a unitary cognitive structure at all (e.g., Klein & Kihlstrom, 1986; for a review, see Higgins & Bargh, 1987), the dominant position in the literature has been that the self, or at least some subset of it, is a rich, highly organized entity with structural properties.

Many self researchers have come to conceptualize the self as an individual's mental representation of her/his own personality, attributes, and standards. As such, the concepts and methods employed by cognitive psychologists to investigate other types of mental representations have been applied to self-knowledge with considerable success, though almost exclusively within the limited domain of verbal encodings of self-knowledge (Markus & Wurf, 1987). When conceived in its broadest sense, self-knowledge includes within its purview representations of personality traits, affective states, motivational states, action orientations, and behaviors (Markus, 1983). Defined in this manner, the self becomes "one's mental representation of oneself, no different in principle from mental representations that a person has concerning other ideas, objects, and events and their implications. In other words, the self is a concept, not unlike other concepts, that is stored in memory as a knowledge structure, not unlike other knowledge structures" (Kihlstrom & Cantor, 1984, p. 2).

The hypothesized organization of the self varies from theorist to theorist. Kihlstrom and Cantor (1984) distinguished between two basic forms of self-representation prevalent in current theories: (1) the self as a *list structure*, meaning features considered characteristic of oneself and organized in a manner similar to that of other social and nonsocial categories of knowledge (e.g., Cantor & Mischel, 1979); and (2) the self as a *memory structure*, meaning the self is viewed either as a node in a network of semantic memory linked to other nodes that represent knowledge about oneself or as a *schema* (Markus & Sentis, 1982). A semantic network is a medium for representing a person's knowledge or beliefs about concepts or events; each concept or event is characterized by its configuration of associations with other concepts or events (hence the popular label "associative network models"). *Schema* is a general term denoting a mental structure for encoding and representing information; a self-schema may be defined as a "cognitive generalization about the self, derived from past experience, that organizes and guides the processing of self-related information contained in the individual's social experiences" (Markus, 1977, p. 63).

There are a number of current theories in which the self is conceived of as a knowledge structure. Theorists conceptualizing the self as a list or category structure generally base their models on the investigations of Cantor and Mischel (1979), which suggest that social knowledge is organized and stored in the form of categories or prototypes. The significance of this finding for social cognition is that (as had already been demonstrated in other knowledge domains; e.g., Bransford & Franks, 1972) people use their knowledge structures to process incoming information, even to the extent that certain features of the stimulus input that are *typically* present are presumed by the perceiver regardless of whether they are *actually* present in the current instance. Kihlstrom and Cantor (1984) proposed that the self-concept is represented by one or more prototypes, or summaries, of a number of specific instances or exemplars. The prototypes that make up the self are said to consist of sets of central and peripheral features, possibly organized in a loose hierarchy at varying levels of abstraction. Since the self is (from a social-psychological perspective) a person within the subject's social world, Kihlstrom and Cantor concluded that the self-concept is embedded in the person's overall hierarchical organization of person and social concepts.

In a similar vein, Rogers (1981) proposed that the self is a cognitive category with an internal hierarchical organization, containing self-descriptive elements such as *traits, values,*and *episodic memories.* Kuiper (e.g., Kuiper & Derry, 1981) also postulated that the self functions as a prototype, or a representation of a central tendency or modal occurrence of some category. This prototype-based conception of the self is consistent with a large body of research investigating *self-reference* effects in memory, in which information encoded with reference to the self is associated with superior memory characteristics (cf. Higgins & Bargh, 1987). By demonstrating that latency and memory effects associated with judgments concerning well-established cognitive prototypes also occur with judgments concerning the self, these investigations support the proposition that the self functions like a cognitive structure. It is clear that in many respects the "top-down" or "theory-driven" properties of social-information processing are also characteristic of self-referential information processing.

Associative network models (e.g., Anderson, 1983) have been utilized by self researchers to conceptualize the representation and processing of self-referential knowledge. According to such a model, information is stored in the form of propositions that link the subject (i.e., the self) with specific concepts, attributes, or memories. Initially, these models depicted the self as a single node within the total memory network, linked to both semantic and episodic knowledge (Kihlstrom & Cantor, 1984). Other theories have emphasized the multidimensionality of the self by construing it as an overarching organization or as a collection of knowledge structures. For instance, Bower and Gilligan (1979) presented an associative-network conception in which a portion of the individual's overall associative memory network is identified with the self. In another example of this trend, Greenwald (Breckler & Greenwald, 1982) offered a view of the self as a multidimensional cognitive space in which social information (e.g., traits) is represented relative to *several* dimensions rather than simply self-referentiality. Linville (1985) developed a model of self-knowledge relating complexity of self-representation to affective and evaluative responses. According to her self-complexity notion, the less complex a person's cognitive representation of the self, the more extreme the person's variability in affect and self-appraisal. Higgins (Higgins, Van Hook, & Dorfman, 1988) reported a series of studies suggesting that although all self-beliefs are not necessarily interconnected, "problematic" self attributes (i.e., self-attributes involved in a within-self inconsistency) did show evidence of structural interconnectedness (see below). All of these models share an emphasis on the self as cognitively represented in terms of multiple aspects, at least some of which are presumed to be interconnected.

The self-schema concept has become popular among some self theorists. Markus (1977, 1983; Markus & Sentis, 1982) views the self as a system of schemas that contain information about past experiences, personal characteristics, and possible future behaviors and attributes ("possible selves"). Each person actively constructs both generalizations and hypotheses about the self from ongoing life events. Self-schemas are postulated to develop around those aspects of the self that become personally significant in the course of social interactions, reflecting domains of enduring salience, investment, or concern (Markus, 1983). The information-processing consequences of self-schemas are profound. Individuals with self-schemas in particular domains (1) can make judgments about the self more easily and with greater certainty, (2) respond more consistently, (3) show facilitated recognition and recall for schema-relevant information, (4) tend to resist information that is inconsistent with the content of the self-schemas, and (5) process new information in terms of its relevance for the existing self-schemas. Self-schemas are thought to provide not only control over individuals' environments, but also control over behavior, since they help to define those domains over which individuals believe they should have control or have claimed as their own responsibility (Markus, 1983).

In addition to focusing on the representation of information, the information-processing perspective in social psychology also emphasizes the manner in which information is utilized in responding to social events and regulating behavior. Accordingly, a number of self theories highlight self-regulatory processes. Duval and Wicklund's (1972) theory of objective self-awareness argued that when self-focused attention increases, an individual's awareness of discrepancies between the actual self and personal standards also increases, resulting in a motivation to reduce the discrepancy. This approach emphasizes both existing self-standards and attentional processes by which standards become salient and influence mood and behavior. Carver and Scheier (1981) have proposed a control-theory approach to self-regulation based on cybernetic principles and an emphasis on feedback loops for the processing of self-relevant information. Their approach postulates that people self-regulate through a discrepancy-reducing negative feedback process whose function is to minimize differences between one value (typically an aspect of the self-concept) and some other reference value or standard for comparison. As with self-awareness theory, this model assumes that self-directed attention leads to an analysis of self-relevant information. If a relevant self-standard is currently active within the system, a "matching-to-standard" operation takes place, with resultant positive or negative emotional and motivational implications.

Carver and Scheier (1981, 1982) suggested that the self is elaborated into an interconnected hierarchy of control systems at progressively higher levels of abstraction, and that discrepancy-reduction operations can occur at any level, with potential impact on associated levels of self-knowledge.

The principle that knowledge-based expectancies can determine an individual's self-evaluation and behavior also has played an important role in social-cognitive self research. A major theoretical statement concerning the role of perceived ability to reach desired end-states was offered by Bandura (1982, 1986) in his theory of self-efficacy. The term *self-efficacy* refers both to an understanding of the self's importance in the regulation of behavior and to the individual's perception of her/his ability to accomplish a certain task. According to this model, perceptions of self-efficacy are determined both by previous learning and contextual factors. Moreover, a person's beliefs regarding efficacy in a particular domain have been shown to predict goal-seeking behavior, degree of persistence and effort, and contents of cognition during and after efficacy-related behaviors.

A final contribution to the current self literature represents an integration of many of the features of the approaches described above. Self-discrepancy theory (Higgins, 1987, 1989) is a model of the relation between self and affect that seeks to explain how different types of within-self discrepancies are related to different kinds of affective and motivational states. The model postulates that a discrepancy between the actual self and an *ideal* self-guide (the representation of an individual's beliefs about someone's hopes, wishes, or aspirations for them) is associated with the negative motivational state of the absence of positive outcomes, as well as dejection-related emotions such as sadness, disappointment, and frustration. In contrast, a discrepancy between the actual self and an *ought* self-guide (the representation of an individual's beliefs about someone's sense of her/his duties, obligations, or responsibilities) is associated with the negative motivational state of the presence of negative outcomes, as well as agitation-related emotions such as apprehension, anxiety, and guilt. Research testing the theory (e.g., Higgins, Bond, Klein, & Strauman, 1986; Strauman & Higgins, 1987) has provided strong support for the predicted discriminant associations of specific self-discrepancies with different types of negative affect, as well as evidence for the view of self-discrepancies as cognitive structures that can be activated without the individual's awareness or intention.

Social-Cognitive Theories of Emotional Disorder with Implications for the Self

Although it is not the purpose of this chapter to focus extensively on the self in psychopathology, it is useful to present representative theory and research illustrating how the self has been implicated in emotional disorders. This section concentrates on theories of depression, since a predominance of clinical application of self theory has occurred with reference to this disorder. The reader is referred to reviews offered by Coyne and Gotlib (1983), Hollon and Kriss (1984), Moretti and Shaw (1989), and Segal (1988).

The best known cognitive theory of depression with implications for the self belongs to Beck (1967, 1976), who introduced three concepts to account for the onset and maintenance of depression: schemas, the cognitive triad, and cognitive distortions. Beck appropriated the *schema* concept from cognitive psychology to signify an organized, cohesive knowledge structure capable of guiding perception, interpretation, appraisal, and behavior. The *cognitive triad* is Beck's term for characteristic negative thought patterns concerning the depressed individual's views of her/himself, the future, and the world. *Cognitive distortions* are thought products resulting from biased perceptions or interpretations that tend to confirm the negative expectancies of the depressed individual; examples include dichotomous ("black or white") thinking, selective abstraction, arbitrary inferences, and personalization. In Beck's theory, the self-schemas of depression-prone individuals are an important source of biased information processing leading to the onset of distress. Beck, Rush, Shaw, and Emery (1979) proposed that early life experiences provide the basis for forming negative concepts about the self and that such self-schemas are activated by current life events to initiate a sequence of depressogenic cognitive processing. Although this hypothesis has proven difficult to test adequately (Segal, 1988), there is considerable indirect support for the proposition that self-schemas can bias social perception and interpretation in such a manner as to increase the likelihood of negative self-evaluation and resultant negative emotional states (Kuiper & Higgins, 1985).

Other investigators have proposed and tested similar models by which self-knowledge can predispose an individual to depression. Following on the research of Rogers, Kuiper, and Kirker (1977), who demonstrated that novel information is better remembered when it is processed in relation to the self than when it is processed in other contexts (the "self-reference effect"), Rogers (1981) and Kuiper and Derry (1981) postulated that the self is a cognitive structure with unique information-processing properties, since in order for self-reference to facilitate remembering, the self must be a uniform, well-structured entity (Rogers et al., 1977). Guidano (1987; Guidano & Liotti, 1983) proposed that self-knowledge is organized into stable, hierarchically ordered mental structures that are derived from emotionally significant life experiences and operated automatically and implicitly to influence both the content of mental operations and the nature of the operations themselves. Borrowing from Bowlby's (1985) knowledge-structure approach to the development of emotion and object relations, Guidano's model implicates cognitive structures representing negative self and relationship themes in the etiology of emotional disorders such as depression and anxiety.

The Present Status of the Social Self: A Summary

Although several decades ago experimental social psychology appeared not to consider the self a worthwhile topic, during the last 15 years the self returned to center stage as a focus of investigation. As can be observed even from the brief review provided, the influence of the "cognitive revolution" on self theory is "self"-evident. Interestingly, however, reviewers (Higgins & Bargh, 1987; Fiske & Taylor, 1984; Kihlstrom & Cantor, 1984) have suggested that important questions remain concerning the status of the self as an information-processing entity. Perhaps the most notable distinction among the theories reviewed above is the extent to which the self is envisioned simply as an "abstraction" in the mind of the investigator (representing a set of independent bits of information or knowledge referring to the individual who "owns" them) as opposed to a unitary, unique, cognitive structure in which the individual elements are organized with a high degree of interrelation. This distinction, which is probably best considered a continuum, carries significant implications for research and, ultimately, for psychology's construal of the self.

As would be expected for an evolving scientific enterprise, the self construct of 1990s social cognition manifests both strengths and weaknesses. Certainly the introduction of information-processing concepts has provided a degree of rigor and experimental sophistication far beyond what was previously available. In addition, the cognitive *Weltanschauung* of present-day behavioral science permits investigators to focus on unobservable processes and hypothetical constructs without risking ridicule from colleagues. Possibly the greatest advantage of the self construct in present-day social cognition lies in the body of evidence demonstrating that self-knowledge profoundly influences the entire sequence of psychological events that make up social perception, from registration of stimuli to propagation of behavior. The clinically derived suppositions of Freud, Adler, Sullivan, and others concerning the power of self processes to determine experience, as well as the sociological observations of Cooley, Mead, Sarbin, and more recent theorists concerning the sway of interpersonal forces in shaping the self, have largely been validated (albeit primarily in laboratory contexts).

Nonetheless, it is important to remember that each successive paradigm to arise within psychology has had its biases and blemishes. As Gergen (1984) and others have noted, the information-processing perspective and its counterpart, the computer metaphor, entail assumptions about the nature of mental phenomena that are more appropriate for some features of the self (e.g., memory) than others (e.g., goal-directed action, emotion).

Though the point has not been lost within social cognition (e.g., Showers & Cantor, 1985; Sorrentino & Higgins, 1986), it will be crucial for self theorists and researchers not to lose sight of other aspects of the essence of self, such as the experience of human agency (James's "I"). In many respects, the self literature of the past 20 years bears the unmistakable mark of the earlier behavioral paradigm: consideration of the self as primarily engendered by environmental influences and passively responding to social stimuli. If the history of the self-perception literature is any indication, the current emphasis on "cold," amotivational explanations for self phenomena will eventually be succeeded by a complementary accent on "hot," motivation-driven models, and, ultimately, "warm," motivation–cognition interface models (Sorrentino & Higgins, 1986).

THE SELF IN THE FUTURE: ISSUES, DIRECTIONS, AND DILEMMAS

There can be little doubt that the self construct in social cognition boasts impressive theoretical and empirical credentials, and that a great deal has been learned. Having attempted to characterize the development and current status of the self construct in social-cognitive psychology, we will now turn to a speculative appraisal of how the construct will evolve. Of course, such conjecture necessitates an emphasis on the issues and questions that remain, rather than on the achievements of the field to date. Our intent is to identify particularly crucial issues for the hypothesized role of the self in emotional disorder. From time to time we also will describe domains of potential integration with psychodynamic approaches. By learning more about *both* the social-cognitive and psychodynamic perspectives on self-representation, investigators will be better able to take full advantage of the unique conceptual and investigative strengths of each approach.

The Self as an Information-Processing Entity: When Past and Future Are Present

Although the cognitive emphasis in psychology is relatively new, in functional terms the capacity of the self to represent information and engender goals has long been recognized. Murray (1943) wrote that "man is a *time-binding* organism. . . . by conserving some of the past and anticipating some of the future, a human being can, to a significant degree, make his behavior accord with events that have happened as well as events that are to come" (p. 49). Murray, like Lewin (1935), is suggesting that beliefs about one's past and future are represented in the present self-system. Although self-beliefs are a subset of people's social knowledge, they include such influential constructs as self-standards (including self-guides), the self-concept, self-expectancies, and perceived self-efficacy (Higgins, 1990). Self-beliefs, as cognitive structures, represent a significant locus for the "time-binding" phenomenon of which Murray and Lewin spoke. Thus, discerning the manner in which self-beliefs about the past, present, and future are acquired and activated is an essential challenge for emerging theories of the self.

Activation and Consequences of Self-beliefs

People's responses to events derive in part from the meaning of their inherent properties, or "affordances," to people in general (Gibson, 1979; McArthur & Baron, 1983). Nonetheless, much of the significance of events derives from how individuals perceive, categorize, and evaluate them. It has long been recognized that knowledge structures built from past experience are a major determinant of how people categorize and appraise external stimuli (e.g., Bartlett, 1932; Kelly, 1955). The so-called "New Look" in perception research that emerged in the 1940s and 1950s proposed that needs, values, and expectancies help to determine perception and result in people going "beyond the information given" (Bruner, 1957a). To capture the general role of expectancies and motivational states on perception, Bruner (1957b) introduced the notion of category *accessibility*, which denoted the ease or speed with which a given stimulus input is coded in terms of a given category under varying conditions. Two general sets of conditions were proposed to affect accessibility: *expectancies* (subjective probability estimates of the likelihood of a given event) and *motivational states* (search sets induced by needs, task goals, etc.). Expectancies and motivational states increase the accessibility of stored knowledge, which in turn increases the likelihood that a stimulus input will be perceived in terms of that category rather than a competing alternative category.

The importance of accessibility effects in determining the motivational and emotional consequences of activating self-knowledge has been demonstrated in a series of studies employing self-discrepancy theory. The theory proposes that it is the relation between and among self-beliefs (e.g., actual self, ideal self, and ought self-guides) that produces emotional/motivational vulnerabilities, rather than the content of each self-belief per se. Relations between different self-beliefs represent different kinds of psychological situations, which in turn are associated with different emotional/motivational states. As mentioned briefly earlier, actual:ideal and actual:ought discrepancies represent distinct, chronic, negative psychological situations (the absence of positive outcomes vs. the presence of negative outcomes), which produce distinct emotional states (dejection vs. agitation). It has been demonstrated that the *magnitude*, *type*, and *accessibility* of self-discrepancies predict the type and intensity of emotional vulnerability that individuals experience (Higgins et al., 1986). The theory proposes that the pattern of self-beliefs comprising a self-discrepancy constitutes a cognitive structure representing a negative psychological situation and associated emotional/motivational state. Therefore, activating a self-discrepancy (by experimentally manipulating features of the immediate context) should activate the negative psychological situation it represents, thereby producing the associated emotional/motivational state. Further, this activation/emotion induction process should occur without (indeed, *despite*) the awareness of the individual. These latter predictions have been supported in laboratory studies of both nonclinical (Strauman & Higgins, 1987) and clinical (Strauman, 1989b) populations.

The self-discrepancy model and its supporting research provide a framework for understanding how past, present, and future-oriented self-beliefs can influence emotional status and increase vulnerability to emotional distress. In addition, the model highlights the importance of a cognitive viewpoint on the self, and more specifically, demonstrates that the influence of the self on the individual's experience and behavior is due, at least in part, to the cognitive-structural status of self-beliefs. We believe these experimental studies are the first to demonstrate unconscious on-line effects on mood, physiology, and behavior from activating self-belief structures. Thus, the self is not simply a critical construct for social and personality theorists; it may also be a *necessary* concept for theories of emotional vulnerability and psychopathology. Self-beliefs are a means by which the past, the present, and the future interact; matches and mismatches among self-beliefs are critical determinants of self-evaluation, and hence, emotional vulnerability. Self-guides, as representations of the emotional and motivational consequences of self–other contingent interactions earlier in life, both summarize an individual's emotionally significant past and influence how he/she construes his/her future. In the ongoing and largely automatic processes of social perception and self-evaluation, individuals manifest the time-binding characteristic described by Murray (1943)—experiencing both the "aftermath" of the past (as represented in self-knowledge) and the anticipation of the future (as embodied in personal goals and expectancies) in the continuing present.

Is the Self a Cognitive Structure?

In the enthusiasm of self researchers to incorporate cognitive principles into their models, the assumption that the self constitutes a unitary cognitive structure became popular. This conclusion was due in large measure to research on the "self-reference effect" first described by Rogers et al. (1977). From a purely clinical perspective, the question of whether the self represents a coherent, stable structure is not momentous, since (for example) cognitive–behavioral therapy is primarily targeted at individual beliefs and attitudes rather than at a hypothetical, deep-structure entity such as the self (e.g., Beck et al., 1979). Nonetheless, the issue is of great significance for theory and research, with implications for a variety of topics (e.g., self-consistency, self-defeating behavior, personality stability vs. change, etc.), and especially for current cognitive theories of psychopathology (Segal, 1988).

As Higgins and Bargh (1987), among others, have pointed out, many of the consequences that have been attributed to the self forming a unitary structure do not require that self-beliefs be structurally interconnected. For example, the self-reference effect (the finding that material is more easily remembered when it is encoded with reference to self than when it is encoded with reference to some other orientation task) is *consistent* with the self being a cognitive structure, but the memory advantage does not depend on the self-descriptive traits themselves being *interconnected* in memory. It would also occur, for example, if each self-descriptive trait were completely separate from the others but highly familiar and emotionally significant (Greenwald & Pratkanis, 1984), since both familiarity and emotional significance lead to increased accessibility and thus should give the traits a retrieval advantage. The more general observation that self-knowledge can have information-processing consequences (e.g., self-knowledge is associated with quick decisions, easily retrievable evidence, confident self-prediction, and resistance to contrary evidence) likewise is not sufficient evidence for unitary structure. Any belief to which a person is committed or in which a person has confidence should have such properties (e.g., Cantril, 1932; Fazio & Zanna, 1981). This latter point suggests a note of caution for cognitive theories of psychopathology that *presume* a structural interconnection among self-related attitudes or beliefs. The cognitive properties associated with depressogenic beliefs, for example, need not be dependent on structural interconnectedness, but may simply be manifestations of properties associated with any significant belief or attitude.

The critical issue here is not whether self-concept attributes reflect *any* kind of cognitive unit or entity. Since the attributes are in some way identified as self-referential, it stands to reason that all self-concept attributes have some common association with the self. Although in a trivial sense this implies a minimal cognitive unit, it does not follow that self-beliefs are structurally interconnected. Such interconnection would have significant ramifications for how the beliefs were activated and for their impact on self-evaluation and affect. If self-knowledge possesses the same organizational property found for knowledge of naturally occurring categories (such as object categories), then activation of one self-belief should *automatically* activate other self-beliefs. If this were so, then emotional responses to events could be said to derive not just from reaction to a single event-related belief (e.g., "I failed my math exam"), but also from activation of structurally linked self-beliefs (e.g., "I'm also a failure in my social life") (Linville, 1985). Such cognitive distortions as global attributions and overgeneralization seen in depressive episodes would then properly be understood as a consequence of automatic, uncontrolled spreading among negative self-beliefs.

In order to convincingly support a conjecture of cognitive structure, experimental tasks capable of demonstrating the automatic (unintentional) activation of one construct by another are needed. In particular, tasks are required where the individual's performance cannot reflect a deliberate strategy on her/his part (as is the case for measures like questionnaires and thought-listing procedures). One such task is Warren's (1972) Stroop test for memory organization of categories. In this task, subjects find it more difficult to ignore the meaning of a colored target word (e.g., "tree" printed in red ink) while trying simply to name its color, when they have been previously exposed to another word closely related in meaning (e.g., "oak"), than when they have been exposed to a word unrelated in meaning. Apparently the meaning of the target word is automatically activated by prior exposure to words with related meanings, and this increases the difficulty of paying attention to the target word's color rather than its meaning.

This technique was used in a series of experiments (Higgins et al., 1988) testing the proposal that self-referential attributes form a cognitive structure. Subjects were presented with a series of slides of target words printed in different-colored inks and were then asked to name the color of each word as quickly as possible. Prior to each slide presentation, subjects were given a memory-load word that they repeated back after naming the color of the target word. The critical manipulation was the relation between the memory load word and the target word. In each study there were self-related target traits preceded either by other self-related traits or by self-unrelated traits, and object category targets primed either by semantically related or semantically unrelated categories. For both the self as a category and object categories, structural interconnectedness among category attributes themselves should produce slower response times for related prime-target pairs than for unrelated ones.

In the first two studies, there was no significant difference in response times between prime-target pairs involving self-related traits (i.e., both prime and target were self-descriptive traits) and pairs involving self-unrelated traits (i.e., only one of the traits was self-descriptive). In contrast, the predicted effect of relatedness was found for object categories. Thus, the first two studies did not support the proposal that self-concept attributes formed a cognitive structure. The investigators, however, went on to consider *when* such attributes might form a structure even if they do not always do so, so the final study used an idiographic measure of self-concept that identifies chronically accessible and personally significant self-beliefs (the Selves Questionnaire; see Higgins et al., 1986). This questionnaire identifies self-congruent and self-discrepant pairs of self-belief attributes.

Actual self/self-guide attribute pairs constitute a "match" when they are close in value along the same dimension, a "mismatch" when they are distant in value along the same dimension, and a "nonmatch" when they are on different dimensions. Because the Selves Questionnaire asks subjects to list spontaneously the attributes of their actual self or self-guides, it is likely that those listed are chronically accessible constructs; moreover, those attributes that are matches or mismatches are emotionally significant because they are related to the respondent's self-guides. Therefore, it was possible to determine whether only the matches and/or mismatches among an individual's self-beliefs were structurally connected (see Higgins, 1989, and Wyer & Gordon, 1984, for further discussion). The third study, was designed to investigate whether various subsets of self-concept attributes were structurally interconnected, consisted of self-related and self-unrelated prime-target pairs that varied, depending on whether the self-descriptive traits were matches, mismatches, or nonmatches. If self-concept attributes in general are interconnected, then a general effect of slower reaction times when self-related target attributes were primed by *any* other self-related attribute should have been found. No such general effect was found; the third study again failed to find evidence of structural interconnectedness among self-concept attributes in general. However, an interaction was found that was consistent with the hypothesis that *mismatching*, or "problematic," self-concept attributes form the basis for structural interconnectedness. Problematic prime-target pairs, defined as a pair where either the prime or the target (or both) were mismatch self-concept attributes, produced slower reaction times suggestive of interference from structural interconnectedness. Since individuals are especially likely to attend to self-attributes that are problematic (Carver & Scheier, 1981; Wiener, 1948), it is likely that discrepant attributes will be repeatedly and concurrently activated, which should lead to structural interconnectedness (Hebb, 1949).

The presence of structure among problematic self-beliefs is important because it has implications for cognitive processes beyond the accessibility or significance of individual attributes. In particular, it means that activation of one attribute or belief can automatically activate other such attributes. There is considerable evidence that depressed individuals possess more mismatches among their self-concept attributes than do nondepressed individuals (e.g., Higgins, 1987; Strauman, 1989b). If mismatch self-concept attributes form a basis for structure whereas match and nonmatch attributes do not, then the self-concept attributes of depressed individuals should be interconnected to a greater extent than for nondepressed ones. This hypothesis was tested in a recent study by Segal, Hood, Shaw, and Higgins (1988). As expected, evidence of structural interconnectedness was found for depressed subjects but not for nondepressed subjects. These results, then, support the proposal that problematic self-beliefs may be structurally interconnected, and that the interconnectedness, by making possible the automatic activation of problematic beliefs, could be a vulnerability factor for emotional distress.

On a more speculative note, it may be recalled that the original description of category accessibility effects (Bruner, 1957b) proposed two sources of increased accessibility: expectancies and motivational states. The aforementioned description of self as a cognitive structure might be considered to be a nonmotivational account of the impact of self-knowledge on self-evaluation. But, it should be noted that the interconnectedness of the problematic self-beliefs was itself a function of motivational factors; that is, what is responsible for the characteristic cognitive biases of depressed individuals, for example, must be understood as self-regulatory activity involving self-guides rather than simply as a structural property of their self-knowledge per se. This view is consistent with psychoanalytic conceptualizations of needs, standards, or goal states (e.g., "drives" and "wishes"; see Holt, 1976). We would suggest that the role of self-knowledge in vulnerability to emotional disorder should not be considered as purely cognitive or purely motivational. We will elaborate on this comment in the next section.

Self and Motivation: Past and Future as Impetus for the Present

A variety of psychological processes have been suggested as factors in determining how people evaluate themselves (Higgins, Strauman, & Klein, 1986). Historically, psychodynamic theories implicated motivational aspects of self-evaluation, that is, seeking pleasure and avoiding pain, as essential determinants of personality (Freud, 1923/1961; Holt, 1976). Individuals were seen as responding not just to events themselves, but also to the anticipation of pain or pleasure as consequences of those events (as in Freud's notion of "signal anxiety"). Unfortunately, the empirical shortcomings of these theories led to their eventual disfavor among many self researchers. The result has been that, with a few exceptions (e.g., Showers & Cantor, 1985), the motivational nature of self-knowledge has not been given its due as an essential property of the self.

Following both classic (Allport, 1943) and contemporary (Epstein, 1980) reviewers, we would argue that what is unique about self-beliefs is not their status as representations of knowledge per se, but rather *their inherent, developmentally derived association with affect and motivation.* That is, what individuals believe about themselves matters in their lives more than other forms of knowledge, even if all types of knowledge were to be structurally equivalent. Thus, while the more recent social-cognitive theories of the self appear preferable to account for certain cognitive properties, motivational considerations appear to favor the contributions of classic self theories, both psychodynamic and phenomenological. In the following paragraphs, we will identify some of what we consider to be particularly important considerations for self theory in accounting for motivational and affective processes.

Cognitive versus Motivational Processes

If it is ever useful to make some distinctions between cognitive and motivational processes, then surely the study of the self provides such an occasion. In a chapter entitled "Motivation and Information Processing," Kuhl (1986) proposed a set of working definitions for the concepts of affect, motivation, and cognition. The term *cognition* was said to refer to processes that mediate the acquisition and representation of knowledge, that is, processes that have a *representative* relation to the world of events, objects, and facts. *Emotion* was defined as referring to the *evaluation* of the personal significance of those events, objects, and facts. Finally, *motivation* was conceptualized as processes that relate to the world in an *intentional* or actional way, that is, that relate to goal states of the individual in an attempt to produce desired changes in her/himself or the environment. Having provided these definitions (which bear an acknowledged resemblance to James's description of the self), Kuhl goes on to describe the complex interactions among the three systems with respect to such phenomena as choice, persistence, and effort.

Our purpose in citing Kuhl's operational definitions is not to imply that they are necessarily superior to other such frameworks, but rather to illustrate the importance of demarcating the role of information processing and knowledge representation in determining affect and behavior. Our impression has been that most cognitive theories of psychopathology are predominantly models of knowledge representation (e.g., Beck, 1967, 1976). As such, while they have provided useful hypotheses and clinical insights regarding the nature of emotional disorders, they are not sufficient descriptions of the psychological processes underlying psychopathology. In other words, it is not enough to postulate that depression-prone individuals have acquired "negative concepts about the self" that "may be latent but can be activated by specific circumstances" (Beck et al., 1979, p. 97). Referring to Kuhl's outline, it is just as important to determine the motivational (i.e., goal states) and affective (i.e., self-evaluative) aspects of depression proneness. There are a number of critical questions to be asked. Is it advisable to concentrate so exclusively on the pathogenic qualities of declarative self-referential knowledge that depressed individuals appear to possess, to the exclusion of other prerepresentational or representational domains (Bowlby, 1985)? Are there characteristic *goals* or *needs* (either temporary or chronic) that differentiate depressed individuals from nondepressed ones (e.g., Blatt & Bers, Chapter 6, this volume)? How might the behavior regulation deficits observed in depression be determined by the manner in which depressed individuals process information about themselves and vice versa?

Kuhl's commentary is not so much critical of cognitively oriented theories as it is endeavoring to make a distinction between knowledge representation and the manner in which information is utilized—to borrow Freud's term, the *vicissitudes* of information. Logically, how and when a particular element of self-knowledge is used is as crucial to its impact on mood and behavior as is the content of the knowledge element itself. Moreover, that processing is controlled by characteristics of the individual that are distinct from the element being processed. As such, it is likely that what distinguishes the self-system of depression-prone individuals is not limited to the content of their self-beliefs (the information represented), but also involves the *conditions* under which certain self-beliefs are activated, as well as and their interaction with each other and with the individual's goals and emotional state (i.e., self-regulatory and self-evaluative systems).

This distinction between the representation of self-knowledge and the processing of that knowledge features prominently in a number of research programs. Cybernetic models such as those formulated by Carver and Scheier (1981) and Guidano (1987) focus on self-evaluation as a system of interconnected information processing loops or hierarchies. Beck (e.g., 1976) depicted various types of cognitive distortions associated with depression, some of which are process-oriented rather than representational. Barlow (1988) and Mathews (e.g., Mathews & MacLeod, 1986) have offered models of cognitive processes relevant to the onset and maintenance of anxiety states. Kuiper and colleagues (e.g., Kuiper, Olinger, MacDonald, & Shaw, 1985) have explored the conditions under which depressogenic attitudes and beliefs are likely to be activated. Our own research is also relevant in this respect. We have demonstrated in a number of laboratory studies how self-discrepancies, as cognitive structures, can be automatically activated through the manipulation of contextual features to induce distinct emotional states without the awareness or intention of the individual (Strauman & Higgins, 1987; Strauman, 1989b). This research instantiates the theory of person–situation relations offered by Higgins (1990), in which the psychological significance of an event is postulated to be a synergistic function of both the person (i.e., "theory-driven processing") and the situation ("data-driven processing" and "context-driven processing").

The Nature of Self-representation

It is likewise important to note that the nature of what is represented within the self needs to be explored more thoroughly. As implied above, most studies of self-beliefs (including our own) have addressed the domain of declarative memory, focusing on such abstract knowledge as self-ratings of personality traits. But it would be naive to presume that everything we know or believe about our selves is abstract and declarative in nature and can be identified accurately and explicitly. Classic self theories abound with examples of self phenomena outside this domain. Freud's notions of transference and repetition compulsion captured the essence of neurosis as implicit perceptual–behavioral patterns that could not be consciously recognized but were unwittingly repeated in everyday life. Sullivan's social-developmental framework for the acquisition of self-knowledge (good me, bad me, not me) implied that critical features of self-representation are procedural, evaluative, and relational rather than semantic, just as early (Mahler, 1968) and contemporary (Bowlby, 1988) object relations theorists focused on aspects of identity that are derived from internalizations of relationship patterns ("identifications"). Even among contemporary theories of emotion and psychopathology as disparate as those of Lang (1984) and Guidano (1987), there is consensus that much of what is represented within the self is not easily characterized as abstract, declarative knowledge.

Strauman (1989a) suggested that the motivational facet of emotionally significant self-representations is a key ingredient in understanding the relation between self and behavior. He suggested a fundamental distinction between two classes of self-referential goals associated with self-beliefs: *survival-related* and *consistency-related* motives. These two classes would be expected to have different developmental origins, to induce different types and intensities of behavior when activated, and to be associated with different interpersonal and emotional problems. In addition, self-inconsistency could involve a discrepancy or conflict between the informational content, or declarative aspects, of two self-beliefs, between the motivational, or goal-directed, aspects of the beliefs, or both; in each case, different affective and behavioral consequences would result (cf. Showers & Cantor, 1985; Sorrentino & Higgins, 1986, for similar views).

Self and Development: The Transcendent Past

In the preceding section we mentioned that one distinction between self-beliefs and other forms of knowledge is the motivational import inherent in the self. Another distinction is the intimate association between self-beliefs and the individual's personal history. Perhaps the most striking aspect of the self is its long-term coherence and constancy, both as experienced by the individual and with regard to self-regulatory patterns across the life span. Most, if not all, self theories postulate that the self is significantly determined by experiences, events, and social interactions that occurred in the past. For many theorists, in fact, the self construct implies a continuing influence of the individual's history on her/his psychological functioning. This general principle can be characterized as a hypothesis of *continuity* of the self. Aspects of significant life experiences—interpretations, appraisals, affective and motivational consequences, opinions of significant others—are often postulated to become represented in the individual's knowledge base; in turn, most theories predict that those representations exert a notable influence on affect, motivation, and behavior. The famous Freudian dictum that "the child is father to the man" poetically illustrates this inherent developmental characteristic of self-beliefs.

However, there has been relatively little emphasis in the self literature on the *nature* of developmental continuity within the self, that is the psychological processes and structures that are responsible for its postulated stability and relative resistance to change (Higgins, 1989; Strauman, 1989a). In some respects it could be asserted that the developmental roots of the self are more prominent within the folk wisdom of people's implicit personality theories than within social-cognitive self theories. Developmental investigators (e.g., Fischer, 1980; Harter, 1983, 1986) have postulated that representations of the self may differ in content and function depending on the circumstances that led to their acquisition, as well as the maturational status of the individual at that point. We will describe below a framework for considering how the continually increasing cognitive sophistication of the individual affects the developmental nature of self-beliefs and on the overall personality.

Developmental Considerations for the Self–affect Relation

The literature on the development of the self-system describes dramatic changes in children's self-beliefs, self-regulatory processes, and self-evaluative processes (see Harter, 1983). Higgins (1989) examined how cognitive-developmental changes in children's mental representational capacities might underlie general changes in aspects of the self-system relevant to the emergence of self-discrepancies and affective vulnerability. These transformations are presented in terms of five major developmental shifts, each of which is associated with distinct changes in children's general capacity to mentally represent events and resultant changes in the nature and emotional consequences of self-beliefs. A brief description of the five general levels follows:

1. *Early sensorimotor development*. By the end of the first year of life, children are capable of representing the relation between two events, such as the relation between a response produced by them and their mother's response to them. This ability permits children to produce and interpret signals and to experience emotions that involve anticipating the occurrence of some event. Even at this early stage, children can experience four basic, emotionally significant psychological situations: the *presence or absence of positive outcomes* (actual or anticipated), and the *presence or absence of negative outcomes* (actual or anticipated). Thus, from the time that chil-

dren begin to form mental representations of social events, those representations are associated with emotional consequences for behaviors.

2. *Late sensorimotor and early interrelational development.* A dramatic shift in children's ability to mentally represent events occurs between 1½ and 2 years of age (Bruner, 1964; Werner & Kaplan, 1963): children become capable of recognizing the higher order relation that exists between two other relations. As a consequence of this change, children can now consider the bidirectional relationship between themselves and another person (Harter, 1983). For instance, they can represent the relation between a particular self-feature (action, mood, etc.) and a particular response by another person. Thus, children can now represent *self–other contingencies*, which are cognitive precursors of mature self-guides. Such contingencies, although not yet true self-evaluative processes, nonetheless can be used to self-regulate so as to avoid or approach different psychological situations. This new capacity for "interiorized compliance" allows children to deal more successfully with social demands, leading to feelings of pride and joy; conversely, the possibility of failure introduces feelings of abandonment and rejection by others.

3. *Late interrelational and early dimensional development.* Between the ages of 4 and 6, children's representational capacity shifts from egocentric to nonegocentric thought (e.g., Piaget, 1965). The intellectual changes at this stage are reflected in children's increased ability to infer the thoughts, expectations, motives, and intentions of others (Shantz, 1983), as well as increased ability to use sources of information beyond the immediate situation (e.g., autobiographical or social comparison information) when judging the actions of self or others (Ruble & Rholes, 1981). These changes make possible a major transformation in children's self-evaluation and self-regulation: They can now regulate and evaluate their behavior in terms of a standard or guide for their self-features that involves another person's viewpoint. Such standards have the important benefit of increasing the range of circumstances under which children can assert self-control and experience positive emotions. In addition, however, this new capacity to appraise themselves in terms of self-guides is likely to contribute to the appearance of new emotional vulnerabilities such as guilt, apprehension, and embarrassment.

4. *Late dimensional and early vectorial development.* Between 9 and 11 years of age children become capable of coordinating values along two distinct dimensions. This advance makes dispositional judgments of self and others possible, so that children's self-concepts can now contain dispositional attributes. A negative or positive psychological situation can therefore be induced not only from the evaluation of a current or recent performance, but also by extraneous activation of a self-congruent or

self-discrepant trait. The self-evaluation process for a single self-feature could now activate a child's overall self-evaluative system because of spreading activation among interconnected elements (Higgins et al., 1988; Hayes-Roth, 1977; Strauman & Higgins, 1987).

5. *Late vectorial development*. Between 13 and 16 years of age, children become capable of interrelating different perspectives on the same object, including the self (Fischer, 1980; Inhelder & Piaget, 1958). Adolescents can now integrate information about distinct traits into higher-order abstractions such as personality types; therefore, at this stage self-concepts and self-guides can include representations of personality and identity types (Harter, 1983). This could further increase the structural interconnectedness among adolescents' self-attributes, with concomitant implications for increased emotional vulnerability. In the case of self-discrepancies, this is likely to increase the probability that adolescents would be vulnerable to new global negative psychological situations, such as the "overgeneralizations" and "global negative self-attributions" described in the depression literature.

As this developmental framework makes clear, the acquisition of self-knowledge is intimately and *necessarily* associated with the emergence of emotional experience. In turn, both of these phenomena are influenced by the ongoing processes of intellectual development, biological maturation, and socialization modes and practices. We would suggest, then, that to consider self-knowledge processes in isolation—that is, without taking into account their inevitable connection with the development of emotional and motivational processes—risks a kind of conceptual sterility in self theory. Based on our own investigations and those of others, however, we are confident that a developmental perspective on the self can serve to facilitate a more comprehensive consideration of the nature of self-knowledge. Such an approach would then be more likely to provide a useful framework for investigating the role of the self in the etiology of emotional disorders such as depression and anxiety.

Self-guides and Childhood Memories

Recently one of us has begun to explore the relation between self-guides and memory for emotionally significant childhood experiences. The research is based on a developmental premise of self-discrepancy theory, that the acquisition of self–other contingency knowledge during childhood—postulated to occur as a function of social-learning experiences—results in the establishment of internalized standards for self-evaluation. Specifically, several studies (Strauman, 1990, 1992) have been conducted to compare the effects of different types of cues (including self-guides) on childhood memories with respect to both ease of retrieval and incidental negative emotional content. The studies were intended to determine whether self-guides would be preferentially associated with memories for emotionally significant childhood experiences, supporting the hypothesized relation between self-guides (as motivationally significant self-knowledge structures) and childhood experiences involving negative emotional states.

Each study was conducted in two ostensibly unrelated sessions approximately 2 months apart. In the initial session, subjects' chronically accessible self-guides were identified using the Selves Questionnaire. Subsequently, they were contacted to participate in a study of childhood memory in which the task was to respond to a list of cue words by verbalizing the first memory of a childhood experience that came to mind following the presentation of each word. Unknown to each participant, the cue word lists contained selected attributes from her/his self-guides as determined by the Selves Questionnaire (*self-referential* attributes), as well as self-guide attributes from other subjects that had not been listed by the target subject (*yoked control* attributes), as well as positive and negative *affect* words. The dependent measures included retrieval time (the average amount of time for subjects to begin verbalizing a memory following cue word presentation) and the incidental negative affect content of the memories that were verbalized.

Taken together, the studies offer two related conclusions. First, the results demonstrated that cues relevant to negative affect represent potent contexts for retrieving memories of emotionally significant childhood events, suggesting that such memories are likely to be encoded in terms of their emotional significance at the time they were experienced. Second—and more important in this context—self-guide cues (and particularly self-discrepant cues) produced more efficient retrieval and greater incidental negative content of memories than other cue types, in addition to specific and discriminable effects of ideal-discrepant versus ought-discrepant cues on retrieval time and negative affect content. This pattern, which was found in all three studies, occurred even though the self-referential cues were always positively valenced and that no subject reported awareness of the self-referential nature of certain cue words. The most recent study exploring the relation between self-guides and childhood memories (Strauman, 1992) showed that among dysphoric, anxious, and control subjects, only responses to self-referential cues discriminated the subject groups clearly—not even negative or positive affect cues.

Overall, the data provide evidence that self-guides, hypothesized to represent chronically accessible constructs in the service of self-regulation and evaluation, may be systematically related to memories of remote life events. The results of the clinical replication study (Strauman, 1992) are particularly significant for the present discussion. Dysphoric individuals did not relate childhood memories that were significantly more sad or depressive in nature in response to depression-related cue words such as "sad," "disappointed," and "dissatisfied." Rather, they were only discriminable from other subjects in that they generated dysphoric memories when responding to self-guide cues, all of which were positively valenced (and hence not semantically associated with depression-related emotional states). Similarly, anxious subjects were not significantly more likely than their counterparts to generate childhood memories high in anxious content in response to anxious-related cue words such as "nervous"; only in response to self-guide cues were the anxious individuals more likely to do so. This pattern suggests that self-knowledge structures of the two emotionally distressed groups may not necessarily be characterized by global tendencies for negative self-evaluation; rather, the difference may lie in the magnitude, type, and accessibility of self-discrepancies from individual to individual. The findings also lend support (albeit in a retrospective study design) to the developmental postulates of self-discrepancy theory, emphasizing both the need to consider the historical origins of emotionally significant self-beliefs and the inherent emotional and motivational implications of self- knowledge.

"Can," "Past," and "Future" as Domains of the Self

Our perspective on the self as a template for the individual's past, present, and future also suggests that the relations among one's temporally identified self-beliefs have important emotional and behavioral implications. James (1890/1948) described how certain aspects of the self were more appropriately characterized as "potential" rather than factual (see also Bandura, 1982). Rogers (1961) was among the first to investigate systematically how an individual's beliefs about her/his present status in relation to what she/he anticipated in the future determined her/his emotional state. Among contemporary investigators, Markus (Markus & Nurius, 1986) has proposed the notion of *possible selves*, defined as elements of the self-concept that represent the individual's goals, motives, fears, and anxieties, and specifically that subset of goals, outcomes, or expectancies that are individualized and given self-referent form or meaning. In this model, possible selves provide a link between the self-concept and motivation, serving to illuminate the significance of events for the individual and providing incentives for future behavior. In one recent investigation using this framework, Oyserman and Markus (1990) observed that delinquent and nondelinquent youths differed significantly in their expected and feared selves but not in their hoped-for selves. These differences were associated with degree of delinquent behavior.

Our own research has also examined emotional and behavioral consequences of the temporal relations among self-beliefs. Recent studies have expanded self-discrepancy theory to include additional domains of the self, including the *past* self (the person's representation of the attributes that she/he believes she/he actually possessed in the past), the *future* self (the person's representation of the attributes that someone, self or other, believes she/he is likely to possess in the future), and the *can* self (the person's representation of the attributes that someone, self or other,, believes she/he can possess). The future self is a representation of the individual's *expectations* about the type of person she/he will become; the can self is a representation of the person's beliefs about her/his capabilities or potential. We have recently conducted two studies examining the psychological significance of self-belief patterns involving three self-beliefs rather than just pairs of self-beliefs, with the larger configurations of self-beliefs contrasting *temporal* aspects of self-knowledge. Both studies tested the proposal that particular patterns of self-beliefs, as psychological entities, have distinct emotional and motivational significance that depends on the interrelations among the self-beliefs and not simply on the beliefs as independent elements.

Higgins, Vookles, and Tykocinsky (in press) examined several self-belief patterns involving an actual–ideal discrepancy, including two in which the future self was implicated—$A < I(>F)$ and $A < I(= F)$, where A is the actual self, I is the ideal self, and F is the future self. The $A < I(>F)$ pattern signifies an actual self-discrepancy with future–ideal discrepancy. A future–ideal discrepancy represents the belief that one will not reach one's ideal in the future, that is, a desired end-state that one does not expect to attain. In this pattern the actual self is perceived as discrepant from the $I > F$ unit, corresponding to the psychological situation of "doing less well than wished for but not less than expected." The $A < I(= F)$ pattern signifies an actual self-discrepancy with future–ideal congruency. A future–ideal congruency represents the belief that one's ideal is a desired end-state that one *does* expect to attain. The actual self is perceived as discrepant from this $I = F$ unit, corresponding to the situation of "chronically unfulfilled hopes." Since both patterns involved an actual–ideal discrepancy, both would be expected to be associated with dejection-related discomfort. As predicted, however, the $A < I(= F)$ pattern ("chronically unfulfilled hopes") was more strongly associated with suffering, and particularly with a sense of despondency.

Strauman and Higgins (1992) examined several forms of actual–ideal discrepancies in which the past self was implicated. The pattern $(A = P) < I$ signifies an actual–past congruency with ideal discrepancy. An actual–past congruency represents the belief that one's actual attributes in the past are also one's attributes in the present. The ideal self is perceived as discrepant from this $A = P$ unit, creating the psychological situation of "lack of progress." Conversely, the $A < I(= P)$ pattern signifies an ideal–past congruency with actual discrepancy. An ideal–past congruency represents the belief that in the past one had achieved one's desired end-states. The actual self (the attributes one possesses at present) is perceived as discrepant from this $I = P$ unit, resulting in the psychological situation of "the loss of a positive past," or "retrogression." Again, since both involve an actual–

ideal discrepancy, both would be expected to lead to dejection-related emotions. The data suggested that the $A < (I = P)$ pattern, "retrogression," was associated with more severe manifestations of depressive symptomatology, whereas the $(A = P) < I$ pattern, "lack of progress," was associated with frustration and the absence of happiness/satisfaction. It was interesting to note that hardly any subjects indicated a substantial overlap (matches or mismatches) between the past self and the *ought* self-standard. This suggests that within the ideal domain, it makes sense to speak about lack of progress and retrogression, but for one's sense of duty and obligations, the issue of progress is less compelling—either one is or is not violating prescriptions. Both studies illustrate the importance of considering how different aspects of the self are linked to different periods of one's history, with resultant positive and negative implications for self-evaluation and behavior.

CONCLUSION: PROSPECTS FOR A THEORY OF SELF IN PSYCHOPATHOLOGY

The self construct has had an interesting and consequential history in social psychology. In part, of course, this history reflects the ubiquity of the self construct, since, as Allport (1955) argued, any theory in which the individual's personal experience or knowledge plays a significant role can be considered a theory of self. Nonetheless, many major conceptual trends in social psychology over the past 50 years either originated in, or were rapidly assimilated into, the study of the self. Moreover, social psychology has been a consistent contributor to significant ideas and research on the self.

In the 1970s and 1980s, social-psychological theories of the self were primarily concerned with issues of knowledge representation and information processing, as would be expected given the observed paradigm shift toward cognitive models and techniques (Baars, 1986). This shift was a useful and appropriate development for self theory, since one hallmark of the cognitive perspective is its inclusion of hypothetical constructs and inductive methods by which to evaluate them. The study of the self almost certainly necessitates such construct-building, and present-day social psychologists have used this recent perspective in proposing and testing a variety of creative and heuristic self theories. As several reviewers (Higgins & Bargh, 1987; Greenwald & Pratkanis, 1984; Kihlstrom et al., 1988) have noted, the self has regained its former prominence and popularity as a construct and as a research topic.

The comments and critiques offered throughout this chapter exemplify our views on the future of the self. In keeping with an emerging trend in social and personality psychology overall, it is conceivable that in the next few years the study of the self will evolve beyond the current tendency to focus on a single mechanism or theoretical emphasis (e.g., information processing, phenomenology, psychodynamics). Certainly there are at present a number of promising examples of such interdisciplinary efforts, as exemplified throughout the present volume. It would be ideal for such strides toward integration to proceed alongside continued efforts to refine and perfect the cognitively oriented models that comprise the most recent additions to the self literature.

The "paradox" of the self (Strauman, 1989a), and its ultimate challenge as a theoretical construct, is that it simultaneously represents and personifies one's past, present, and future. This paradox, which was clearly identified by James, has significant implications for our understanding of the self as structure, as process, and as a source of vulnerability to emotional distress. In highlighting our own research alongside the work of other investigators, we hope to illustrate our contention that the self construct is a natural locus for inquiry regarding the manner in which an individual's identity, experience, and regulatory processes may predispose her/him to emotional vulnerability and, ultimately, emotional disorders.

The eventual direction in which this consequential and challenging research area evolves should entail a deliberate effort to appreciate more fully each historical perspective on the self. In reviewing the conceptual and empirical trends within the self literature, it is striking and encouraging to consider the wealth of ideas and observations that have accumulated, even if to date there has been less integration and cross-fertilization than might be desired. Investigators and theorists should take full advantage of the unique emphases of psychodynamic, phenomenological, and social-cognitive models of the self—their approaches to the experiential, motivational, emotional, and representational facets of the self construct—and in doing so acknowledge the relative strengths and weaknesses of each school. If the present volume with its creative format of dialogue and contrast is any indication, we anticipate a new era of integration and progress in the psychological study of the self.

REFERENCES

Allport, G. W. (1937). *Personality: A psychological interpretation*. New York: Holt, Rinehart & Winston.

Allport, G. W. (1943). The ego in contemporary psychology. *Psychological Review*, *50*, 451–478.

Allport, G. W.(1955). *Becoming*. New Haven, CT: Yale University Press.

Anderson, J. (1983). *The architecture of cognition*. Cambridge, MA: Harvard University Press.

Aronson, E. (1969). The theory of cognitive dissonance: A current perspective. *Advances in Experimental Social Psychology*, *4*, 1–34.

Baars, B. J. (1986). *The cognitive revolution in psychology*. New York: Guilford Press.

Bandura, A. (1982). Self-efficacy mechanism in human agency. *American Psychologist*, *37*, 122–147.

Bandura, A. (1986). *Social foundations of thought and action: A social cognitive theory*. Englewood Cliffs, NJ: Prentice-Hall.

Barlow, D. H. (1988). *Anxiety and its disorders*. New York: Guilford Press.

Bartlett, F. C. (1932). *Remembering*. Cambridge: Cambridge University Press.

Beck, A. T. (1967). *Depression: Causes and treatment*. Philadelphia: University of Pennsylvania Press.

Beck, A. T. (1976). *Cognitive therapy and the emotional disorders*. New York: Basic Books.

Beck, A. T., Rush, A. J., Shaw, B. F., & Emery, G. (1979). *Cognitive therapy of depression*. New York: Guilford Press.

Bower, G. H., & Gilligan, S. G. (1979). Remembering information relating to one's self. *Journal of Research in Personality*, *13*, 420–461.

Bowlby, J. (1985). The role of childhood experience in cognitive disturbance. In M. J. Mahoney & A. Freeman (Eds.), *Cognition and psychotherapy* (pp. 181–199). New York: Plenum Press.

Bowlby, J. (1988). *A secure base*. New York: Basic Books.

Bransford, J. D., & Franks, J. J. (1972). The abstraction of linguistic ideas: A review. *Cognition*, *1*, 221–249.

Breckler, S. J., & Greenwald, A. G. (1982). Charting coordinates for the self-concept in multidimensional cognitive space. In *Functioning and measurement of self-esteem*. Symposium conducted at the meeting of the American Psychological Association, Washington, DC.

Bruner, J. S. (1957a). Going beyond the information given. In H. Gruber, R. Blake, & G. Ramsey (Eds.), *Contemporary approaches to cognition* (pp. 121–147). Cambridge, MA: Harvard University Press.

Bruner, J. S. (1957b). On perceptual readiness. *Psychological Review*, *80*, 307–336.

Bruner, J. S.(1964). The course of cognitive growth. *American Psychologist*, *19*, 1–15.

Bugental, J. (1964). Investigations into the self-concept: 3. Instructions for the W-A-Y method. *Psychological Reports*, *15*, 643–650.

Cantor, N., & Kihlstrom, J. F. (1986). *Personality and social intelligence*. Englewood Cliffs, NJ: Prentice-Hall.

Cantor, N., & Mischel, W. (1979). Prototypes in person perception. In L. Berkowitz (Ed.), *Advances in experimental social psychology* (Vol. 12, pp. 75–122). New York: Academic Press.

Cantril, H. (1932). General and specific attitudes. *Psychological Monographs*, *192*.

Carver, C. S., & Scheier, M. F. (1981). *Attention and self-regulation: A control theoryapproach to human behavior*. New York: Springer-Verlag.

Carver, C. S., & Scheier, M. F. (1982). Control theory: A useful conceptual framework for personality-social, clinical, and health psychology. *Psychological Bulletin*, *92*, 111–135.

Cooley, C. H. (1964). *Human nature and the social order* (rev. ed.). New York: Schocken Books. (Original work published 1902)

Coyne, J. C., & Gotlib, I. H. (1983). The role of cognition in depression: A critical appraisal. *Psychological Bulletin*, *94*, 472–505.

Duval, S., & Wicklund, R. A. (1972). *A theory of objective self-awareness*. New York: Academic Press.

Epstein, S. (1973). The self-concept revisited, or a theory of a theory. *American Psychologist*, *28*, 404–416.

Epstein, S. (1980). The self-concept: A review and a proposal of an integrated theory of personality. In E. Staub (Ed.), *Personality: Basic issues and current research* (pp. 82–132). Englewood Cliffs, NJ: Prentice-Hall.

Erikson, E. H. (1963). *Childhood and society* (2nd ed.). New York: W. W. Norton. (Original work published 1950)

Fazio, R. H., & Zanna, M. P. (1981). Direct experience and attitude-behavior consistency. *Advances in Experimental Social Psychology*, *14*, 161–202.

Festinger, L. (1957). *A theory of cognitive dissonance*. Evanston, IL: Row, Peterson.

Fischer, K. W. (1980). A theory of cognitive development: The control and construction of hierarchies of skills. *Psychological Review*, *87*, 477–531.

Fiske, S. T., & Taylor, S. E. (1984). *Social cognition*. Reading, MA: Addison-Wesley.

Freud, S. (1961). The ego and the id. In J. Strachey (Ed. and Trans.), *The standard edition of the complete psychological works of Sigmund Freud* (Vol. 19, pp. 3–66). London: Hogarth Press. (Original work published 1923)

Gergen, K. J. (1984). Theory of the self: Impasse and evolution. *Advances in Experimental Social Psychology*, *17*, 49–115.

Gibson, J. J. (1979). *The ecological approach to visual perception*. Boston: Houghton Mifflin.

Gordon, C. (1968). Self-conceptions: Configurations of content. In C. Gordon & K. Gergen (Eds.), *The self in social interaction: Vol. 1. Classic and contemporary problems* (pp. 121–149). New York: Wiley.

Greenwald, A. G., & Pratkanis, A. R. (1984). The self. In R. Wyer & T. Srull (Eds.), *Handbook of social cognition* (Vol. 3). Hillsdale, NJ: Lawrence Erlbaum.

Guidano, V. F. (1987). *Complexity of the self: A developmental approach to psychopathology and therapy*. New York: Guilford Press.

Guidano, V. F., & Liotti, G. (1983). *Cognitive processes and emotional disorders: A structural approach to psychotherapy*. New York: Guilford Press.

Harter, S. (1983). Developmental perspectives on the self-system. In P.H. Mussen (Ed.), *Handbook of child psychology: Vol. 4. Socialization, personality, and social development* (pp.275–385). New York: Wiley.

Harter, S. (1986). Cognitive-developmental processes in the integration of concepts about emotions and the self. *Social Cognition*, *4*, 119–151.

Hayes-Roth, B. (1977). Evolution of cognitive structures and processes. *Psychological Review*, *84*, 60–278.

Hebb, D. O. (1949). *The organization of behavior*. New York: Wiley.

Higgins, E. T. (1987). Self-discrepancy: A theory relating self and affect. *Psychological Review*, *94* (3), 319–340.

Higgins, E. T. (1989). Knowledge accessibility and activation: Subjectivity and suffering from unconscious sources. In J. Uleman & J. A. Bargh (Eds.), *Unintended thought* (pp. 75–123). New York: Guilford Press.

Higgins, E. T. (1990). Personality, social psychology, and person-situation relations: Standards and knowledge activation as a common language. In L. Pervin (Ed.), *Handbook of personality: Theory and research* (pp. 301–338). New York: Guilford.

Higgins, E. T., & Bargh, J. A. (1987). Social cognition and social perception. *Annual Review of Psychology, 38*, 369–425.

Higgins, E. T., Bond, R., Klein, R., & Strauman, T. (1986). Self-discrepancies and emotional vulnerability: How magnitude, type and accessibility of discrepancy influence affect. *Journal of Personality and Social Psychology, 51*(1), 5–15.

Higgins, E. T., Strauman, T. J., & Klein, R. (1986). Standards and the process of self-evaluation: Multiple affects from multiple stages. In R. Sorrentino & E. T. Higgins (Eds.), *Handbook of motivation and cognition: Foundations of social behavior* (Vol. 1, pp. 23–63). New York: Guilford Press.

Higgins, E. T., Van Hook, E., & Dorfman, D. (1988). Do self attributes form a cognitive structure? *Social Cognition, 6*, 177–207.

Higgins, E. T., Vookles, J., & Tykocinsky, O. (in press). Self and health: How "patterns" of self-beliefs predict types of emotional and physical problems. *Social Cognition.*

Hollon, S. D., & Kriss, M. R. (1984). Cognitive factors in clinical research and practice. *Clinical Psychology Review, 4*, 35–76.

Holt, R. R. (1976). Drive or wish? A reconsideration of the psychoanalytic theory of motivation. In M. M. Gill & P. S. Holzman (Eds.), Psychology versus metapsychology: Psychoanalytic essays in memory of George S. Klein. *Psychological Issues, 9*, 158–197.

Horney, K. (1950). *Neurosis and human growth*. New York: W. W. Norton.

Inhelder, B., & Piaget, J. (1958). *The growth of logical thinking from childhood to adolescence*. New York: Basic Books.

James, W. (1948). *The principles of psychology*. New York: World. (Original work published 1890)

Kelly, G. A. (1955). *The psychology of personal constructs*. New York: W. W. Norton.

Kihlstrom, J. F., & Cantor, N. (1984). Mental representations of the self. *Advances in Experimental Social Psychology, 17*, 1–47.

Kihlstrom, J. F., Cantor, N., Albright, J. S., Chew, B. R., Klein, S. B., & Niedenthal, P. M. (1988). Information processing and the study of the self. *Advances in Experimental Social Psychology, 21*, 145–178.

Klein, S. B., & Kihlstrom, J. F. (1986). Elaboration, organization, and the self-reference effect in memory. *Journal of Experimental Psychology: General, 115*, 26–38.

Kuhl, J. (1986). Motivation and information processing: A new look at decision making, dynamic change, and action control. In R. Sorrentino & E. T. Higgins (Eds.), *Handbook of motivation and cognition: Foundations of social behavior* (Vol. 1, pp. 404–434). New York: Guilford Press.

Kuiper, N. A., & Derry, P. A. (1981). The self as a cognitive prototype: An application to person perception and depression. In N. Cantor & J. F. Kihlstrom (Eds.), *Personality, cognition and social interaction* (pp. 120–159). Hillsdale, NJ:Lawrence Erlbaum.

Kuiper, N. A., & Higgins, E. T. (1985). Social cognition and depression: A general integrative perspective. *Social Cognition*, *3*, 1–15.

Kuiper, N. A., Olinger, L. J., MacDonald, M. R., & Shaw, B. F. (1985). Self-schema processing of depressed and nondepresed content: The effects of vulnerability to depression. *Social Cognition*, *3*, 77–93.

Lang, P. J. (1984). Cognition in emotion: Concept and action. In C. Izard, J. Kagan, & R. Zajonc (Eds.), *Cognition, emotion, and behavior* (pp. 192–226). New York: Cambridge University Press.

Lecky, P. (1961). *Self-consistency: A theory of personality*. New York: McGraw-Hill.

Lewin, K. (1935). *A dynamic theory of personality*. New York: McGraw-Hill.

Linville, P. W. (1985). Self-complexity and affective extremity: Don't put all your cognitive eggs in one basket. *Social Cognition*, *3*, 94–120.

Mahler, M. S. (1968). *On human symbiosis and the vicissitudes of information*. New York: International Universities Press.

Markus, H. (1977). Self-schemata and processing information about the self. *Journal of Personality and Social Psychology*, *35*, 63–78.

Markus, H. (1983). Self-knowledge: An expanded view. *Journal of Personality*, *51*, 544–565.

Markus, H., & Nurius, P. (1986). Possible selves. *American Psychologist*, *41*, 954–969. Markus, H., & Sentis, K. (1982). The self in social information processing. In J. Suls (Ed.), *Psychological perspectives on the self* (Vol. 1, pp. 38–79). Hillsdale, NJ: Lawrence Erlbaum.

Markus, H., & Wurf, E. (1987). The dynamic self-concept: A social psychological perspective. *Annual Review of Psychology*, *38*, 299–337.

Mathews, A. M., & MacLeod, C. (1986). Discrimination of threat cues without awareness in anxiety states. *Journal of Abnormal Psychology*, *95*, 131–138.

McArthur, L. Z., & Baron, R. M. (1983). Toward an ecological theory of social perception. *Psychological Review*, *90*, 215–235.

McGuire, W. J., & McGuire, C. V. (1982). The spontaneous self-concept as affected by personal distinctiveness. In M. Lynch, A. Norem-Hebeisen, & K. Gergen (Eds.), *Self-concept: Advances in theory and research* (pp. 179–229). Cambridge, MA: Ballinger.

Mead, G. H. (1934). *Mind, self and society*. Chicago: University of Chicago Press.

Moretti, M. M., & Shaw, B. F. (1989). Automatic and dysfunctional cognitive processes in depression. In J. Uleman & J. A. Bargh (Eds.), *Unintended thought* (pp. 383–421). New York: Guilford Press.

Murray, H. A. (1943). *Explorations in personality*. New York: Oxford University Press.

Oyserman, D., & Markus, H. R. (1990). Possible selves and delinquency. *Journal of Personality and Social Psychology*, *59*, 112–125.

Piaget, J. (1965). *The moral judgment of the child*. New York: Free Press. (Original translation published 1932)

Rogers, C. R. (1961). *On becoming a person*. Boston: Houghton Mifflin.

Rogers, T. B. (1981). A model of the self as an aspect of the human information processing system. In N. Cantor & J. Kihlstrom (Eds.), *Personality, cognition, and social interaction* (pp. 165–198). Hillsdale, NJ: Lawrence Erlbaum.

Rogers, T. B., Kuiper, N. A., & Kirker, W. S. (1977). Self-reference and the encoding of personal information. *Journal of Personality and Social Psychology, 35*, 677–688.

Ruble, D. N., & Rholes, W. S.(1981). The development of children's perceptions and attributions about their social world. In J. D. Harvey, W. Ickes, & R. F. Kidd (Eds.), *New directions in attribution research* (Vol. 3, pp. 3–36). Hillsdale, NJ: Lawrence Erlbaum.

Sarbin, T. R.(1952). A preface to a psychological analysis of the self. *Psychological Review, 59*, 11–22.

Secord, P. F., & Backman, C. W. (1964). *Social psychology*. New York: McGraw-Hill.

Segal, Z. V. (1988). Appraisal of the self-schema construct in cognitive models of depression. *Psychological Bulletin, 103*, 147–162.

Segal, Z. V., Hood, J.E., Shaw, B. F., & Higgins, E. T. (1988). A structural analysis of the self-schema construct in major depression. *Cognitive Therapy and Research, 12*, 471–485.

Shantz, C. U. (1983). Social cognition. In J. H. Flavell & E. M. Markman (Eds.), *Cognitive development*, Vol. 3 in P. H. Mussen (Ed.), *Carmichael's manual of child psychology*, (4th ed., pp. 495–555). New York: Wiley.

Showers, C. J., & Cantor, N. (1985). Social cognition: A look at motivated strategies. *Annual Review of Psychology, 36*, 275–305.

Sorrentino, R. M., & Higgins, E. T. (1986). Motivation and cognition: Warming up to synergism. In R. Sorrentino & E. T. Higgins (Eds.), *Handbook of motivation and cognition: Foundations of social behavior* (Vol. 1, pp. 3–19). New York: Guilford Press.

Steele, C. M., & Liu, T. J. (1983). Dissonance processes as self-affirmation. *Journal of Personality and Social Psychology, 45*, 5–19.

Strauman, T. J. (1989a). The paradox of the self: A psychodynamic and social-cognitive integration. In R. Curtis (Ed.), *Self-defeating behaviors: Experimental research, clinical impressions, and practical implications* (pp. 263–299). New York: Plenum Press.

Strauman, T. J. (1989b). Self-discrepancies in clinical depression and social phobia: Cognitive structures that underlie emotional disorders? *Journal of Abnormal Psychology, 98*, 14–22.

Strauman, T. J. (1990). Self-guides and emotionally significant childhood memories: A study of retrieval efficiency and incidental negative content. *Journal of Personality and Social Psychology, 59*, 869–880.

Strauman, T. J. (1992). Self-guides, autobiographical memory, and anxiety and dysphoria: Toward a cognitive model of vulnerability to emotional distress. *Journal of Abnormal Psychology, 101*, 87–95.

Strauman, T. J., & Higgins, E. T. (1987). Automatic activation of self-discrepancies and emotional syndromes: When cognitive structures influence affect. *Journal of Personality and Social Psychology, 53*, 1004–1014.

Strauman, T. J., & Higgins, E. T. (1988). Self-discrepancies as predictors of vulnerability to distinct syndromes of chronic emotional distress. *Journal of Personality*, *56*, 685–707.

Strauman, T. J., & Higgins, E. T. (1992). *Self present and past: The psychological significance of self-belief patterns involving actual, past, and ideal self-states.* Unpublished manuscript.

Stryker, S., & Statham, A. (1985). Symbolic interaction and role theory. In G. Lindzey & E. Aronson (Eds.), *Handbook of social psychology* (Vol. 1, pp. 311–378). New York: Random House.

Sullivan, H. S. (1953). *The interpersonal theory of psychiatry*. New York: W. W. Norton.

Swann, W. B., Jr. (1983). Self-verification: Bringing social reality into harmony with the self. In J. Suls & A. Greenwald (Eds.), *Social psychological perspectives on the self* (Vol. 2, pp. 33–66). Hillsdale, NJ: Lawrence Erlbaum.

Warren, R. E. (1972). Stimulus encoding and memory. *Journal of Experimental Psychology*, *94*, 90–100.

Werner, H., & Kaplan, B. (1963). *Symbol formation*. New York: Wiley.

Wicklund, R. A., & Gollwitzer, P. M. (1982). *Symbolic self-completion*. Hillsdale, NJ: Lawrence Erlbaum.

Wiener, N. (1948). *Cybernetics: Control and communication in the animal and the machine*. Cambridge, MA: MIT Press.

Wyer, R. S., Jr., & Gordon, S. E.(1984). The cognitive representation of social information. In R. S. Wyer, Jr., & T. K. Srull (Eds.), *Handbook of social cognition* (Vol. 2, pp. 73–150). Hillsdale, NJ: Lawrence Erlbaum.

Wylie, R. C. (1979). *The self-concept*. Lincoln: University of Nebraska Press.

2

The Self Construct in Psychoanalytic Theory: A Comparative View

STEVEN H. COOPER
Harvard Medical School
and Boston Psychoanalytic Society
and Institute

LIKE MANY PSYCHOANALYTIC terms, the concept of the self has been used in varying ways and with reference to differing levels of theoretical discourse. In early psychoanalytic theory (e.g. Freud, 1923/1961), the term *ego,* as a construct within Freud's structural theory, was used synonymously with the self. At times the self concept has been used synonymously with identity and a sense of personal continuity, that is, the enduring characteristics of an individual as revealed in roles and behaviors. Some authors refer to the self as a superordinate, regulatory system that is either coordinate or subordinate to the system's id, ego, and superego within Freud's structural theory of the mind. In other contexts, the self has been called a superordinate concept when it refers to an overall intrapsychic constitution. In still other theoretical treatments of the subject, the self has been referred to in more exclusively experiential terms as relating to an individual's collective (past and present) affective experience. In other words, there has been little consensus regarding the use of the term *self.*

Overall, probably the most significant source of confusion in the use of the terms *self* and *self-representation* centers around whether they are is used as an abstract, metapsychological terms or experiential ones. Most contemporary psychoanalytic theorists fail to take a systematic stand concerning the self as distinguished from the self-representation. Generally, the term *self* is a nontheoretical concept that people use in talking and reflecting about themselves. As will be outlined in this chapter, some metapsychological treatments of the concept of the self provide clarity, whereas others add to conceptual confusion. Some authors, for example, have confused self-representations with the ego system by attributing systemic properties to representations. Usually, however, the term *self-representation* has followed Schafer's (1968) suggested usage as referring to contents of subjective experience. Schafer defined the term as an idea that the subject has about his own person. Within this usage, the self refers to the aggregate of the more general or schematic self-representations. As will be detailed later, highlighting the self-representation as an idea is not meant to minimize the primarily affective and somatic experiential referents of many self-representations. Rather, this definition is meant to distinguish between raw experience versus the subjectively conceptualized nonverbal way in which these experiences are organized.

My purpose here is to explicate and differentiate among several of the major competing models for understanding the concept of the self and the individual's development of the concept of self. I will also attempt to contrast some of the major differences among contemporary psychoanalytic theorists regarding conceptualizations of psychopathology of the self, namely, "self disorders" and "narcissistic personality disorders."

OVERVIEW: CONTRIBUTIONS TO THE UNDERSTANDING OF NARCISSISM AND THE SELF

In 1914 in his paper "On Narcissism," Freud introduced the concept of narcissism as an important principle in psychoanalytic theory. Part of the impetus for this paper was Freud's attempt to apply his formulations of drive theory and his developmental view of psychosexuality to the study of schizophrenia. He hypothesized a stage of "autoeroticism," or autoerotic instincts, in the earliest stage of infancy. Freud (1914/1957) argued in this paper that prior to the extension of libido to objects, there is "an original libidinal cathexis of the ego, from which some is later given off to objects, but which fundamentally persists and is related to the object-cathexes much as the body of an amoeba is related to the pseudopodia which it puts out" (p. 75). Freud described schizophrenic symptomotology as the product of the period before to the earliest stage of object relations involving a libidinal regression. This regression is related to a movement of libido, from infantile attachments to parental figures back to a stage of "primary narcissism," in which the infant or child views others and the external world as an extension of the self. In positing a stage of primary narcissism, Freud implied that libido directed toward the self occupies a position prior to the capacity for object love; thus, Freud viewed narcissism as a stage that is intermediate between autoeroticism and object love. During Freud's historic period in psychoanalytic theory building the concepts of self and ego were not clearly distinguished and defined. Freud (1923/1961) believed the ego was one of the three agencies of the mind, along with the id and superego, that made up the tripartite personality structure. Freud's definition of ego (1923/1961) was described as an organization with constant cathexis, and he assigned to it the functions of perception, memory, defense, reality testing, attention, and judgment. Freud (1923 Ä1, p. 26) stated that "the ego is first and foremost a bodily ego." By this statement he meant that the ego develops out of the id in contact with reality. Many psychoanalytic theorists and infant researchers (e.g., Spitz, 1964) have questioned this notion in the sense that the body ego, or the body or corporeal self, if you will, can only exist when differentiation between self and object representations is consolidated or at least well along. In other words, in the earliest period of infancy most researchers would say that there is not yet an awareness of the maternal object, and little or no awareness of the body as an entity.

Subsequent psychoanalytic theory has been keenly interested in detailing how the identificatory process leads to the formation of self-representations as well as object representations. For example, Hartmann and Lowenstein (1962) attempted to clarify the concept of the self, and in so doing they differentiated it from the ego. Hartmann, often regarded as the father of ego psychology, attempted to revise Freud's concept of ego, particularly elaborating ego functions beyond defense. He emphasized the ego as an organ of adaptation and accommodation that has access to the use of defense, among a variety of ego functions, to cope with exigencies of the external world as well as drive demands (Cooper, 1989). Hartmann referred to the ego as an organized system of functions and structures within the personality. He referred to the self as an intersystemic unit that serves as the "reservoir of narcissism" (Meissner, 1981). The self was viewed as the entity that becomes the object of libidinal cathexis in the development of secondary narcissism. Thus, Hartmann and Loewenstein (1962) did not consider the self as a separate psychic system to be conceptualized in the same manner as the ego, id, and superego. In contrast, Kohut (1971) argued that the self is a structure within the mind, since it is cathected with instinctual energy and it has continuity in time. He believed that the self is a psychic structure, although it is not conceptualized as an agency of the mind, unlike the ego, id, and superego within Freud's structural theory of the mind.

Jacobson (1964) attempted to clarify and distinguish among the concepts of ego, self, and self-representation. Her distinction between the self and self-representation lent theoretical precision for many subsequent theorists delineating the concept of the self. Jacobson used the term *self-representation* to stress the notion of the self and object as they were experienced, as distinguished from external objects. She stated that the ego is a structure in contrast to the self, which is the totality of the bodily and psychic person, and defined self-representations as "the unconscious, preconscious, and conscious endopsychic representations of the bodily and mental self in the system ego" (p. 19).

Jacobson attempted to modify Freud's (1914/1957) theory of narcissism, which presented a rather confusing and in some ways contradictory picture of ego formation and the development of self-representations. Freud (1914) had hypothesized a stage of "primary narcissism" in which libidinal cathexis, or aggression, is turned against the ego. Jacobson argued that in the early months of life, before the ego has developed and before there is a distinction between self and object, both the libidinal and aggressive drives are undifferentiated and are discharged through physiological channels. She maintained that it is meaningless to describe turning libido or aggression toward the ego before the ego has been differentiated. Dispensing with the notion of primary narcissism, suggested that it is not the ego that becomes cathected with these drives. Instead, she argued that at the stage of development when the self and object begin to be differentiated from one another, the mental representations of the self and object begin to be cathected with aggressive or libidinal drives. She posited that the ever-increasing memory traces of satisfying and unsatisfying instinctual, emotional, and ideational experiences with objects are what lead to the "bodily and psychic self." Jacobson (1964) stated: "Vague and variable at first, they gradually expand and develop into consistent and more or less realistic endopsychic representations of the object world and of the self" (p. 19). She contrasted infantile identifications in which self–object boundaries are, to some degree, fused (a stage referred to by some authors such as Kernberg as introjection) with later identifications, which involve "—the child's ego assuming characteristics of his love objects. As the inner concept of his self becomes a more faithful mirror of his ego, he can now achieve a partial blending between self and love-object representations on the basis of realistic likeness" (pp. 242–243).

Throughout his early writing, Kohut (1971, 1977) attempted to conceptualize the formation of psychological structure (self development) in early development. Kohut (1971) adopted Hartmann's (1958) conceptualization of internalization as processes by which regulation supplied by the environment is gradually replaced by autonomous self-regulation. "Optimal frustration"—inevitable, empathic failures—were said to provide the motivation for the withdrawal of cathexis from the object and the redirection of these cathexes in the gradual formation of psychic structure. Kohut (1971) argued that "optimal frustration" leads to "transmuting internalization"; thus, the child learns to perform psychological functions previously performed by the object. As many have pointed out (e.g., Stolorow, Brandchaft, & Atwood, 1987), Kohut's notion of optimal frustration is not far removed from Freud's (1923/1961) proposal that the ego develops and is modified through frustrating experiences (conflict with the reality principle) in the external world: "the ego is that part of the id which has been modified by the direct influence of the external world" (p. 25).

SCHAFER'S CONTRIBUTIONS TO THE CONCEPT OF THE SELF

Schafer (1968) attempted to describe and differentiate among several concepts related to the self and self representation. He defined the self-representation as an idea that the subject has about his/her own person. It is the subjective conceptualization of nonverbal (somatic, affective, and ideational) phenomena. Schafer assumed that the self-representation may fall anywhere along the continuum of primary process (drive organization of thinking) to secondary process (more abstract conceptual thinking). In other words, the self-representation may refer to any aspect of the subject's body or personality and may be organized on any level of abstractness. More broadly, it may refer to the subject's concept of his/her personality, or more specifically, to an aspect of the subject's body. The self-representation is invariably related to an individual's feelings and attitudes toward his/he person and others. The degree to which self-representation is organized, chaotic, disjointed, and consistent is highly variable in terms of how realistic, self-aggrandizing, idiosyncratic (including autistic), somatic, contemplative (self-reflective), or self-critical it is.

Clinically, the self-representation is related to the ways in which individuals feel about themselves, undergoes change over the course of psychodynamic psychotherapy. For example, individuals who enter psychotherapy with a deep sense of shame attached to the way they feel about themselves may learn a great deal about the unconscious determinants of this self representation. They may learn that underlying their experience of shame about presenting their work is an unconscious fantasy that involves competitive and hostile feelings toward others' work. As these unconscious fantasies are elucidated during psychotherapy, the shame attached to their self-representation may be modified, yielding greater acceptance of these hostile and competitive feelings, with accompanying reductions in the degree to which the self-representation is burdened with feelings of shame.

Schafer continually emphasized that the self-representation is not a major motivating or regulatory psychic system, thus distinguishing the self-representation from the system's id, ego, and superego within Freud's structural theory of the mind. Self-representations, however, do serve as a source of information or "guide-posts" to behavior. Schafer termed the representation of oneself as thinker of thoughts, the "reflective self representation." In psychosis, the capacity for reflective self-representation is particularly compromised. The psychotic individual demonstrates a limited capacity to move back and forth between primary- and secondary-process thought. In primary process ideation, thinking is essentially equivalent to the action. In contrast, fantasy involves the ability to suspend the reflective self-representation, but then to return to secondary process in which the ideation is distinguished from the action. According to Schafer (1968, p. 106), reflective self-representations "bear the hallmark of ego function, superego function, or both." He posits that to the extent that reflective self-representations ensure proper reality testing, "they express the ego system's objective perception of the workings of the psychic apparatus" (p. 107). To the extent that the reflective self-representation pertains to oneself as the thinker of thought and observer of oneself as the thinker of thought, it has its origins in superego functions. Thus, Schafer's conceptualizations of the self-representation and the reflective self representation are clarifying because he resisted the notion of attributing to such concepts systemic properties (regulatory and motivational forces and pressures).

Schafer also resisted referring to the self as an abstract concept in the mind of the observer. Instead, he adhered more exclusively to the use of the term *subjective self,* by which he meant an experiential reservoir or datum. The subjective self is what is referred to when the subject says "I" or "me," so the self-representation includes the cumulative experiences of the subjective self. The work of clinical psychoanalysis and psychoanalytic psychotherapy involves the exploration and understanding of the subjective self and the self-representation.

WINNICOTT'S CONTRIBUTIONS TO THE CONCEPT OF THE SELF

Winnicott (1960) detailed how the child, with the interacting environment, develops or fails to develop a sense of self, a "true self." His theory, albeit never systematically set forth, brilliantly foreshadowed much of the focus of contemporary psychoanalysis on the self as a basis for psychology, the self and object as intertwined and reciprocally influencing agents, the self as an experientially defined entity, and psychoanalysis as a mode of investigation for understanding the vicissitudes of self-development and defensive processes that are invoked to protect the self.

Winnicott (1960) defined the "true self" as a "theoretical position from which comes the spontaneous gesture and the personal idea" (p. 589). It appears as soon as there is any mental organization of the individual, and it refers simply to the summation of sensorimotor experiences; thus, for

Winnicott the true self collects together the details of the experiences of being alive and includes the working of body functions, the organization of the experiential self. Winnicott linked the "true self" with Freud's division of the self into an ego powered by instincts and sexual drives, and the "false self" with the part of the individual that is related to the external world. Winnicott sought to detail a period of the infant's development in which instincts are not yet clearly defined as internal for the infant—a period in which "id demands" are not yet felt as part of the self. Winnicott postulated that id excitements can be traumatic when the ego is not ready to include them. This results when the caretaker is unable emotionally to protect or hold the demands of the infant, so that the infant does not need to learn to tolerate extreme frustration or longing. When the infant is met with a "good enough" maternal response, the child is able (through ego functions) to experience id tensions as a part of the self.

Winnicott proposed that during the earliest stage of development the infant is not yet able to achieve a cohesion of the various sensorimotor elements. As the infant begins to express "the spontaneous gesture"—an expression of a need or impulse—the "good enough" mother meets this need much of the time. She holds the child physically or figuratively in such a way that the child can experience satisfaction rather than anxiety regarding the expression of her/his impulse life. These experiences of satisfaction are what constitute what Winnicott (1960, p. 145) referred to as the child's "infantile omnipotence." The "not good enough mother" fails to meet the child's infantile omnipotence (spontaneous expressions of need or impulse) and instead tacitly or explicitly communicates that the child's impulse life is dangerous to her; this communication, in turn, leads to anxiety and the psychological basis for the development of the false self. The false self is essentially a defense of compliance with the external world, which hides the true self in the context of environmental demands. If the mother is good enough, the child begins to accept and believe in external reality because it does not necessarily clash with the desires of the infant. So the child learns eventually and nontraumatically (and authentically) to abrogate infantile omnipotence. Play and illusion are capacities that the child is able to learn to enjoy in the context of the external world and the reality principle. The child learns very quickly that play and imagination are illusory but provide ways of omnipotently creating and controlling his/her environment for periods of time. The child learns to enjoy and delight in her/his new-found ability to go back and forth between experiencing the self in the context of reality (including the limitations of others) and in visiting and revisiting the world of illusion and omnipotence through play (and later through fantasy as a more parsimonious version of play).

Winnicott (1951) discovered the child's use of "transitional objects," which lie in an intermediate zone between viewing the other as an extension of the self, on the one hand, and the capacity for a self that relates to objects as separate entities, on the other. Winnicott defined the transitional object as an object that exists in the real world (e.g., a teddy bear) but that the infant believes owes its existence to the needs arising for the object. As a result, the child learns to extend his/her experience of omnipotent control into the world of reality, in which real objects, such as parents, disappoint, even in the best of circumstances. Within this formulation of optimal development, the child's self begins as a set of sensorimotor experiences, moves to a period of infantile omnipotence in which needs (id tensions) are met with a satisfactory environmental response much of the time, to a stage in which the child begins to accept that his/her needs cannot be met all of the time. The child deals with the latter circumstance by using transitional objects to deny and magically mitigate painful experiences in the environment, such as separation with parental figures.

Winnicott's vast theoretical contributions to psychoanalysis advanced the notion that the self and not just psychological structures such as the ego, id, and superego within Freud's structural model were the basis of psychoanalytic investigation. The false self as a massive defensive organization invoked to mitigate and protect the self from painful environmental disappointment shifted the psychoanalyst's clinical perspective from a view of the environment as the sum of the patient's projections. Instead, Winnicott tried to delineate the vicissitudes of interaction between the instinctual life of the infant and the environmental response that made it possible for the individual to develop and defend against impulses and needs. But when the environmental response failed, the outcome was a true self (the authentic instinctual experience of the individual) that was buried and covered with a patina of compliance—in essence, the false self. Winnicott's theory lay the groundwork for later contributors such as Klein and Kohut, who attributed motivational properties to constructs such as self-continuity, self-consistency, and self-cohesion. Later, developmental theorists such as Lichtenberg, Stern, and Stechler built on Winnicott's formulations regarding the inherently interpersonal and mutually effecting nature of the infant–parent dyad, in their theory and observations related to the child's development for the capacity of a sense of self. When Winnicott (1960) stated that "there is no such thing as an infant," he revolutionized, through a broadening of the canvas, our understanding that the child's sense of a developing self can never be observed or understood without reference to the other.

KERNBERG'S CONTRIBUTIONS TO THE CONCEPT OF THE SELF

Kernberg (1976) described the concept of self-image, or self-representation, as a component of the processes of internalization. It is one of three such components, the others being object images, or object representations, and dispositions to affective states, which he terms *drive derivatives.* The three processes of internalization include introjection, identifications and ego identity and correspond roughly to developmental processes involving the acquisition of experiences and behaviors that reflect an individual's self-image, or self-representation, as well as object representations.

Introjection is the most basic level in the organization of the internalization process and involves the reproduction (involving perception and memory) of an interaction with the environment by means of the clustering of memory traces attached to the self-image, the object image, the interaction of the self and object images, and the "affective colorations" of these interactions between self and object images. According to Kernberg, the process of affective coloring occurs under the influence of drives and drive derivatives at the time of these interactions, that is, that affective coloring follows from experiences that are either gratifying ("libidinal") or frustrating ("aggressive"). Kernberg's theory related to a process borrowed from Jacobson (1964) and held that self and object images are not yet distinguishable from each other during the earliest stages of introjection. In Kernberg's view, the "reciprocal smiling response" noted by Spitz (1964) at 3 months of age is suggestive of the beginning of the differentiation between self and object images.

In contrast, identification is predicated on the child's cognitive ability to recognize the variety of role dimensions in interactions with others. Identification, in Kernberg's terms, involves the individual's capacity to model the self after an object. Implicit in this modeling are the abilities to differentiate the self from the other, and to experience the self as interacting with the other. Kernberg would suggest that the perceptions of the object, the roles of the object, and the interaction between the self and the object are always influenced by the impact of fantasy and drive derivatives. It is also the drives and affective states of the individual that partly determine or motivate the process of identification. For example, Freud (1914/1957) described how the boy's identification with the father and the formation of the superego are partly motivated by frustrated wishes to have what the father has (mother) and that this identification partly involves a vicarious opportunity for gratification of otherwise frustrated wishes. This example illustrates how Kernberg viewed the process of internalization of actual interpersonal interactions as implying the accrual of self-representations linked to particular affects within the ego and the superego. Thus, the individual's experiences of gratification and frustration have bearing on the degree to which one's self-representation is flexible, veritable, and complex as a function of identification. Implicit here, too, is the notion that the process of identification involves the way in which the self-representation is modified and influenced by the actual experiences with the object and the gradually internalized object representation.

Kernberg (1976) referred to the concept of ego identity (Erikson, 1956) as the overall organization of introjections and identifications under the guiding principle of the synthetic functions of the ego (Hartmann, Kris, & Loewenstein, 1946). He referred to such concepts as the individual's overall and enduring conceptualization of the "world of objects," a sense of the continuity of the self, and the ability to recognize consistency in interactions between the self and others.

Kernberg has made extensive clinical contributions related to the self-representation concept as it unfolds in the psychotherapeutic situation. In Kernberg's (1983) view, intrapsychic conflict always involves a constellation of self and object representations directed against an opposite (usually affectively contrasting) set of self and object representations. These competing self and object representations are manifested in the transference, with the therapist and patient usually assigned to one or another of these representations. Kernberg's writing emphasized the degree to which the self-representation is comprises of many unconscious and repressed or split-off aspects that can be integrated over the course of psychoanalytic treatment.

KLEIN'S CONTRIBUTIONS TO THE CONCEPT OF THE SELF AND SELF-INTEGRITY

Klein (1976) posited an overriding, or superordinate, need for the individual to maintain a coherent and integrated self. His work, like that of other psychoanalytic theorists such as Fairbairn and Kohut, was aimed at reformulating psychoanalytic theory as a psychology of the self, emphasizing the maintenance of "self-integrity" as having key motivational properties. In contrast to other contemporary self psychologists such as Kohut (1971, 1977) Klein attempted to integrate his conceptualization of self and object relations within an intrapsychic context and, in essence, a psychology of intrapsychic conflict.

Klein (1976) began his theoretical revisions with the notion that the individual is always trying to maintain and preserve her/his sense of self, or "self-conception." A primary task for any individual, according to Klein, is to preserve the self-structure by splitting off meaning schemas that cause conflict. He termed this phenomenon *fractionation*. Within his reformulations of many psychoanalytic phenomena, conflict was defined not as the opposition between two forces but rather as some meaning that is in conflict with a self-conception. For example, he defined repression as "a meaning scheme that is dissociated from the person's self-conception" (Klein, 1976, p. 241). Repression was viewed as an example of fractionation in that meanings become separated from understanding and thus dissociated from the self. Klein redefined the notion of ego as experiences and actions related to the self, and the id as actions and experiences occurring without a reflective self. Another means by which the individual seeks continuity of the self is through "identification." The process of identification is, for Klein, a means to preserve the continuity of the self by changing the self-schema (in Piagetian terms, this is somewhat akin to the process of assimilation).

Klein also sought to reconceptualize sexuality and sexual gratification as phenomena that maintain the unity of the self. He regarded as sexual tension the failure to accomplish self-worth or the maintenance of self-continuity, which in some circumstances comes to be symbolized through sexual gratification. The need for cohesiveness of the self therefore takes precedence over the opportunity for drive discharge or sexual gratification. Klein also minimized the role of psychosexual aims and their relation to anxiety. Within Klein's theory, anxiety results from any incompatibility between self-continuity and incompatible aims. In agreement with Eagle (1984), Klein's theory remains compatible with a basic psychology of intrapsychic conflict to the extent that he viewed the individual as involved in a constant psychological struggle to resolve and reconcile incompatible aims with the self-conception.

KOHUT'S CONTRIBUTIONS TO THE THEORY OF THE SELF

Although Kohut's early work (Kohut, 1971) the self was conceptualized as a component of ego structure, in his later writings (1977–1984) the self was regarded as a superordinate structure (with drives and defenses as constituent parts of the self structure). Kohut (1971, 1977, 1984) posited that the main developmental achievement for any individual pertains to the attainment of a "cohesive self." One of his primary points of divergence from much of psychoanalytic theory (and other theorists who developed the notion of the self as a superordinate structure, such as Klein) involved his hypothesis of a separate line of narcissistic development, separate from psychosexual and object relations development.

Kohut viewed drives and defenses as secondary or subordinate components, in contrast to the self as a superordinate structure. For example, it is the "enfeebled self" (Kohut, 1977) that turns defensively toward pleasure aims via the erotogenic zones (drives), and then secondarily involves the ego in managing drive aims (defenses). Within Kohut's theory of self psychology, consequently, drives are viewed as disintegration or breakdown products of disappointments to the self, usually involving failures in emotional attunement of "selfobjects" (other people who in varying stages of development are experienced as a part of the self). For example, Kohut (1977, p. 116) noted that rage is "always motivated by an injury to the self." Like Fairbairn (1952) then, Kohut viewed aggression not as a primary drive but as a disintegration product—a reaction to environmental disappointment or limitation.

I will later review in more depth Kohut's formulation of self-development in describing his view of narcissistic psychopathology, but I should point out here some of the primary developments he believed as necessary for the accomplishment of a cohesive self. (It is important to remember that the development of a cohesive self is hypothesized as involving a separate line of development, that of object relations, in contrast to the theories of Freud, Kernberg, and Klein.) Kohut (1971) hypothesized an early stage of development called "autoeroticism" in which only a "fragmented self" exists. During this period, the child's infantile omnipotence is said to be met with inevitable maternal disappointments, which lead to the child's developing two new ways of maintaining narcissistic equilibrium: developing a "grandiose" self, which includes exhibitionistic components, and giving over the previous perfection of the developing self to an admired and omnipotent parent, the "idealized parental imago" (p. 25). If the child is able to retain a sense of connection and union with the idealized parent through age-appropriate mirroring and opportunities for idealization of the parent (i.e., if the parent is not too disappointing), archaic grandiosity and exhibitionism are tamed or neutralized, leading to "heathy narcissism" and a cohesive self. As will be detailed later in this chapter, in pathological development, the cohesive self fails to develop, leading to wishes for perfection and a compromised ability for the regulation of self-esteem.

For Kohut, then, self-cohesion is the primary motivational property guiding human behavior; inevitable rather than traumatic disappointments to the child's grandiosity and exhibitionistic needs and the need for an idealized parent lead to the psychological capacity for self-cohesion. Kohut (1971) argued that in early development, the child relies on others ("selfobjects") to regulate psychological functions such as the maintenance of self-esteem. In his later writings, Kohut (1984) claimed that all individuals rely on selfobjects throughout the life cycle to help in the maintenance of self-cohesion, but that in healthy development there is more of a diminution and flexibility in the degree to which the self relies on selfobjects for these functions. Throughout Kohut's writing, he distinguished between two types of objects as counterposed to the self-concept. He termed "selfobjects," objects experienced as part of oneself or serving to maintain the organization of the self. He contrasted selfobjects with "objects," the latter being the target of desires emanating from a more demarcated self-concept. The two types of objects emanated from Kohut's notion that narcissistic libido and object-instinctual energies follow their own separate developmental courses. Even after Kohut (1977) abandoned the notion that we ever outgrow our need for selfobject ties, he retained the essential dichotomy between the two types of objects, which ultimately formed, in his view, the basis for a complementarity between self psychology and a conflict psychology (Stolorow et al., 1987).

Kohut placed the individual's (self's) relation to her/his own grandiosity and exhibitionism to values and ideals of perfection as a linchpin to psychological health. Many have criticized Kohut's relative deemphasis on other aspects of optimal psychological functioning, such as the capacity for intimacy, mutuality, and reciprocity in interpersonal relationships, and the ability to experience spontaneity and satisfaction.

Another line of important criticism directed to Kohut's self psychology has involved the question of whether his theory relates to a general psychology of the individual or, instead, to the understanding of particular types of pathology, namely patients with self disorders, or in the terms of DSM-III (American Psychiatric Association, 1980), Narcissistic Personality Disorder. For example, at different points in the development of his theory, Kohut asserted that traditional drive theory was more relevant to understanding the etiology of neurosis and that self psychology as a theory was more relevant to the understanding of patients with self disorders. However, some of Kohut's associates such as Goldberg (1973), have attempted to discuss Kohut's self psychology as a general psychology, specifically, that the separate line of narcissistic development is a basic aspect of personality, distinct from the development of ego functions and psychosexual development. This observation or hypothesis, depending on one's perspective and degree of skepticism regarding the theory, requires considerably more clinical and theoretical investigation. At the level of theory, however, several theorists (e.g., Mitchell, 1979) have cogently criticized Kohut for some of the problems in retaining a bifurcated model for understanding people, one that applies to neurotics and the other that applies to patients with narcissistic disorders. Mitchell (1979, p. 181) highlighted some of the internal inconsistency in Kohut's theory: "If drives are disintegration products reflecting a breakdown of primary relational configurations, how can 'structural neuroses' contain at one and the same time no self pathology and conflicts concerning drives which, by definition, reflect severe self pathology?"

Like Klein, Kohut attempted to take a number of phenomena explained by traditional psychoanalytic theory regarding the vicissitudes of drive and redefine such phenomena in terms of self-cohesion . With regard to anxiety, for example, Kohut differentiated between anxiety related to danger situations described by Freud (1923/1961), such as the fear of instinctual gratification meeting with self-reproach, castration, or object loss, and anxiety related to the fear of disintegration of the self. For Kohut and a number of contemporary theorists, the threat to the self is a result of the self's experience of defect or enfeeblement within the structure of the self. Kohut, like Freud, believed that anxiety is ultimately the greatest threat to the individual, but the sources of threat related less to blocked discharge of drive tensions than to the individual's experience of a lack of cohesiveness and continuity in the sense of self.

CONTRIBUTIONS OF STOLOROW AND ATWOOD: THE INTERSUBJECTIVE APPROACH

Strongly influenced by Kohut's self psychology, Stolorow et al. (1987) attempted to define more precisely the experiential nature of the self concept. Stolorow and Atwood (1984) noted the confusion within the psychoanalytic literature regarding the use of the term *self* to refer both to the self as an existential agent or initiator of action, on the one hand, and as a psychological structure or organizer of experience, on the other. They suggested that the term *self* is a specific concept referring to the structure of a person's experience to him/herself. They argued that "psychoanalysis can only illuminate the experience of personal agency or its absence in specific contexts of meaning" (Stolorow & Atwood, 1984, p. 34). In addition, they proposed that the concept of the person as an experiencing subject and agent who initiates action lies outside the bounds of psychoanalytic inquiry. Stolorow and Atwood defined the self as a psychological structure through which self-experience acquires continuity, cohesion, and enduring organization, referring to their experiential orientation in psychoanalysis as an "empathic-introspective perspective" that focuses on the structuralization of experience rather than the acquisition of abilities as judged by an external observer.

Stolorow et al. (1987) criticized Kohut (1977) for confusing the two notions of self as structure, and the person as agent. In particular, they felt that Kohut's view of the self as a supraordinate structure to a mental apparatus offered another variety of mechanistic thinking and reification in psychoanalytic conceptualizations of the self. In their view, the self-concept and drive axis (or drive–discharge apparatus) exist on different levels of theoretical discourse. From their experiential perspective, what is most problematic in Kohut's formulations is his conceptualization of the bipolar self. Kohut suggested that the self is composed of two basic components: guiding ideals and nuclear ambitions, which are internalized from the idealizing and mirroring functions of others (selfobjects). Psychological activity, according to Kohut, is described by the metaphor of a "tension arc"; all activity is said to flow between these two poles of the self. Stolorow and his colleagues argued that the metaphor of the tension arc introduces a new motivational construct to psychoanalysis that is not accessible to an experiential focus in clinical analytic work. Instead, they asserted that the two poles of the bipolar self are better regarded and conceptualized as systems of affective meanings that are intrinsically motivational. Stated another way, they argued that Kohut's concept of the supraordinate self moves psychoanalysis back to a focus on metapsychology and away from an experiential focus of the self. Their own work has concentrated on studyine the degree to which a sense of self (ranging from poorly to firmly established or demarcated) guides the organization of a person's subjective experiences. In parallel to this revision in Kohut's theory, Stolorow et al. (1987) argued for a movement away from the selfobject–object dichotomy proposed by Kohut (1971) and suggested, instead, that the term *selfobject* refer only to a class of psychological functions, a dimension of experiencing an object.

SOME PERSPECTIVES ON THE DEVELOPMENT OF A SENSE OF SELF

Peterfreund (1978) criticized what he viewed as a dominant trend in some sectors of psychoanalytic developmental research, namely, to "adultomorphize" infancy. This adultomorphization involves the tendency to describe early states of normal development in terms of hypotheses about later states of psychopathology. Peterfreund (1978) pointedly questioned the veracity of many such psychoanalytic descriptions of the development of a sense of self:

> Early infancy is described as a state of fusion, narcissism, and omnipotence. The terms autism and symbiosis . . . are used to characterize normal infantile states. We hear of "hallucinatory wish-fulfillments" and other hallucinatory experiences, and of the existence of a stimulus barrier in infancy. Finally, the infant is described as disoriented and even as delusional, e.g., as having a delusion of a common boundary between self and mother. (p. 427)

Stechler and Kaplan (1980), in agreement with Peterfreund, suggested that there is insufficient empirical evidence to support these claims and, furthermore, very few ways to test these hypotheses.

Stechler and Kaplan (1980), Lichtenberg (1975), Sander (1962), and Stern (1985) among many others in recent years, have attempted, through empirically based, longitudinal studies of infants and their families, to elucidate the pathways that lead to the child's development of the sense of self. This work essentially attempted to characterize and draw conclusions about the infant's and child's subjective experience based on the observation of their evolving behavior. Although these contributions are enormously complex, deserving a chapter in their own right, I will merely summarize a few of their major conclusions.

Stechler and Kaplan's (1980) view of the developing sense of self, like Stern's (1985)—the outcome of infant observation—began with the premise that the capacity to function in accordance with an "internal self-regulating organization is a developmental acquisition originating in innumerable attempts to resolve experienced breaches of expectancy" (p. 87). In contrast to Freud's view that conflict in the unity of the self arises as a result of conflict among opposing systems (e.g., id, ego, and superego), Stechler and Kaplan suggested that the sense of self emerges through a series of syntheses, which are the active resolutions of experienced conflict. "Breaches of expectancy" may or may not be a result of conflict; they may involve failures of integration as a result of developmental crises, environmental failures, or a clash of mutually exclusive aims and desires. Stechler and Kaplan proposed an initial stage of development they called the "preself," which reflects the observations of the infant's early capacities to organize his/her experiences (Lichtenberg, 1979; Stern, 1985).

Lichtenberg (1975), for example, observed the neonate's capacities to screen perceptual input with reference to information stored from daily experience, as well as to exert preferences for particular stimuli. In the second stage, the "preawareness self" is exemplified by the infant's abilities to take the initiative in establishing areas of reciprocity between mother and father, including the ability for differentiated responses toward each parent as observed by Sander (1962). In this stage, the infant's experience of the self is facilitated by pleasure in practicing and repeating new skills and in the infant's experience of effecting his/her surroundings (usually, the parents). Finally, in the third stage, "the self," the child moves toward the experience of the self as the locus of experience, in which language (the utterance of "me") marks the growing awareness of the self.

Stern (1985) argued that there are four discernable senses of self that occur during development: a sense of an "emergent self," from birth to 2 months of age; a sense of a "core self," which forms between 2 and 6 months of age; a sense of a "subjective self," between 7 and 15 months; and a sense of "verbal self," which forms after that. Stern's observational research led him to the conclusion that the infant never experiences a stage of total self–other undifferentiation. The infant is designed to be selectively responsive to external social events (emergent self), in contrast to Mahler and Furer's (1968) hypothesis of a stage of infantile autism in which there is no self–other differentiation. Between the ages of 2 and 9 months, Stern maintained, that the infant consolidates a sense of core self as a separate, cohesive unit with a sense of agency, affectivity, and continuity in time (subjective self). During the ages of 9 to 18 months of age, the child is not only involved with the developmental task of independence (rapprochement, in Mahler's terms) but also to the task of "seeking and creating an intersubjective union with another" (Stern, 1985, p. 10). After 18 months of age, the child moves into a process by which the self serves as the primary subjective perspective that organizes a variety of social experiences (verbal self). In Stern's view, the infant's gradual acquisition of new senses of self partly bring about major developmental changes in social experience. This view contrasts with the notion that the changes in the infant's subjective world result from shifts in specific developmental tasks (e.g., orality, attachment, autonomy, and trust) that move from one phase to the next.

In most contemporary infant research related to the emergence of a sense of self, what is perhaps of greatest importance is a shift to viewing the contextual unit for observation and research away from an infant in isolation (strictly intrapsychic mechanisms) to one that involves the infant and caretakers. Winnicott's (1960) startling statement—"there is no such thing as an infant"—established the new contextual unit for infant research as one involving an infant interacting with the emotional surround. In this way, psychoanalytic theory, in general, has moved from an encapsulated model (or closed-system model) of the self–object polarity, to include the self and other in a continual, interactional pattern.

"SELF" PATHOLOGY IN CONTEMPORARY PSYCHOANALYTIC THEORY

The diagnosis of Narcissistic Personality Disorder (NPD) has been defined as a discrete diagnostic category in the DSM-III, yet the diagnosis and the concepts that underlie it remain poorly defined and variously employed. The DSM-III marked the first major attempt to delineate diagnostic criteria for NPD, which involve enduring character traits, not just episodic behaviors. These characteristics included the following: (1) a grandiose sense of self-importance; (2) exhibitionism requiring attention and admiration from others; (3) marked feelings of shame, humiliation, or rage in response to criticism from others; (4) preoccupation with fantasies of success, brilliance, or power; and (5) at least two of the following characteristics of impairment in interpersonal relationships: entitlement, exploitation, lack of empathy, and the prominence of idealization or devaluation, or fluctuations between the two in interpersonal relationships.

The attempt to discuss narcissistic pathology runs throughout the history of psychoanalytic writings. Although Freud (1914/1957), in his first paper dealing with narcissism, did not write about character pathology per se, he did offer clinical descriptions of individuals whose narcissistic features were prominant. These descriptions come close to some contemporary definitions of narcissistic disturbances. Freud (1914) described what he termed the "narcissistic character type" in a manner that was strikingly similar to many contemporary psychoanalytic descriptions of narcissistic character pathology:

> The subject's main interest is directed to self-preservation; he is independent and not open to intimidation. His ego has a large amount of aggressiveness at its disposal, which also manifests itself in readiness for activity. In his erotic life, loving is preferred above being loved. People belonging to this type impress others as being "personalities";they are especially suited to act as a support for others, to take on the role of leaders, and to give a fresh stimulus to cultural development or to damage the established state of affairs. (p. 100)

Waelder (1925) described "narcissistic personalities" as prone toward a lack of concern and empathy toward others and intense preoccupation with their self-esteem. Waelder, in emphasizing these individuals' maintenance of adequate adaptation to external demands, spoke of the "libidinization of thinking" and a "narcissistic mode of thought," by which he meant an overestimation of their capacities for thought or mental processes.

Kohut (1968) introduced the terms "narcissistic personality disorder" and the "grandiose self." Since that time, a major debate between Kernberg (1967, 1975, 1976) and Kohut (1971, 1977, 1984) has ensued regarding both the diagnosis and developmental formulation of narcissistic disorders and self pathology.

Kernberg has made substantial contributions to our understanding of the psychopathology of the self, which he refers to, in crystalized form, as "narcissistic personality structure" (Kernberg, 1967). He attempted to describe the clinical characteristics and bases for diagnosis of narcissistic personality and observed that these patients often display an overreliance on acclaim, grandiose fantasies, intense ambition, and extreme self-absorption. He described their behavior as superficially adaptive, but said that their pathology is most apparent in an inability to love, including a lack of empathy, a tendency to exploit others, feelings of emptiness, and a proclivity toward boredom. Kernberg (1975) also noted that these patients' defenses often include devaluation, omnipotence, and withdrawal, particularly when trying to cope with or mitigate envy of others. He noted that while such patients have a capacity for consistent work, and even success, their work is often focused around opportunities for exhibitionism. Even in their work, there is a lack of depth for genuine intellectual or professional involvements, which he referred to as "pseudosublimatory" tendencies. In contrast to mature forms of activity and productivity, the values and conscience of such patients are corruptible and subject to shifts in order to win praise.

Kernberg proposed an etiology for the narcissistically disturbed individual in which the child, disappointed by a cold or rejecting mother or caretaker, is left with few resources to rely on outside the self. The child's primary defense and adaptation is to fall back on the self, or as he called it, the "grandiose self." Whatever resources are available to the child in the form of parental caretaking (i.e., to whatever extent the parents are emotionally, positively valenced) is further compromised by the child's tendency to project rage and frustration on to the parents. This projection eventuates in the parents' being perceived as even less likely to meet the child's needs, which, in turn, requires the child to fall back even more on the grandiose self. In essence, "self-sufficiency" (Modell, 1975) becomes the only resource for soothing, comfort, and withdrawal in the context of mitigating both the child's rage and longings for another.

The term *grandiose self* is one that Kohut (1968) originated and used in a very different manner than Kernberg, as will be outlined later in the chapter. For Kernberg the grandiose self has three primary psychic structures: (1) the admired aspects of the child; (2) the fantasied version of the child, compensatory in nature, which defends against feelings of disappointment, rage, and envy directed toward parental figures; and (3) the fantasied image of a loving, empathic mother. The grandiose self allows the needy parts of the individual to remain dissociated or separated from his/her experience. Kernberg believed that over the course of analytic treatment, the grandiose self becomes increasingly manifest in the transference and thus becomes a point of beneficial analytic exploration. The patient is viewed as having major resistances to this analytic development. Treatment of such patients involves the analysis and understanding of these major resistances, including their adaptive value for maintaining self-esteem and a sense of self-preservation in the context of overwhelming feelings of rage and helplessness.

Modell (1975) provided a model of formulating and treating these patients, which developed and added to some of the elements from Kernberg's formulations. For example, Modell proposed that narcissistic individuals are essentially traumatized by parents who radically fail the child's needs for mirroring and validation of reality testing. He argued that many such patients are highly intelligent and capable at an early age of perceiving the parents' emotional limitations or specious capacities for adequate reality testing. Modell posited that such children begin to fall back on a compensatory self-structure to avoid relying on the parents. By so doing, they achieve a modicum of reality testing for themselves and mitigate the painful feelings that ensue from relying on parents who are highly compromised in their abilities to help the child's development. Essentially, the child develops a sense of self-sufficiency (Modell, 1975) or precocious autonomy (pseudoautonomy, to be more precise), which is roughly equivalent to the grandiose self described by Kernberg. Modell's treatment formulations follow Kernberg's in his emphasis on the eventual need, however carefully and tactfully, to help the patient confront this defensively invoked position of self-sufficiency in order to overcome it (Modell, 1975).

Kohut (1971, 1977, 1984) wrote extensively on the treatment of patients with Narcissistic Personality Disorder, although he explicitly avoided the enterprise of making a diagnosis based on presenting symptomatology. Instead, Kohut (1971) argued that the diagnosis should only be made based on the development and unfolding of particular kinds of transferences within psychoanalytic treatment: "the crucial diagnostic criterion is based not on the evaluation of the presenting symptomatology or even the life history, but on the nature of the spontaneously developing transference" (p. 23).

Despite Kohut's position that self disorders are not easily or usefully diagnosed based on symptomotology, Akhtar and Thomson (1982) cogently extracted and summarized some of the behavioral features of the NPD culled from Kohut's writings. These features include a proneness toward rage as a reaction to self-esteem (Kohut, 1966), as well as the need for revenge, difficulty in forming and maintaining relationships, a lack of empathy, a limited capacity for humor, and hypochondriacal concerns.

Kohut believed that Narcissistic Personality Disorder was best conceptualized as a form of developmental arrest, arguing that "primary infantile narcissism" is inevitably impinged upon by maternal and parental disappointments. The grandiose self is seen as a defensive structure to help the child minimize and deny parental disappointments. It is essentially a grandiose or megalomanic self-image that the child employs to restore and regain narcissistic equilibrium in the face of parental disappointments. Kohut also posited that the child defensively idealizes the parents and that self-esteem is regained by the attempt to merge or associate with these idealized "parental imagos" (Kohut, 1971). He saw the emergence of the grandiose self as a normal part of development, which, in healthy progression, is made more realistic by age-specific mirroring responses by the parental figures. This allows for the affective neutralization of the grandiose self and the idealized parental imagos. In healthy development. the child internalizes the inevitable (nontraumatic) disappointments in the parents (the parents' realistic limitations), and these internalizations are eventually integrated into the child's own system of values and ideals.

According to Kohut, in the development of Narcissistic Personality Disorder, this normal sequence of nontraumatic disappointment is disrupted in a number of ways. The grandiose self persists in unneutralized form if the child is not met with age-appropriate mirroring responses. So, too, the child may not be able to internalize the idealized parental images if the parent has either been unable to help the child appreciate the parent's real limitations or, conversely, if the parent has disappointed the child in a more massive (in contrast to an inevitable) manner. As described earlier in the chapter, Kohut's developmental formulation of self pathology rests squarely on his resolve that narcissistic libido exists independent of one's object attachments. In contrast, Kernberg's model views narcissistic libido as falling on the same developmental line as that of the development of object relations.

The differences proposed by Kernberg and Kohut regarding their theories of child development and the etiology of NPD have substantially influenced their recommended therapeutic stances in the analytic treatment of such individuals. It follows that since Kernberg saw the grandiose self as purely defensive and pathological, rather than as a form of developmental arrest, his therapeutic technique revolves around the interpretation of the defensive nature of this grandiosity. He attempted to help the patient explore the dissociated or split-off, needy elements of the self and their attendant affective colorations and components in order to help the individual integrate disparate self-representations.

As stated earlier, Kohut hypothesized a line of narcissistic libido that is separate from the developmental line of object relations (the latter is determined by libidinal and aggressive drives). Kohut's treatment approach followed from his belief that the narcissistic disorder is best understood as a form of developmental arrest. He espoused the merits of allowing patients to express both their idealization of the therapist and their own grandiosity without necessarily interpreting these phenomena as defenses used to mitigate rage. Instead, Kohut viewed these spontaneously occurring clinical phenomena as the naturalistic resumption of the individual's attempt to have the grandiose self met with empathic responses from another, in this case the analyst. The analyst inevitably (not intentionally) disappoints the patient, and it is the interpretation of these failures in empathy that allows the patient to resume the developmental tasks of neutralizing both the grandiose self and the idealizations (compensatorily determined) of the parental figures. In contrast to Kernberg, Kohut viewed the patient's rage as it manifests itself in treatment as reactive or secondary to empathic failures.

The controversy surrounding Kernberg's and Kohut's formulations regarding both the etiology and treatment of patients with self disorders requires that considerably more clinical and empirical testing be done. It is possible, as some such as Spruiell (1975) have suggested, that part of this controversy involves the possibility of both etiological and diagnostic heterogeneity regarding this patient population.

Horowitz (1975) proposed a new model for conceptualizing Narcissistic Personality Disorder that combined the contributions of psychoanalytic theorists (chiefly Kernberg and Kohut) and information-processing theory. He viewed the individual described as having the disorder as perceiving and integrating the meaning of events in such a way as to aggrandize the self or to see her/himself in as positive a way as possible. Horowitz described these patients' tendency to be vigilant to sources of praise and criticism in terms of "sliding meanings," which essentially serve to defend against ubiquitous threats to self-esteem; thus he offered a cognitive and defensive style that accompanies some of the object-relational tendencies advanced by Kernberg and Kohut.

CONCLUDING REMARKS

Not surprisingly, the concept of the self, variously defined, reflects the diversity of current psychoanalytic theory in general. Since Freud, definitions and formulations of the concept of the self reveal a tension between understanding the self as one or several of the following: a theoretical construct such as ego, with motivational properties; a term or idea that represents the sum or organization of a person's experience; a person, a corporeal and emotional self.

Freud focused on constructing a psychology that could elucidate the ways in which concepts of unconscious and psychic determinism were primary motivational factors in the choices we make, the psychopathology of everyday life, and all psychopathology. He attempted to explain the motivational and organizing principles for how the mind works and how the individual survives psychologically. His psychology was a theory of mind, and particularly the psychological and biological determinants that dictate the functioning of the mind; within this theory, the ego was essentially synonymous with the self. It is of note that in 1894, Freud wrote that the concept of defense was the "cornerstone on which the whole structure of psychoanalysis rests." In my view, Freud's early implicit theory of self involved the elucidation of how impulses break through and are titrated by the mind. Within Freud's psychology, the self is a concept that, de facto, refers to the mental content and the processes of cathexis and countercathexis (impulse and defense). These processes, in turn, regulate the degree to which mental content expresses itself (becomes conscious). In some ways, then, it might be said that Freud's theory of self was, in essence, a theory of conflict between self-expression (gratification) and self-titration (defense), always occurring in the context of self-preservation.

Hartmann, Kris, and Loewenstein (1946) underscored the ego's broader functions, as an organ of adaptation and accommodation that had access to the use of a variety of ego functions to cope with exigencies of the external and internal world. Again, the ego was regarded as essentially synonymous with the concept of self, but the ego's functions were extended to include capacities beyond the primary function of defense.

Although contemporary theories differ regarding the degree to which drives and drive demands are viewed as primary, most consist of extended definitions of the self beyond the biological matrix that Freud developed. In contemporary psychoanalytic theory, particularly "relational theory" (Mitchell, 1988), the self is generally a concept that is viewed as a component within a relational configuration. The dynamic properties of this configuration vary, but the components usually remain the same: the self, the object, and "the space between the two" (Mitchell, 1988, p. 33). This configuration translates into the notion that it is impossible to define or conceptualize the self except in relation to another self (object), and that it is further necessary to consider the psychic space in which self and object interact.

Psychoanalysts have always been interested in the way in which an individual regulates the self in the context of others. Winnicott (1960) extended Freud's revolutionary descriptions of self-preservation to include the individual's continual interaction with another, the primary caretaker. Homeostasis was now regarded as something that is achieved not only with reference to an internal state, but between two individuals (the space between). As Winnicott described it, the self can go to great lengths to hide and protect itself in the face of external trauma. Here, defense is extended beyond the realms of cathexis and countercathexis (impulse and defense), to a new and revolutionary frame of reference for the concept of the self: the self with the other. Winnicott was referring to self-experience (the self's experience with itself and with another), not just a level of discourse related to a process of fragmentation of the self. The individual who displays a "false self" cannot experience him/herself as real and authentic. The experiential self has been described by a number of theorists who have been detailed in this chapter, including Klein, Schafer, Stolorow and Atwood, and Kohut.

Regardless of a particular theoretical model, psychoanalysis as a science of observation and a therapy has moved increasingly to an experientially based perspective—one that, functionally, emphasizes the individual's experience of being with others and with the analyst during the process of analytic work (e.g., Kohut, 1971; Loewald, 1986; Gill, 1982; Schwaber, 1983; Schafer, 1983; Stolorow et al., 1987). Functionally, the contemporary psychoanalyst is interested in collaborating with a patient to examine the process involved in expressing, developing, and preserving the sense of self. And although there are enormous differences in theoretical preferences among analysts, particularly relating to the degree to which drives are considered an important aspect of functioning, a greater experiential focus has become a more common axis across theories. For example, Gill (1976) functionally defines transference as the patient's experience of the analyst, as do Stolorow et al. (1987), but other aspects of their theoretical approaches are quite different. There is a very strong movement away from helping patients to understand "objective reality" through psychoanalytic treatment, and much more emphasis on helping patients to observe, understand, and integrate their experiences of "psychic reality" (McLaughlin, 1981; Michaels, 1985; Loewald, 1986; Wolf, 1986) . The self's subjectivity is no longer seen as something in opposition to the analyst's "objective reality." Instead, subjectivities of both participants are elicited and become part of a transference–countertransference matrix that partly constitute the analytic context.

Models of psychopathology, as well as issues related to the assessment of analyzability (the ability to benefit from analysis), have also been effected by changes in our understanding of the self concept. While psychoanalysis is still a treatment approach that is chiefly interested in ameliorating and treating symptoms, there is an increased movement to augment our more objectified descriptions of clinical entities such as "narcissism," with descriptions that emphasize how people experience conflict, pain, and disappointment. Many analysts have found that affect tolerance is often more helpful as a tool in assessing analyzability than some of the more traditional categorizations of patients, according to diagnostic criteria.

The evolution of the concept of self permits a window on some of the most important transitions in general concept development through the history of psychoanalytic theory. Within the last 20 years in particular, there has been a movement away from a closed-system approach within psychoanalytic theory, to one in which the concept of self implies a more open-system approach. This, suggests a movement away from a theory based on a machine model in which the self is explained through the theoretical ego, to one in which a concept of self implies an experiential base, with a sense of curiosity about, and adaptation to, multiple levels of reality, engaged in a process of constant mutual influence with others. Patients in analytic treatment express themselves through multiple levels of experiential reality, especially as indicated through the examination of transference (Modell, 1990). Infant–caretaker interactions are also regarded as mutual influencing systems governed by their own psychological organizations (internal homeostasis) and the interaction of the infant and the caretaker. Psychoanalytic theorists of the self are still interested in explicating how past experience expresses itself in current behavior through the cornerstone concept of repetition. There is an additional emphasis, however, within contemporary viewpoints relating to the self—namely, that the self is constantly in the position of discovering itself as it expresses itself. The self is more than the unfolding of aggregate experience (i.e., the unfolding of internalized self and object representations) during analytic therapy or outside relationships. The self is also the organizer of new experience and experience yet to come.

REFERENCES

Akhtar, S., & Thomson, J. (1982). Overview: Narcissistic personality disorder. *American Journal of Psychiatry, 139,* 12–21.

American Psychiatric Association (1980). *Diagnostic and statistical manual of mental disorders* (3rd ed.). Washington, DC: Author.

Cooper, S. (1989). Recent contributions to the theory of defense mechanisms. A comparative view. *Journal of the American Psychoanalytic Association, 37*(4), 865–891.

Diagnostic and Statistical Manual of Mental Disorder. American Psychiatric Association, 1980. Washington, DC.

Eagle, M. (1984). *Recent developments in psychoanalysis: A critical evaluation.* New York: McGraw-Hill.

Erickson, E. (1956). The problem of ego identity. *Journal of the American Psychoanalytic Association, 4,* 56–121.

Fairbairn, W. (1952). *Psychoanalytic studies of the personality.* London: Routledge & Kegan Paul.

Freud, S. (1957). The neuro-psychoses of defense. In J. Strachey (Ed. and Trans.), *The standard edition of the complete psychological works of Sigmund Freud* (Vol. 3, pp. 45–52). London: Hogarth Press. (Original work published 1894)

Freud, S. (1961). The ego and the id. In J. Strachey (Ed. and Trans.), *The standard edition of the complete psychological works of Sigmund Freud* (Vol. 19, pp. 3–66). London: Hogarth Press. (Original work published 1923)

Freud, S. (1957). On narcissism. In J. Strachey (Ed. and Trans.), *The standard edition of the complete psychological works of Sigmund Freud* (Vol. 14, pp. 67–104). London: Hogarth Press. (Original work published 1914)

Gill, M. M. (1982). *Analysis of transference* (Vol. 1). New York: International Universities Press.

Hartmann, H. (1958). *Ego psychology and the problem of adaptation.* New York: International Universities Press.

Hartmann, H., & Lowenstein, R. (1962). Notes on the superego. *Psychoanalytic Study of the Child, 18,* 42–81.

Hartmann, H., Kris, E., & Lowenstein, R. (1946). Comments on the formation of psychic structure. *Psychoanalytic Study of the Child, 2,* 11–38.

Horowitz, M. (1975). Sliding meanings: A defense against threat in narcissistic personalities. *International Journal of Pschoanalysis, 4,* 167–185.

Jacobson, E. (1964). *The self and the object world.* New York: International Universities Press.

Kernberg, O. (1975). *Borderline conditions and pathological narcissism.* New York: Jason Aronson.

Kernberg, O. (1976). *Object relations theory and clinical psychoanalysis.* New York: Jason Aronson.

Kernberg, O. (1960). Object relations theory and character analysis. *Journal of the American Psychoanalytic Association, 31,* 247–271.

Klein, G. (1976). *Psychoanalytic theory: An exploration of essentials.* New York: International Universities Press.

Kohut, H. (1966). Forms and transformations of narcissism. *Journal of the American Psychoanalytic Association, 14,* 243–272.
Kohut, H. (1968). The psychoanalytic treatment of narcissistic personality disorders. *Psychoanalytic Study of the Child, 23,* 86–113.
Kohut, H. (1971). The analysis of the self. New York: International Universities Press.
Kohut, H. (1977). The restoration of the self. New York: International Universities Press.
Kohut, H. (1984). How does analysis cure? New York: International Universities Press.
Lichtenberg, J. (1975). The development of the sense of self. *Journal of the American Psychoanalytic Association, 23,* 453–483.
Loewald, H. (1986). Transference-countertransference. *Journal of the American Psychoanalytic Association, 34,* 275–288.
Mahler, M., & Furer, M. (1968). *On human sybiosis and the vicissitudes of individuation.* New York: International Universities Press.
McLaughlin, J. (1981). Transference, psychic reality and countertransference. *Psychoanalytic Quarterly, 50,* 639–664.
Meissner, W. (1981). *Internalization in psychoanalysis.* New York: International Universities Press.
Michels, R. (1985). Perspectives on the nature of psychic reality: Panel introduction. *Journal of the American Psychoanalytic Association, 33,* 515–525.
Mitchell, S. (1979). Twilight of the idols: Change and preservation in the writings of Heinz Kohut. *Contemporary Psychoanalysis, 15,* 170–189.
Mitchell, S. A. (1988). *Relational concepts in psychoanalysis: An integration.*Cambridge, MA: Harvard University Press.
Modell, A. (1975). A narcissistic defense against affects and the illusion of self-sufficiency. *International Journal of Psycho-Analysis, 56,* 275–282.
Modell, A. (1990). *Other times, other realities.* Cambridge, MA: Harvard University Press.
Peterfreund, E. (1978). Some critical comments on psychoanalytic conceptualizations of infancy. *International Journal of Psycho-Analysis, 59,* 427–441.
Sander, L. (1962). Issues in early mother-child interaction. *Journal of the American Academyh of Child Psychiatry, 3,* 231–264.
Schafer, R. (1968). *Aspects of internalization.* New York: International Universities Press.
Schafer, R. (1983). *The analytic attitude.* New York: Basic Books.
Schwaber, E. (1983). Psychoanalytic listening and psychic reality. *International Review of Psycho-Analysis, 10,* 379–392.
Spitz, R. (1964). Stimulus overload, action cycles, and the completion gradient. *Journal of the American Psychoanalytic Association, 12,* 752–772.
Spruiell, V. (1975). Three strands of narcissism. *Psychoanalytic Quarterly, 44,* 557–579.
Stechler, G., & Kaplan, S. (1980). The development of the sense of self: A psychoanalytic perspective. *Psychoanalytic Study of the Child, 35,* 85–105.
Stern, D. (1985). *The interpersonal world of the human infant.* New York: Basic Books.

Stolorow, R., & Atwood, G. (1984). Psychoanalytic phenomenology: Toward science of human experience. *Psychoanalytic Inquiry, 4,* 87–104.

Stolorow, R., Brandchaft, B., & Atwood, G. (1987). *Psychoanalytic treatment: An intersubjective approach.* Hillsdale, NJ: Analytic Press.

Waelder, R. (1925). The psychoses, their mechanisms and accessibility to influence. *International Journal of Psycho-Analysis, 6,* 259–281.

Winnicott, D. (1951). Transitional objects and transitional phenomena. In *Through paediatrics to psycho-analysis* (pp. 229–242). New York: Basic Books.

Winicott, D. (1960).The theory of the parent-infant relationship. *International Journal of Psycho-Analysis, 41,* 585–597.

Winnicott, D. (1965). *The maturational process and the facilitating environment.* New York: International Universities Press.

Wolf, E. (1986). Discrepancies between analysand and analyst in experiencing the analysis. In A. Goldberg (Ed.), *Progress in self psychology* (Vol. 2, pp. 84–94). New York: Guilford Press.

II

Anxiety

3

Self-representation in Post-traumatic Stress Disorder: A Cognitive Perspective

RICHARD J. MCNALLY
Harvard University

COGNITIVE INTERPRETATIONS OF emotional disorders have abounded for the past 15 years (e.g., Beck, 1976), but few have been based on research and theory in cognitive psychology. Although clinical theorists have often used cognitive concepts (e.g., schema), few have employed them with the precision of their experimental counterparts. Indeed, cognition has often been equated with conscious thought rather than broadly conceived as information processing in the brain.

But the gap between clinical theory and cognitive psychology is closing. Cognitively oriented psychopathologists increasingly rely on paradigms drawn from experimental psychology to test hypotheses about emotional disorder (McNally, 1990; Segal, 1988; Williams, Watts, MacLeod, & Mathews, 1988). These paradigms promise to isolate specific defects in cognitive structures and processes that give rise to the signs and symptoms of mood (e.g., Williams & Nulty, 1986; Gotlib & Cane, 1987), anxiety (e.g., MacLeod, Mathews, & Tata, 1986; McNally, Foa, & Donnell, 1989), and eating disorders (e.g., Channon, Hemsley, & de Silva, 1988; Schotte, McNally, & Turner, 1990). In contrast to early approaches to cognitive assessment, as reviewed by Hollon and Bemis (1981), these laboratory-based paradigms are not restricted to subjective reports of conscious states. Accordingly, they enable inferences about cognition that are not accessible to self-report. For example, Mathews and MacLeod (1986) used a dichotic listening paradigm to demonstrate that patients with Generalized Anxiety

Disorder (GAD) exhibit attentional shifts toward threat cues of which they are unaware. Such attentional biases are inaccessible to self-report and therefore lie beyond the ken of traditional cognitive methods.

Among the phenomena recently subjected to the rigors of the laboratory is self psychopathology, the topic of the present volume. Long in the domain of personology (Baumeister, 1987), the self has been studied with increasing sophistication by students of social cognition (Higgins & Bargh, 1987; Markus & Wurf, 1987). Methods devised by these scholars have been applied to psychopathological manifestations of self phenomena in depression (Segal & Vella, 1990) and social phobia (Strauman, 1989).

This chapter concerns self-representation in Post-traumatic Stress Disorder (PTSD), as viewed from a cognitive perspective. It contains much speculation because cognitive research on PTSD has scarcely begun (Litz & Keane, 1989). Although this research was not designed to elucidate self-representation, it may have indirect implications for self pathology in PTSD.

The first section of this chapter provides a brief phenomenological overview of PTSD, as conceptualized in the DSM-III-R (American Psychiatric Association [APA], 1987); the second covers cognitive theory and research on PTSD; and the third outlines possible applications of cognitive-experimental methods for investigating self pathology in PTSD. The chapter closes with a discussion of conceptual issues in studying the traumatized self from a cognitive perspective.

PTSD: A PHENOMENOLOGICAL OVERVIEW

PTSD comprises a characteristic cluster of symptoms that develop following exposure to an extremely stressful event (APA, 1987). Such events produce distress in nearly everyone, are experienced with terror and helplessness, and are exemplified by rape, combat, horrific accidents, and natural disasters. The characteristic symptoms include (1) reexperiencing the traumatic event, (2) avoidance of reminders of the trauma or emotional numbing, and (3) increased arousal. A DSM-III-R diagnosis requires the presence of symptoms for at least one month.

The traumatic event can be reexperienced in several ways. Traumatized individuals usually have recurrent intrusive recollections of the event and recurrent distressing dreams in which the event is relived. Occasionally they may reexperience the event during "flashbacks," acting and feeling as if the trauma were recurring. The duration of these dissociative episodes may range from seconds to days. Finally, traumatized persons typically become intensely distressed when they encounter reminders of the trauma, such as anniversaries of the event.

Avoidance symptoms include attempts to avoid stimuli associated with the trauma, and attempts to suppress thoughts or feelings about it. Psychogenic amnesia for aspects of the event may occur. Among the symptoms of emotional numbing are the inability to experience positive emotions, to feel close to others, or to enjoy pleasurable activities. Finally, symptoms of elevated arousal include exaggerated startle, hypervigilance, sleep disturbance, concentration difficulties, irritability, and physiological reactivity in response to reminders of the trauma.

To what extent does the phenomenology of PTSD suggest alterations in self-representation? To what extent do the signs and symptoms of the disorder arise from disturbances in self-related structures and processes rather than from other mechanisms? On the one hand, representations of the *world* rather than of the self seem most dramatically altered by trauma. The conception of the world as a safe, predictable, and perhaps controllable place is shattered following exposure to trauma. Yet it is not merely a representation of the world that is transformed by trauma, but the world in reference to oneself. Indeed, most people live under the illusion that trauma can happen to others but not to themselves, an illusion that promotes mental health (Taylor & Brown, 1988). But a sudden, terrifying encounter with death can destroy this illusion and alter the representation of the self as secure and invulnerable. Several PTSD symptoms implicitly reflect such a change in self-representation. Fears of recurrence of the trauma, chronic anxiety, hypervigilance, and a sense of foreshortened future all reveal a sense of one's helplessness in the face of sudden, unpredictable, catastrophic stressors. Although a representation of the self as vulnerable to threat characterizes the anxiety disorders in general, in no case is it more dramatic than in PTSD.

In addition to anxiety and depression, PTSD patients experience other emotional disturbances that suggest alterations in self-representation (Horowitz, 1986). Following a traumatic event, individuals may experience survivor guilt about emerging relatively unscathed when others did not. Conversely, they may feel guilty about their anger toward those who died and therefore abandoned them. Soldiers who kill noncombatants or participate in atrocities often experience intense guilt about performing acts profoundly inconsistent with their self-concept as a moral being (March, 1990). Finally, rape survivors may experience shame about their victimization (Steketee & Foa, 1987).

In summary, chronic post-traumatic emotional disturbances imply that cognitive representations of the self are pathologically altered in several ways. Unfortunately, apart from clinical observations and speculations, there is little research directly bearing upon altered self-representation in PTSD. In the next section, I review cognitive research that indirectly has implications for altered self-representations in PTSD.

COGNITIVE THEORY AND RESEARCH ON PTSD

The ratification of PTSD as a diagnostic entity has greatly stimulated research on psychological trauma (APA, 1980), as exemplified by the founding of the International Society for Traumatic Stress Studies and the establishment of the *Journal of Traumatic Stress*. Most of this research has concerned descriptive and biological psychopathology, epidemiology, and to some extent, treatment. These studies have largely supported the syndromal validity of PTSD as a discrete entity (March, 1990; McNally, in press).

Despite increasing scientific interest in PTSD, theory and research conducted within a cognitive framework has been scarce. Only very recently have theorists advanced information-processing conceptualizations of the disorder (Chemtob, Roitblat, Hamada, Carlson, & Twentyman, 1988; Foa, Steketee, & Rothbaum, 1989; Litz & Keane, 1989).

Experiments involving the application of cognitive psychology paradigms have been equally scarce. In their review of information-processing research on anxiety—with special reference to PTSD—Litz and Keane (1989) cited only two experiments involving such paradigms (McNally et al., 1987; Trandel & McNally, 1987). Since the publication of Litz and Keane's paper, however, researchers have been increasingly applying these methods to study information-processing biases in PTSD (Cassiday, McNally, & Zeitlin, 1992; Foa, Feske, Murdock, Kozak, & McCarthy, 1991; Kaspi & McNally, 1991; McNally, English, & Lipke, in press; McNally, Kaspi, Riemann, & Zeitlin, 1990; Zeitlin & McNally, 1991). Moreover, Pitman's research on the psychophysiology of traumatic imagery might also be classified under this rubric (Pitman et al., 1990; Pitman, Orr, Forgue, de Jong, & Claiborn, 1987).

Cognition and PTSD

Information-processing theories of emotional disorder explain psychopathology in terms of dysfunctional cognitive processes and structures. Though instantiated in neural tissue, such dysfunctions are not reducible to disturbances in the underlying biological substrate. Similarly, errors in a computer program are not reducible to defects in the computer running the program. Candidates for the cognitive dysfunction in PTSD include pathological memory organization and ease of activation of threatening episodic memories.

Memory Organization

Anxiety disorders are usually related to future threats; thus, the obsessive–compulsive checker ritualizes to prevent possible disasters, the panic-disordered patient lives in dread of the next attack, and the GAD patient worries continually about a variety of impending threats. Unique among the anxiety disorders, PTSD has a focus on past rather than future threats. The trauma of a past threat is relived again and again during involuntary recollections, flashbacks, and nightmares. More than the other anxiety disorders, PTSD is a disorder of memory.

Several cognitive theorists have situated the psychopathology of PTSD in the organization of memory (Chemtob et al., 1988; Foa et al., 1989; Litz & Keane, 1989). These theorists have appealed to Lang's (1985) bio-informational theory of emotion as a basis for explicating pathological memory organization. According to Lang, emotional information is represented in memory as a network of stimulus, response, and meaning propositions. Information about the context of emotion is embodied in stimulus propositions; information about physiological, motoric, and verbal behavior is embodied in response propositions; and information interpreting the significance of stimulus and response information is embodied in meaning propositions. For example, a traumatic memory for a combat veteran might include stimulus propositions incorporating information about the hot, humid jungle in which the patient accidentally killed a noncombatant; response propositions encoding the physiological arousal (e.g., heart pounding, nausea) associated with the event; and meaning propositions elucidating its meaning (e.g., "I'm a murderer"). Such fear networks can be activated as a unit when a critical number of propositions are accessed through a match to input information, internal association, or both (Lang, 1985).

Although PTSD theorists working in the Langian tradition (e.g., Foa et al., 1989) have not addressed self-representation per se, their theories imply that the self is represented in memory as a network of interlocking propositions referring to the person himself or herself. Rather than being simply a single node in memory, the self arises emergently as the common feature of response and meaning propositions expressing a variety of facts about the person.

Trauma networks in PTSD are presumably large and coherent and therefore readily activated by a variety of inputs (Foa et al., 1989). Because propositions are tightly interconnected, activation emanating from some propositions spreads automatically to others. For example, a Vietnam veteran may instantly recall memories of combat trauma when he hears a helicopter flying overhead. Full activation of the trauma network is most dramatic during flashbacks in which the patient not only remembers the event but seems to reexperience it as well.

Barring amnesia, all traumatized persons "remember" the trauma. What, then, distinguishes the memory representations of those who develop PTSD from those who do not? Presumably for the former, the representation of the event is linked in memory to many other representations such that activation of a variety of concepts can trigger recall of the trauma, as exemplified by the rape victim who involuntarily recalls the assault whenever she encounters any man, not merely one resembling her assailant. Foa et al. (1989) also suggest that cognitive representations of the probability of subsequent trauma are higher for those who fail to recover from trauma than for those who do. Finally, connections between declarative knowledge about the trauma and procedural knowledge controlling emotional response programs are much stronger in PTSD patients than among recovered trauma victims. In contrast to PTSD patients, recovered trauma victims can recollect the event without engaging programs for emotional expression. Accordingly, they can *remember* the trauma without *reliving* it (Pitman et al., 1987).

Pitman and his associates have applied Lang's (1985) imagery paradigm to study memory organization in combat veterans with and without PTSD (Pitman et al., 1987; Pitman et al., 1990). In this paradigm, subjects are exposed to audiotaped scripts that describe their personal traumatic events and to control tapes that describe events unrelated to trauma. The scripts include stimulus, response, and meaning propositions, and are written in the second person, present tense. Network activation is presumably reflected by increases in physiological arousal and by emotional self-reports that match the semantic content of the script.

In contrast to healthy combat veterans, those with PTSD exhibit elevations in heart rate, skin conductance, and electromyogram activity when exposed to imagery scripts describing their personal traumatic events (Pitman et al., 1987). When imagining these events, PTSD patients also report more subjective distress than do their healthy counterparts. That verbal input engages the physiological system of PTSD patients suggests that semantic representations of trauma are closely linked to response programs governing the expression and experience of emotion.

Lang's imagery paradigm was not designed to elucidate self-representation per se, but its success in activating affect seems tied to processing of self-referent information. For example, textual prompts require that subjects place themselves in the scene as if it were actually happening, thus implying a crucial self-focus. Response propositions always reference the self (e.g., "Your heart begins to pound as the enemy approaches"), and meaning propositions often do as well (e.g., "You have just killed the child. You say to yourself, 'I'm a murderer!'"). Finally, combat scripts that describe personal traumatic events are more evocative than combat scripts that describe generic combat traumas (Pitman et al., 1990); that is, episodic information processing is more emotionally evocative than is semantic information processing.

Ease of Accessibility of Representations of Trauma

Not only may the organization of memory distinguish PTSD patients from recovered survivors, but ease of accessibility of cognitive representations of trauma seems especially characteristic of the disorder. Indeed, some consider involuntary retrieval of distressing episodic memories, as evinced by intrusive thoughts, nightmares, and flashbacks, to be the hallmark of the disorder (Pitman, 1989). These reexperiencing phenomena suggest that cognitive representations of trauma reside in a primed or partially activated state in memory (McNally et al., 1987).

If their traumatic memories are, indeed, primed, PTSD patients should exhibit delayed color-naming of trauma-related words in the modified Stroop (1935) paradigm. In this paradigm, subjects are shown words of varying emotional significance and asked to name the colors in which the words are printed while ignoring the meanings of the words (Mathews & MacLeod, 1985). Delays in color-naming (i.e., Stroop interference) occur when the meaning of the word automatically attracts the subject's attention despite the subject's effort to focus on the color of the word. Because color-naming delays reflect involuntary semantic activation (Williams et al., 1988, p. 65), interference produced by trauma-related words may provide a quantitative index of intrusive cognitive activity—the hallmark of PTSD. A further strength of this method for assessing intrusive activity is that it does not rely on patients' subjective self-report.

To evaluate the Stroop paradigm as a means for assessing intrusive cognition, McNally et al. (1990) had Vietnam combat veterans with and without PTSD color-name PTSD words related to the Vietnam War (e.g., "bodybags"), positive words (e.g., "love"), words related to another anxiety disorder (Obsessive–Compulsive Disorder [OCD] e.g., "germs"), and neutral words (e.g., "input") matched to the PTSD words in terms of frequency of usage in American English.

Results indicated that PTSD patients took significantly longer to color-name PTSD words than other words, and took significantly longer to name PTSD words than did control subjects. Differential responding did not occur for the other word types, thus indicating the specificity of the effect for trauma-related information in patients with PTSD. Correlational analyses indicated that Stroop interference scores for PTSD words were related to severity of PTSD ($r = .64$) (Mississippi Scale for Combat-Related Posttraumatic Stress Disorder [M-PTSD]) (Keane, Caddell, & Taylor, 1988), but not to the extent of combat exposure ($r = .14$) (Combat Exposure Scale [CES]) (Keane et al., 1989). Moreover, the correlation between interference for PTSD words and severity of the disorder remained significant even when the effects of combat exposure were partialled out ($r = .59$). These patterns of Stroop interference were replicated in another sample of Vietnam veterans with PTSD (McNally et al., in press). Taken together, the data suggest that delayed color-naming of trauma-related material may constitute an objective, quantitative index of intrusive cognitive activity.

In a subsequent experiment, Cassiday et al. (1992) developed a computerized version of the Stroop paradigm that enables precise measurement of color-naming latencies in response to single words that appear on the screen one at a time. This procedure contrasts with the traditional Stroop format in which all words of a single type (e.g., PTSD words) appear on the same card, and in which the dependent measure is the total time taken to color-name items on the entire card. There were three groups of subjects in this experiment: rape victims with PTSD, rape victims without PTSD, and nontraumatized normal control subjects. Subjects named the colors of high-threat words related to rape (e.g., "rape"), moderate-threat words related to rape (e.g., "crime"), positive words (e.g., "loyal"), and neutral words (e.g., "typical"). High-threat rape words had received higher threat ratings than moderate-threat rape words by rape victims who were not participants in this study. If Stroop interference is a function of the threat-relevance of the material processed, high-threat words should produce more interference relative to moderate-threat words.

In contrast to both control groups, rape victims with PTSD were slower to color-name high-threat rape words than moderate-threat rape words, positive words, and neutral words. This suggests that the threat-relevance of a stimulus may, indeed, be the key determinant of interference. Interference, however, was not restricted to rape victims with PTSD; those without the disorder exhibited more interference for high-threat rape words than did nontraumatized control subjects. Although these victims did not qualify for a DSM-III-R diagnosis of PTSD, most still had residual PTSD symptoms, thus suggesting an incomplete recovery. The degree of interference associated with high-threat rape words paralleled the degree of clinical impairment.

Surprisingly, rape victims with PTSD also exhibited greater interference for positive words than for neutral words, perhaps because these nominally positive words (e.g., "loyal" and "love") had negative connotations for them. Unlike other traumatic events (e.g., combat), rape closely intermingles themes of sexual intimacy with those of terror and violence. Accordingly, presentation of certain presumptively positive words may have readily activated threat-related concepts, thus producing Stroop interference. On the other hand, individuals with PTSD, or any other anxiety disorder, may simply exhibit selective processing of *any* emotional information, as suggested by Martin, Williams, and Clark (1991).

Finally, interference for high-threat rape words was significantly related ($r = .41$) to the intrusion subscale of the Impact of Events Scale (IES) (Horowitz, Wilner, & Alvarez, 1979), but not to the avoidance/numbing subscale of the IES. These findings further suggest that delayed color-naming of trauma-related words is an index of intrusive cognitive activity.

Using a similar computerized Stroop paradigm, Foa et al. (1991) had rape victims with and without PTSD and nontraumatized control subjects color-name rape words (e.g., "rape"), general threat words (e.g., "coffin"), neutral words (e.g., "apple"), and nonwords (e.g., "scroam"). Consistent with the aforementioned findings, Foa et al. found that rape victims with PTSD exhibited greater interference for rape words than for other words, and greater interference for rape words than did subjects in either of the control groups. Unlike Cassiday et al.'s (1992) non-PTSD rape victims, Foa et al.'s non-PTSD rape victims exhibited no tendency to process rape words selectively. Foa et al.'s subjects, however, had recently received successful cognitive–behavioral treatment for PTSD, whereas Cassiday et al.'s subjects were community volunteers who had never received more than palliative medication or brief emergency-room counseling, and who still experienced residual symptoms of PTSD. Accordingly, Cassiday et al.'s non-PTSD rape victims exhibited a degree of interference intermediate between victims with full-blown PTSD and Foa et al.'s treated rape victims, and the nontraumatized control subjects in both studies.

Kaspi and McNally (1991) modified the computerized Stroop paradigm to investigate the effects of personal relevance, threat, and emotionality on selective processing. Subjects were Vietnam combat veterans with PTSD, and healthy medical students who were about to take the National Boards medical examination. This examination constitutes a major, albeit nontraumatic, stressor because those who fail cannot become licensed as physicians.

Immediately before the experimental session, each subject rated the personal emotional significance of a long list of words on a 7-point scale that ranged from +3 (very positive emotional significance), through 0 (neutral emotional significance), to −3 (very negative emotional significance). The list comprised words likely to be rated as either neutral, positive, or negative. In addition, medical students rated a set of words related to academic failure, and PTSD patients rated a set of words related to Vietnam. For each subject, we selected five words receiving a 0 rating, five words receiving a +3 rating, and five words receiving a −3 rating, and loaded them into the computer as neutral, positive, and general threat words, respectively. Finally, for each medical student (or PTSD patient), we selected five academic (or Vietnam) words receiving a −3 rating, and loaded them into the computer as personal threat words. This "idiographic" Stroop paradigm enabled us to determine whether Stroop interference occurs only to personally threatening material or whether it occurs to generally threatening material as well, and whether positive information of equivalent emotional magnitude (but opposite valence) produces the effect.

Results indicated that PTSD patients exhibited substantial Stroop interference for Vietnam words, and some interference for generally negative words, relative to neutral and positive words. Inconsistent with Martin et al.'s (1991) hypothesis that anxious patients selectively process *any* emotional information, PTSD patients actually exhibited somewhat greater interference for neutral words receiving an idiographic emotionality rating of 0 than for positive words receiving an idiographic emotionality rating of +3. Medical students exhibited no differential Stroop interference, even for academic words having negative personal emotional valence. Taken together, these findings suggest that Stroop interference is strongest for threatening information having strong self-reference—but only in anxiety-disordered individuals (e.g., PTSD patients).

The Stroop data are consistent with the hypothesis that information about trauma is primed in individuals with PTSD. These findings parallel phenomenological reports of the ease with which traumatic memories involuntarily "come to mind" for patients with PTSD. If traumatic memories are, indeed, primed and readily accessible, other paradigms may also triangulate the phenomenon. For example, PTSD patients should exhibit both explicit and implicit memory biases favoring information about trauma. *Explicit* memory tasks include conventional free recall, cued recall, and recognition tasks where memory for previously presented material is revealed by the subject's conscious recollection of being exposed to the item. *Implicit* memory, on the other hand, is inferred when the subject's behavior shows evidence of having been exposed to certain information even though the subject does not consciously recall being exposed to it. Implicit memory is commonly assessed by word-completion tasks. For example, subjects may be presented with a list of words containing the item "forest," and later be asked to complete word stems such as "for____." Implicit memory is inferred when subjects complete such stems with "-est" rather than, say, "-get" after having been exposed to "forest." Implicit memory is believed to be relatively automatic, and it does not rely on elaborative encoding or effort or conscious recollection at testing. The automaticity of implicit memory would seem to render it especially relevant for understanding involuntary activation of traumatic episodes.

Based on the assumption that traumatic memories are chronically primed in PTSD, Zeitlin and McNally (1991) hypothesized that combat veterans with PTSD, but not those without PTSD, ought to exhibit both explicit and implicit memory biases for words related to Vietnam. Subjects were exposed to combat words (e.g., "bodybags"), social threat words (e.g., "humiliated"), positive words (e.g., "charm"), and neutral words (e.g., "predict"). In counterbalanced order, subjects were given a cued recall test and a word completion test. For the former, they were told that the word stem constituted the first three letters of a word to which they had recently been exposed. For the latter, they were simply told to complete the word stem with the first word that came to mind.

Results indicated that on the explicit memory test, PTSD patients exhibited a greater bias than did control subjects for relative recall of combat words (e.g., number of combat words recalled minus number of neutral words recalled). In contrast to control subjects, PTSD patients also exhibited an implicit memory bias for combat words. The memory biases for combat information exhibited by the patients was especially striking insofar as they tended to exhibit impaired memory for nonthreat information relative to controls. These findings provide further objective evidence that information about trauma is, indeed, primed in memory for PTSD patients.

What relevance do these cognitive psychology experiments have for self-representation in PTSD? Although none of these experiments was conducted to investigate the self, they nevertheless indicate that only *personally* threatening information is preferentially processed. Only disorder-specific threat information is associated with physiological activation (Pitman et al., 1987), Stroop interference (McNally et al., 1990), and preferential recall (Zeitlin & McNally, 1991). Moreover, information threatening for obsessive–compulsives (McNally et al., 1990) or social phobics (Zeitlin & McNally, 1991) is not preferentially processed by PTSD patients.

Connections between the aforementioned cognitive research and self-representational issues are indirect. Accordingly, elucidation of self pathology in PTSD will be advanced by application of cognitive paradigms that directly target the self. In the following section, I outline strategies used to study the self in depression and in social phobia. These approaches may prove useful in the investigation of PTSD.

STRATEGIES FOR STUDYING SELF-REPRESENTATION IN PTSD

Self-representation has been studied more in depression than in other emotional disorders (Segal, 1988). Investigators have endeavored to test Beck's (1976) hypothesis that depressed patients are characterized by a negative self-schema that biases information processing in ways that maintain depressed mood. The negative self-schema constitutes a cognitive structure in memory comprising a set of interlocking negative attributes. Though considerable evidence has been adduced in support of this structure, much of it can be interpreted otherwise (Higgins & Bargh, 1987; Segal, 1988). Interpretive ambiguity has arisen because researchers have often failed to use paradigms based on automatic cognitive processing. Segal quotes Posner and Warren (1972) on this point:

> When we say a structure exists in memory we are really saying that one item will activate another in a quite direct and simple way even perhaps when the subject does not intend for it to occur. If we had methods to tap structure uninfluenced by conscious search, we might reflect the structure of memory more simply . . . How can we study automatic processes as distinguished from those that involve conscious search? Even the definition of "automatic" is a difficult matter, and yet without such a distinction it appears impossible to develop a meaningful analysis of structure. (p. 34)

These methodological guidelines for documenting memory structure have been observed in recent research on depression (Segal, Hood, Shaw, & Higgins, 1988; Segal & Vella, 1990) and, accordingly, have relevance for the study of self-representation in PTSD. For example, Segal and Vella (1990) devised a priming version of the modified Stroop paradigm to test the hypothesis that self-descriptive negative attributes cohere as a structure in memory for patients with major depression. Subjects were asked to color-name personal adjectives that had been rated in terms of their self-descriptiveness. Each trial consisted of the presentation of a prime word followed by a target word printed in color. The subject's task was to name the color of the target as quickly as possible and then state the prime. If the prime and target are related for the subject, semantic activation originating from the cognitive representation of the prime ought to activate the semantic activation of the target, thereby delaying color-naming of the target. Consistent with this hypothesis, Segal and Vella found that color-naming of self-descriptive negative (target) adjectives was delayed when preceded by another self-descriptive negative (prime) adjective. These findings suggest that negative attributes do, indeed, cohere as a structure in memory for patients with major depression. The self-attributes of PTSD patients could be studied similarly to determine whether they cohere as a negative self-schema in memory.

Higgins's (1987) research on self-discrepancies provides additional methods for elucidating pathological self-representations in PTSD. According to self-discrepancy theory, specific types of discrepancy between self-states are related to vulnerability for specific negative emotions. Underlying these self-state representations are two cognitive dimensions: domains of the self and standpoints on the self. The three basic self domains are the *actual* self, which constitutes one's representation of the attributes that someone (oneself or another) believes one has; the *ideal* self, which constitutes one's representation of the attributes that someone (oneself or another) would like one to possess (e.g., attributes one wishes to possess); and the *ought* self, which constitutes one's representation of the attributes that someone (oneself or another) believes one should possess (e.g., representation of someone's sense of one's responsibilities). Standpoints on the self can be either one's own or that of some significant other (e.g., a parent). Six basic self-state representations result from crossing each of the domains of the self with each of the standpoints: actual/own, actual/other, ideal/own, ideal/other, ought/own, and ought/other. Actual/other, and especially actual/own, are the self-state representations that constitute the self-concept. The remaining four self-state representations constitute self-guides or standards.

Discrepancies between self-concept attributes and personally significant self-guides have specific emotional consequences. For example, guilt results from an actual/own versus ought/own discrepancy. Such feelings arise when people believe they have violated a personally accepted moral standard. Shame results from an actual/own versus ideal/other discrepancy in which people believe that they have failed to meet the expectations of others. Fear or feeling threatened results from an actual/own versus ought/other discrepancy when people believe that they have violated the standards of others. Fear involves anticipating sanctions from others for having broken their rules, whereas guilt involves self-chastisement for having violated one's own standards for conduct. In summary, the greater the magnitude and accessibility of a certain type of self-discrepancy, the more one will suffer the kind of emotional distress associated with that type of discrepancy.

Several studies suggest that activation of certain self-discrepancies can produce increases in specific negative emotions (e.g., Strauman, 1989; Strauman & Higgins, 1987). For example, Strauman (1989) used a questionnaire to identify mismatches among the self-states of normal control subjects and patients with either depression or social phobia. Approximately 10 days later, subjects participated in an ostensibly unrelated study in which they were presented with audiotaped questions of the form "Why is it important for a person to be ______?" The blanks were filled by trait attributes, of which some were ideal self-guides and some were ought self-guides. Subjects responded orally to the questions, and skin conductance and self-report measures of mood were taken. As Strauman predicted, when subjects were primed with attributes that mismatched their actual self-representation, changes in affect, arousal, and behavior occurred that fit the predicted mood change. These findings suggest that self-discrepancies constitute a self-evaluative cognitive structure that when activated can induce specific types of negative affect.

The Higgins–Strauman approach to elucidating structural self pathology has yet to be applied to PTSD. There are aspects of the disorder, however, that lend themselves well to this approach. Self-schematic relations underlying guilt, for example, should be revealed by the priming of actual/own versus ought/own, and cognitive structures underlying shame should be revealed by the priming of actual/own versus ideal/other discrepancies. On the other hand, it is unclear whether the cognitive self-structures underlying fear are entirely relevant for PTSD. Higgins (1987) holds that fear is related to actual/own versus ought/other discrepancies. But this discrepancy applies best to interpersonal situations in which censure is delivered by others, contingent upon one's failing to meet one's obligations. The fear and anxiety associated with PTSD is not this everyday sort of social anxiety. Indeed, anxiety can be produced in ways other than solely through actual/own versus ought/other discrepancies. A self-representational construal of panic disorder, for instance, would emphasize a self perpetually on the verge of annihilation resulting from fatal heart attacks, imminent insanity, and so forth.

Indeed, Higgins's self-structural construal of fear best fits those anxiety disorders driven by concerns about the approval of others, such as social phobia and some forms of OCD. Social phobia, especially the generalized subtype, is the prototypical anxiety disorder in which negative self-referential cognition predominates; the self as an object of critical scrutiny by others is the hallmark of the disorder.

Some OCD patients experience the anxious self-discrepancies described by Higgins. Examples include obsessive–compulsive checkers who retrace their driving routes to determine whether they have struck any pedestrians, and those with "harming obsessions" who remove sharp knives from their sight to prevent themselves from stabbing their children. In contrast, other manifestations of OCD (e.g., contamination obsessions and washing compulsions) appear related to concerns about self-preservation and only secondarily about the disapproval of others.

The Higgins–Strauman paradigm involves the provocation of momentary emotional syndromes congruent with the activation of specific self-discrepancies. This may prove problematic in the study of PTSD because PTSD patients tend to exhibit chronically high levels of guilt, anger, depression, and anxiety (APA, 1987). Accordingly, a ceiling effect may prevent any further increases in negative affect associated with the activation of self-discrepancies. These potential problems notwithstanding, experimental assessment of self-discrepancies is warranted in PTSD.

TREATMENT ISSUES

Cognitive–behavioral approaches to the therapeutic alteration of pathological self-representation in the anxiety disorders takes much the same form as the alteration of other maladaptive beliefs. Consistent with Bandura's (1977) dictum that enactive procedures are the surest method to produce cognitive change, cognitive–behavior therapists devise ways to generate experiences for patients that refute aspects of their pathological self-representations.

In the treatment of panic disorder (Clark & Beck, 1988), the therapist has the patient conduct behavioral experiments that are designed to alter the patient's representation of his or her own bodily sensations of arousal. For example, patients who believe that dizziness will produce collapse are asked to hyperventilate while sitting, and then to stand up quickly. That fainting does not occur serves to refute the patient's prediction that he or she will collapse if dizzy. The cumulative effect of such tests can alter the representation of the self as vulnerable to unpredictable and dangerous bodily sensations. Similarly, in vivo exposure for social phobics, often involving generation of the feared symptom (e.g., blushing in public), produces innocuous results, thereby modifying the patient's self-representation as being forever exposed to the critical scrutiny of others.

Cognitive–behavioral treatment research on PTSD has scarcely begun, and none of it directly addresses therapeutic alteration of pathological self-representation (e.g., Keane, Fairbank, Caddell, & Zimering, 1989; Shapiro, 1989). Unlike other anxiety disorders that clearly involve exaggerated estimates of personal vulnerability (e.g., panic disorder) or unrealistically negative self-conceptions (e.g., social phobia), PTSD is less obviously "neurotic." After having been exposed to serious personal threats, PTSD patients may entertain representations of the self as vulnerable that have more than a grain of truth to them, and combat veterans may be justifiably guilt-ridden over atrocities they committed during warfare. Accordingly, veridical aspects of distressing self-representations in PTSD create challenges for the therapist that are relatively uncommon in the other anxiety disorders.

PTSD AND SELF-REPRESENTATION: GENERAL ISSUES

A premise of this volume is that specific disorders are associated with specific disturbances in self-representation. That is, greater similarity in self-representation should obtain within diagnostic groups than between diagnostic groups. This is consistent with Beck's (1976) view that emotional disorders are cognitively distinguishable, at least at the level of self-report. Thus, he notes that the self of anxious patients is characterized by a sense of vulnerability, whereas the self of depressed patients is characterized by a sense of worthlessness.

It remains to be seen, however, whether distinctions apparent at the level of self-report persist at the level of underlying cognitive structure. The self-representations of emotionally disturbed individuals may be more similar than different. For example, PTSD patients as well as depressed patients are often characterized by guilt, sadness, and anxiety. And low self-esteem is associated not only with depression but also with most emotional disorders. Accordingly, an important task for future research is to determine whether variations in self-representational disturbance isomorphically correspond to our nosological categories.

Although PTSD is the primary focus of this chapter, pathologies of self-representation are likely in at least some of the other anxiety disorders. Conceptions of the self as helpless, incompetent, and vulnerable ought to be most common in those disorders marked by pervasiveness of disability, such as agoraphobia, and severe OCD. As mentioned above, the hallmark of generalized social phobia is a representation of the self as an object of other people's critical scrutiny. In contrast to these anxiety disorders, circumscribed simple phobias are unlikely to be associated with much self pathology.

Another important task is to determine when self pathology contributes to the etiology and maintenance of anxiety disorders. Self-representational disturbances may merely constitute epiphenomena with no causal import. Although panic disorder, for example, may develop in persons whose self-representations are marked by characterizations of personal vulnerability, representations of the self as vulnerable may solely be a cognitive consequence of a fundamentally biological disease, as implied by Klein (1981). Indeed, some patients subscribe to a purely biological conceptualization of their disorder, perhaps to counteract the stigmatizing self-representations that often accompany mental illness. It remains to be seen whether self pathology in anxiety disorders is more cause or consequence of the emotional and behavioral problems. This is especially important given related studies that suggest that negative thinking in depression results from temporary mood disturbances rather than from stable underlying negative self-schemas (e.g., Dohr, Rush, & Bernstein, 1989).

The negative impact of trauma on the development of healthy self-representations is perhaps most apparent in children with PTSD. Child psychiatrists have noted that traumatized children are especially likely to see themselves as having a foreshortened future in which they do not expect to achieve a normal lifespan, establish a career, get married, have children, and so forth (Pynoos, 1990; Terr, 1979). Traumatized adults who have already achieved these developmental goals are presumably less likely than children to experience themselves as having a foreshortened future.

An assumption guiding recent work on the self is that inferences about cognitive structure require experimental paradigms based on automatic cognitive processing (e.g., Segal, 1988). This methodological principle, however, raises a potentially thorny problem insofar as controversy has erupted concerning the concept of automaticity itself (Bargh, 1989). According to the received view, automatic cognitive processes are rapid, difficult to suppress, and can occur without intention, awareness, or consumption of attentional resources. Moreover, each instance of automatic processing ought to be characterized by all of these properties because the unitary nature of automaticity is what distinguishes it from each of its defining attributes (Bargh, 1989). But as Bargh (1989) emphasized in his penetrating analysis of the concept of automaticity, the consensus view is crumbling. Experimental tasks long thought to be automatic have been found to require attentional resources and adoption of certain intentional processing goals. Accordingly, Bargh suggests that there may be varieties of automaticity, and that different cognitive processes may be more or less automatic. Because the concept of automaticity is not as clear as it once was (e.g., Shiffrin & Schneider, 1977), the documentation of disturbances in self-representation may be unexpectedly complex, if demonstrations of structure must be based on automatic cognitive processing.

Although the concept of the self is phenomenologically compelling to those reared in the Western tradition (Baumeister, 1987; Weintraub, 1978), it is drawn from the discourse of everyday life, an idiom criticized by some cognitive scientists (e.g., Churchland, 1988). Indeed, one influential doctrine in cognitive science, *eliminative materialism*, holds that "folk psychology" concepts such as the self, belief, and desire will not survive the development of the cognitive and neurosciences. This view states that "folk psychology is a hopelessly primitive and deeply confused conception of our internal activities" (Churchland, 1988, p. 45). Accordingly, folk psychology will share the fate of folk physics, folk biology, and other prescientific disciplines whose concepts (e.g., phlogiston, *élan vital*) were not translated or reduced to the concepts of mature science, but were simply eliminated because they lacked existential status within the new framework. Thus, scientists have not sought to determine the referent for the *élan vital* within the conceptual framework of molecular biology, and have not attempted to translate phlogiston into the terminology of modern physics. Similarly, eliminative materialists believe that the concept of the self will have no place in a mature cognitive science.

The jury is still out on eliminative materialism. Even if concepts such as the self are destined for obsolescence, the abolition of folk psychology is not imminent. The wisest policy, therefore, may be to explore the explanatory potential of self-representation with as much rigor and imagination as possible.

CONCLUSIONS

In this chapter, I have endeavored to survey cognitive research and theory on PTSD, with special reference to self-representational issues. The application of cognitive-experimental methods to the study of anxiety disorders in general, and PTSD in particular, is a relatively new development (Williams et al., 1988). Accordingly, the ratio of speculation to data is uncomfortably large in this review. But new methods for studying self pathology in depression (Segal & Vella, 1990) and social phobia (Strauman, 1989) may prove useful in determining the extent to which the self is implicated in PTSD. The further interpenetration of cognitive psychology and psychopathology is the surest route for addressing such issues.

ACKNOWLEDGMENT

Preparation of this chapter was supported in part by National Institute of Mental Health Grant #MH43809 awarded to the author.

REFERENCES

American Psychiatric Association. (1980). *Diagnostic and statistical manual of mental disorders* (3rd ed.). Washington, DC: Author.

American Psychiatric Association. (1987). *Diagnostic and statistical manual of mental disorders* (3rd ed., rev.). Washington, DC: Author.

Bandura, A. (1977). Self-efficacy: Toward a unifying theory of behavioral change. *Psychological Review, 84*, 191–215.

Bargh, J. A. (1989). Conditional automaticity: Varieties of automatic influence in social perception and cognition. In J. S. Uleman & J. A. Bargh (Eds.), *Unintended thought* (pp. 3–51). New York: Guilford Press.

Baumeister, R. F. (1987). How the self became a problem: A psychological review of historical research. *Journal of Personality and Social Psychology, 52*, 163–176.

Beck, A. T. (1976). *Cognitive therapy and the emotional disorders.* New York: Meridian.

Cassiday, K. L., McNally, R. J., & Zeitlin, S. B. (1992). Cognitive processing of trauma cues in rape victims with post-traumatic stress disorder. *Cognitive Therapy and Research, 16*, 283–295.

Channon, S., Hemsley, D., & de Silva, P. (1988). Selective processing of food words in anorexia nervosa. *British Journal of Clinical Psychology, 27*, 259–260.

Chemtob, C., Roitblat, H. L., Hamada, R. S., Carlson, J. G., Twentyman, C. T. (1988). A cognitive action theory of post-traumatic stress disorder. *Journal of Anxiety Disorders, 2*, 253–275.

Churchland, P. M. (1988). *Matter and consciousness.* Cambridge, MA: MIT Press.

Clark, D. M., & Beck, A. T. (1988). Cognitive approaches. In C. G. Last & M. Hersen (Eds.), *Handbook of anxiety disorders* (pp. 362–385). Elmsford, NY: Pergamon Press.

Dohr, K. B., Rush, A. J., & Bernstein, I. H. (1989). Cognitive biases in depression. *Journal of Abnormal Psychology, 98*, 263–267.

Foa, E. B., Feske, U., Murdock, T. B., Kozak, M. J., & McCarthy, P. R. (1991). Processing of threat-related information in rape victims. *Journal of Abnormal Psychology, 100*, 156–162.

Foa, E. B., Steketee, G., & Rothbaum, B. O. (1989). Behavioral/cognitive conceptualizations of post-traumatic stress disorder. *Behavior Therapy, 20*, 155–176.

Gotlib, I. H., & Cane, D. B. (1987). Construct accessibility and clinical depression: A longitudinal investigation. *Journal of Abnormal Psychology, 96*, 199–204.

Higgins, E. T. (1987). Self-discrepancy: A theory relating self and affect. *Psychological Review, 94*, 319–340.

Higgins, E. T., & Bargh, J. A. (1987). Social cognition and social perception. *Annual Review of Psychology, 38*, 369–425.

Hollon, S. D., & Bemis, K. M. (1981). Self-report and the assessment of cognitive functions. In M. Hersen & A. S. Bellack (Eds.), *Behavioral assessment: A practical handbook* (pp. 125–174). Elmsford, NY: Pergamon Press.

Horowitz, M. J. (1986). *Stress response syndromes.* Northvale, NJ: Jason Aronson.

Horowitz, M., Wilner, N., & Alvarez, W. (1979). The Impact of Events Scale: A measure of subjective stress. *Psychosomatic Medicine, 41*, 209–218.

Kaspi, S. P. & McNally, R. J. (1991, November). *Selective processing of idiographic emotional information in PTSD*. Paper presented at the meeting of the Association for Advancement of Behavior Therapy, New York, NY.

Keane, T. M., Caddell, J. M., & Taylor, K. L. (1988). Mississippi Scale for Combat-Related Posttraumatic Stress Disorder: Three studies in reliability and validity. *Journal of Consulting and Clinical Psychology, 56*, 85–90.

Keane, T. M., Fairbank, J. A., Caddell, J. M., & Zimering, R. T. (1989). Implosive (flooding) therapy reduces symptoms of PTSD in Vietnam combat veterans. *Behavior Therapy, 20*, 245–260.

Keane, T. M., Fairbank, J. A., Caddell, J. M., Zimering, R. T., Taylor, K. L., & Mora, C. A. (1989). Clinical evaluation of a measure to assess combat exposure. *Psychological Assessment: A Journal of Consulting and Clinical Psychology, 1*, 53–55.

Klein, D. F. (1981). Anxiety reconceptualized. In D. F. Klein & J. Rabkin (Eds.), *Anxiety: New research and changing concepts* (pp. 235–263). New York: Raven Press.

Lang, P. J. (1985). The cognitive psychophysiology of emotion: Fear and anxiety. In A. H. Tuma & J. D. Maser (Eds.), *Anxiety and the anxiety disorders* (pp. 131–170). Hillsdale, NJ: Lawrence Erlbaum.

Litz, B. T., & Keane, T. M. (1989). Information processing in anxiety disorders: Application to the understanding of post-traumatic stress disorder. *Clinical Psychology Review, 9*, 243–257.

MacLeod, C., Mathews, A., & Tata, P. (1986). Attentional bias in emotional disorders. *Journal of Abnormal Psychology, 95*, 15–20.

March, J. S. (1990). The nosology of posttraumatic stress disorder. *Journal of Anxiety Disorders, 4*, 61–82.

Markus, H., & Wurf, E. (1987). The dynamic self-concept: A social psychological perspective. *Annual Review of Psychology, 38*, 299–337.

Martin, M., Williams, R. M., & Clark, D. M. (1991). Does anxiety lead to selective processing of threat-related information? *Behaviour Research and Therapy, 29*, 147–160.

Mathews, A., & MacLeod, C. (1985). Selective processing of threat cues in anxiety states. *Behaviour Research and Therapy, 23*, 563–569.

Mathews, A., & MacLeod, C. (1986). Discrimination of threat cues without awareness in anxiety states. *Journal of Abnormal Psychology, 95*, 131–138.

McNally, R. J. (1990). Psychological approaches to panic disorder: A review. *Psychological Bulletin, 108*, 403–419.

McNally, R. J. (in press). Psychopathology of post-traumatic stress disorder (PTSD): Boundaries of the syndrome. In M. Başoğlu (Ed.), *Torture and its consequences: Current treatment approaches*. Cambridge: Cambridge University Press.

McNally, R. J., English, G. E., & Lipke, H. J. (in press). Assessment of intrusive cognition in PTSD: Use of the modified Stroop paradigm. *Journal of Traumatic Stress.*

McNally, R. J., Foa, E. B., & Donnell, C. D. (1989). Memory bias for anxiety information in patients with panic disorder. *Cognition and Emotion*, *3*, 27–44.

McNally, R. J., Kaspi, S. P., Riemann, B. C., & Zeitlin, S. B. (1990). Selective processing of threat cues in post-traumatic stress disorder. *Journal of Abnormal Psychology*, *99*, 398–402.

McNally, R. J., Luedke, D. L., Besyner, J. K., Peterson, R. A., Bohm, K., & Lips, O. J. (1987). Sensitivity to stress-relevant stimuli in posttraumatic stress disorder. *Journal of Anxiety Disorders*, *1*, 105–116.

Pitman, R. K. (1989). Post-traumatic stress disorder, hormones, and memory. *Biological Psychiatry*, *26*, 221–223.

Pitman, R. K., Orr, S. P., Forgue, D. F., Altman, B., de Jong, J. B., & Herz, L. R. (1990). Psychophysiologic responses to combat imagery of Vietnam veterans with posttraumatic stress disorder versus other anxiety disorders. *Journal of Abnormal Psychology*, *99*, 49–54.

Pitman, R. K., Orr, S. P., Forgue, D. F., de Jong, J. B., & Claiborn, J. M. (1987). Psychophysiologic assessment of posttraumatic stress disorder imagery in Vietnam combat veterans. *Archives of General Psychiatry*, *44*, 970–975.

Posner, M. I., & Warren, R. E. (1972). Traces, concepts and conscious constructions. In A. W. Melton & E. Martin (Eds.), *Coding processes in human memory* (pp. 25–43). Washington, DC: Winston.

Pynoos, R. S. (1990). Post-traumatic stress disorder in children and adolescents. In B. D. Garfinkel, G. A. Carlson, & E. B. Weller (Eds.), *Psychiatric disorders in children and adolescents* (pp. 48–63). Philadelphia: Saunders.

Schotte, D. E., McNally, R. J., & Turner, M. L. (1990). A dichotic listening analysis of bodyweight concern in bulimia nervosa. *International Journal of Eating Disorders*, *9*, 109–113.

Segal, Z. V. (1988). Appraisal of the self-schema construct in cognitive models of depression. *Psychological Bulletin*, *103*, 147–162.

Segal, Z. V., Hood, J. E., Shaw, B. F., & Higgins, E. T. (1988). A structural analysis of the self-schema construct in major depression. *Cognitive Therapy and Research*, *12*, 471–485.

Segal, Z. V., & Vella, D. D. (1990). Self-schema in major depression: Replication and extension of a priming methodology. *Cognitive Therapy and Research*, *14*, 161–176.

Shapiro, F. (1989). Efficacy of the eye movement desensitization procedure in the treatment of traumatic memories. *Journal of Traumatic Stress*, *2*, 199–223.

Shiffrin, R. M., & Schneider, W. (1977). Controlled and automatic human information processing: II. Perceptual learning, automatic attending, and a general theory. *Psychological Review*, *84*, 127–190.

Steketee, G., & Foa, E. B. (1987). Rape victims: Post-traumatic stress responses and their treatment: A review of the literature. *Journal of Anxiety Disorders*, *1*, 69–86.

Strauman, T. J. (1989). Self-discrepancies in clinical depression and social phobia: Cognitive structures that underlie emotional disorders? *Journal of Abnormal Psychology*, *98*, 14–22.

Strauman, T. J., & Higgins, E. T. (1987). Automatic activation of self-discrepancies and emotional syndromes: When cognitive structures influence affect. *Journal of Personality and Social Psychology*, *53*, 1004–1014.

Stroop, J. R. (1935). Studies of interference in serial verbal reactions. *Journal of Experimental Psychology*, *18*, 643–661.

Taylor, S. E., & Brown, J. D. (1988). Illusion and well-being: A social psychological perspective on mental health. *Psychological Bulletin*, *103*, 193–210.

Terr, L. C. (1979). Children of Chowchilla: A study of psychic trauma. *Psychoanalytic Study of the Child*, *34*, 547–623.

Trandel, D. V., & McNally, R. J. (1987). Perception of threat cues in post-traumatic stress disorder: Semantic processing without awareness? *Behaviour Research and Therapy*, *25*, 469–476.

Weintraub, K. J. (1978). *The value of the individual.* Chicago: University of Chicago Press.

Williams, J. M. G., & Nulty, D. D. (1986). Construct accessibility, depression and the emotional Stroop task: Transient mood or stable structure? *Personality and Individual Differences*, *7*, 485–491.

Williams, J. M. G., Watts, F. N., MacLeod, C., & Mathews, A. (1988). *Cognitive psychology and emotional disorders.* Chichester, UK: Wiley.

Zeitlin, S. B., & McNally, R. J. (1991). Implicit and explicit memory biases for threat in post-traumatic stress disorder. *Behaviour Research and Therapy*, *29*, 451–457.

Commentary

TRACY D. EELLS
University of Louisville

BRAM FRIDHANDLER
CHARLES H. STINSON
MARDI J. HOROWITZ
University of California, San Francisco

WE WILL ORGANIZE our commentary on Dr. McNally's chapter around themes suggested by the editors for each chapter in this book. These include the definition of the self, the relevance of the self for the particular emotional disorder, developmental processes and outcomes of self-representation, measurement issues, and the role of affect in self-representation. In each area we will draw comparisons between the cognitive perspective of Post-traumatic Stress Disorder (PTSD) discussed by Dr. McNally and the person schemas approach to PTSD as well as other anxiety disorders.

DEFINITION OF THE SELF

As Dr. McNally notes, psychopathologists have only begun to study emotional disorders, and particularly anxiety disorders, from the context of dysfunctional cognitive processes and structures. Very little of this work has focused on self-representations; thus, definitions of the self have not been precisely articulated by researchers in this area. McNally extends Lang's (1985) bio-informational model of anxiety to suggest that the self is represented in memory as

> a network of interlocking propositions referring to the person himself or herself. Rather than being simply a single node in memory, the self arises emergently as the common feature of response and meaning propositions expressing a variety of facts about the person. (p. 10)

This view is similar to the person schemas theory assumption that the self is an organized meaning structure, but differs in that it does not explicitly presume that each individual has a repertoire of multiple self-schemas. Another distinction is that our view of self includes a self-in-relationship-to-other. We propose, in other words, that in some states of mind, the self arises in contrast to another. The self as an emergent property is also consistent with parallel distributed processing (PDP) theory, which we described as a cognitive model that may underlie schematic organization. According to PDP, the self as well as other schemas emerges from simpler processing units and activation states of these units.

McNally also mentions Higgins's (1987) self-discrepancy theory as a cognitive model by which research of anxiety disorders can be guided. Higgins's model assumes multiple selves viewed from the perspective of either the self or the other. This comes closer to our view, although our emphasis is not only exclusively on discrepant views of the self, but also on sets of relations between self and other, whether discrepant or concordant.

RELEVANCE OF THE SELF FOR ANXIETY DISORDERS

McNally questions the relevance of the self for various anxiety disorders, suggesting it may have more relevance for social phobia—the hallmark of which is anxiety related to the self and the potentially harsh scrutiny of it by others, or for agoraphobia and severe Obsessive–Compulsive Disorder, both of which involve views of the self as vulnerable and helpless—than for simple phobias, which are more circumscribed. He points out that in PTSD, more than in other anxiety disorders, it is the world, rather than the self, that appears to undergo change; that is, a severe trauma may break down the illusion of a safe, predictable, and nonthreatening world and replace it with a view of the world as persistently dangerous, unpredictable, and threatening. As he also points out, it is the world in relation to the self that makes the changed representation of the world significant and threatening.

The person-schemas approach typically models anxiety in terms of self-representations. The role of self-representations is particularly suggested by the guilt, shame, and feelings of personal weakness sometimes experienced by those with PTSD, but these feelings cannot be explained soley by a changed representation of the world. Although it is an important feature of PTSD, we agree with McNally, and perhaps emphasize more than he, that the *self in relationship to the world*, not simply a changed perception of the world, is the critical feature in PTSD.

DEVELOPMENTAL PROCESSES AND OUTCOMES OF SELF-REPRESENTATION

McNally does not so much address the developmental processes involved in PTSD as he does the outcomes, specifically, the dysfunctional cognitive organization of the individual who has PTSD. His only statement that relates to developmental processes is the acknowledgment that "chronic post-traumatic emotional disturbances imply that cognitive representations of the self are pathologically altered in several ways" (p. 73). He does not explain how this occurs, but he does discuss two areas where the developmental outcomes may be dysfunctional: memory organization and the "ease of accessibility of representations of trauma" (p. 76). In essence, he argues that individuals with PTSD have a "trauma network" that is "large and coherent" (p. 75) and that these individuals are therefore more susceptible to painful memories of the trauma. McNally cites several studies supporting these propositions and suggests that self-representations may also be pertinent.

A key developmental question is, Why do some develop PTSD and others not? McNally answers this question as follows: "Presumably for [those who do develop PTSD], the representation of the event is linked in memory to many other representations such that activation of a variety of concepts can trigger recall of the trauma" (p. 75). This does not address developmental processes, but developmental outcomes. That is, the *outcome* for those with PTSD is a greater number of links between trauma-related representations and other representations, but we are not told how, why, or through what mechanisms these differences come to exist between those with and those without PTSD. Processes that are involved may relate to the role played by *inhibitory* representations that ward off stress-related memories.

Person schemas theory is consistent with the view that memory organization and ease of accessibility to trauma-related material are altered in the individual with PTSD. Clearly, strong and multiple links must exist between existing schemas and incoming information to provoke the symptoms experienced by those with PTSD. However, while McNally stresses the *match* between "fear networks" and "input information, internal association, or both" (p. 75), we also emphasize a *mismatch* between schemas and incoming information. For example, with PTSD, mismatches between incoming information (external or internal) and a strong self-schema of the individual as invulnerable lead to repeated activation of trauma-relevant memories as the individual attempts to integrate the two. Mismatches are also involved when the incoming information is misinterpreted as being relevant to a dreaded weak self-schema. When this occurs, the individual is likely to invoke control processes to ward off the dreaded self-schema. As this mechanism indicates, a key feature of the person schemas model is of an active individual who is motivated to resolve these discrepancies.

Person schemas theory also addresses the question of why some people are more susceptible to PTSD than others. Presumably, when an individual experiences a trauma, schemas related to previous traumas are more readily activated. If the individual experienced childhood traumas, or previous adult traumas, he/she would thus be more susceptible to PTSD. An additional influence would be the individual's resilience to withstanding such assaults to the self-concept that is involved when a trauma is experienced. This is why we emphasize control processes, which, of course, may be adaptive or maladaptive.

MEASUREMENT OF SELF-REPRESENTATIONS

Within the framework of the quasi-experimental controlled study, McNally describes four basic methods for measuring dysfunctional cognitive structures and processes. These are (1) exposure to personally traumatic imagery scripts with self report and peripheral nervous system correlates as dependent measures, (2) modified Stroop paradigms with delayed color-naming as the dependent variable, (3) explicit (e.g., free recall, cued recall, recognition tasks) and implicit (e.g., sentence completion) memory tasks, and (4) paradigms designed to test Higgins's self-discrepancy theory with self-report measures and peripheral nervous system correlates as dependent variables. As McNally notes, few of these paradigms have been utilized specifically to test self-representations in individuals with PTSD or other anxiety disorders; however, studies suggest that such research may be fruitful. For example, McNally reports research suggesting that disorder-specific information is processed differently by individuals with a particular disorder than is nondisorder-specific information, and that such information is processed differently by individuals without the disorder. These studies suggest, further, that schema-specific attributes appear to cohere as a self-schema, at least a negative self-schema in those with major depression (Segal & Vella, 1990).

These paradigms may also be useful for testing hypotheses generated by the person schemas model of anxiety disorders. To take PTSD as an example, we conjectured that incoming information may threaten to instantiate a dreaded self-schema of the individual as weak, assaulted, and overwhelmed. We could test this hypothesis by exposing individuals with PTSD to personally threatening information that is ostensibly unrelated to the PTSD-inducing trauma, thus priming the dreaded self-schema. The purpose in choosing a prime that is personally threatening but not outwardly related to the trauma is to test for the influence of a dreaded self-schema that is more general than one specifically related to the topic of the trauma, but is nevertheless cognitively linked to it. We would then present a Stroop task in which the individual is asked to color-name words that were hypothesized to be characteristic of the dreaded schema. One set might refer to general characteristics of the schema (e.g., "weak," "assaulted") and another specifically to the PTSD-inducing trauma (e.g., "bodybag," "Charlie"). We would compare delayed color-naming of these words with sets of control words, for example, neutral words or dreaded components of a schema for a different disorder. If individuals with PTSD exhibit delayed color-naming to trauma-related and weak-self-schema-related words, we would have evidence to support the existence of the weak self-schema and its cognitive link to the trauma. The Stroop test might also be used to test hypotheses about obligatory linkages between desired and dreaded role-relationship models (RRMs). Memory tasks and other methodologies from cognitive science might also be adapted to test person schemas theory.

There are limitations associated with these paradigms, however, one of which is presented by the laboratory setting itself. The analogue studies discussed by McNally may not accurately represent the pattern of an anxiety disorder as it occurs outside the lab. To use the Higgins self-discrepancy paradigm as an example, imagine a social phobic with an "actual/own" attribute of "weak" and an "ideal/own" attribute of "powerful." Following Strauman's (1989) design, if we then ask the individual, "Why is it important for a person to be powerful?" with the goal of tapping an actual/own–ideal/own self-discrepancy, we might generate a pattern of schematic activation that is attenuated and different in form from what is generated when the individual is in a personally significant performance situation. A setting that is more naturalistic, yet also allows for controls and measurement, may facilitate study of anxiety disorders as they naturally occur. One such setting is the psychotherapy session. If the problematic behavior that motivated the individual to seek psychotherapy is reenacted in the consulting room, and if we are able to monitor it closely, we may discover patterns that more controlled experiments do not allow.

Studying individuals in the context of psychotherapy addresses two other limitations posed by traditional laboratory experiments. These are the problems of the temporal patterning of emotional disorders and the effect of multiple variables contributing to a disorder. As an individual regulates access to anxiety-provoking stimuli, whether they come from internal or external sources, and as such stimuli themselves vary in terms of their presence or absence, the individual will experience variations in the extent to which the disorder influences his/her life. Even the most anxious individual is not anxious all the time, but experiences some variability in the activity of the anxiety disorder. Such variations, through time, may offer valuable insights into mental representations involved in the disorder, and they cannot be studied except temporally and individually. The identification and measurement (e.g., by frequency counts) of such patterns may provide persuasive evidence of their presence and underlying organization.

The multiple variable problem involves the notion that the products of anxiety disorders—for example, intrusive thoughts or images, excessive physiological arousal, hypochondriacal alarm at physical sensations, anxious forgetting—may reflect the operation of multiple variables acting in concert. Shifts from desired to dreaded to compromise RRMs, for instance, may be reflected in several variables and only under certain conditions. Such variables may include verbal behavior (e.g., sudden topic shifts, use of particular words or word combinations, occurrence of dysfluencies, stuttering), nonverbal behavior (e.g., gaze aversion or frozen gaze, shoulder shrugs, idiosyncratic gestures), and by patterns of physiological arousal. Patterns characterizing anxiety may only emerge when certain conditions are met, such as when the interpersonal tone between therapist and patient is of a particular quality for the patient. Modeling these patterns may provide a useful means of inferring self-representational activity and may also lead to more controlled experiments in which certain variables are isolated and their effects measured under different conditions.

A third limitation is that individual patterns in the onset of an anxiety experience may go undetected in controlled experiments such as those described by McNally. Hints of these could be found by looking at the data of individuals for whom the aggregate (i.e., group) effect (e.g., delayed color-naming in Stroop paradigms) did *not* occur. These exceptions may not be due to random "error," but to processes of central importance in understanding the role of self-representation in emotional disorders. For example, an individual may employ control (i.e., defensive, regulatory) processes to inhibit the priming of a self-schema and thus circumvent the Stroop interference that is characteristic of the group.

The use of multiple methodologies and attempts to establish convergent validity across them will provide the greatest support for hypotheses about the role of self-representation in anxiety. Other than quasi experiments, these methodologies may include analysis of psychotherapy dialogue, cluster analysis, and experience sampling. In addition, findings based on what occurs in the psychotherapy setting may be more relevant and persuasive to practicing clinicians.

ROLE OF AFFECT IN SELF-REPRESENTATION OF ANXIETY DISORDERS

McNally takes his lead from Lang (1985) and Higgins (1987) in discussing the role of affect and self-representation in PTSD. As he explains, in Lang's bio-informational approach, emotion

> is represented in memory as a network of stimulus, response, and meaning propositions. Information about the context of emotion is embodied in stimulus propositions; information about physiological, motoric, and verbal behavior is embodied in response propositions; and information interpreting the significance of stimulus and response information is embodied in meaning propositions. (p. 75)

For Higgins, negative emotional states arise as a function of discrepancies between self-schemas. In the person schemas approach, we view complex affective states emerging as a function of relational configurations (i.e., RRMs) and in the interrelations of sets of RRMs (Horowitz, 1986).

These views need not be incompatible. Each sees emotion as a function of a network of meaning, motoric, verbal, and physiological activity. One difference is the apparent emphasis of Lang's model on a behavioristic, stimulus-organism-response model. This suggests a view of the organism as a passive recipient of stimuli, to which it responds with emotion. In contrast, the person schemas model assumes a "wishing" individual who initiates action on the world, but inhibits or attenuates the satisfaction of wishes when they are countered by possible fearful scenarios.

CONCLUSION

Taken together, we think Dr. McNally's chapter and our own suggest that fruitful collaboration and, perhaps, theoretical convergence between cognitive and psychodynamic perspectives of the anxiety disorders is possible. Methodological and theoretical hurdles must be passed before this happens, however. Methodologically, a reconciliation must be achieved between the data from controlled laboratory experiments, the psychotherapy hour, and the suffering individual's experience in the world. A research strategy that aims at convergent validity based on studies using multiple methodologies is a promising direction to go toward this end. Primary areas of theoretical divergence pertain to the motivational, regulatory, and developmental processes involved in producing and maintaining an anxiety disorder.

ACKNOWLEDGMENT

Support for this chapter was provided by the Program on Conscious and Unconscious Mental Processes of the John D. and Catherine T. MacArthur Foundation.

REFERENCES

Higgins, E. T. (1987). Self-discrepancy: A theory relating self and affect. *Psychology Review*, *94*, 319–340.

Horowitz, M. J. (1986). *Stress response syndromes* (2nd ed.). New York: Plenum Press.

Lang, P. J. (1985). The cognitive psychophysiology of emotion: Fear and anxiety. In A. H. Tuma & J. D. Maser (Eds.), *Anxiety and the anxiety disorders* (pp. 131–170). Hillsdale, NJ: Lawrence Erlbaum.

Segal, Z. V., & Vella, D. D. (1990). Self-schema in major depression: Replication and extension of a priming methodology. *Cognitive Therapy and Research*, *14*, 161–176.

Strauman, T. J. (1989). Self-discrepancies in clinical depression and social phobia: Cognitive structures that underlie emotional disorders? *Journal of Abnormal Psychology*, *98*, 14–22.

4

Self-representation in Anxious States of Mind: A Comparison of Psychodynamic Models

TRACY D. EELLS
University of Louisville
MARDI J. HOROWITZ
CHARLES H. STINSON
BRAM FRIDHANDLER
University of California, San Francisco

IN FREUD'S (1894/1962) early psychodynamic model, the repression of threatening memories, ideas, and impulses played the most important role in explaining anxious states of mind. In later writings (1923/1961, 1926/1959), the role of psychic structures was emphasized, as well as repression. Since Freud, object relational (e.g., Fairbairn, 1941; Klein, 1948/1975; Jacobson, 1964; Kohut, 1971, 1977, 1984; Sandler & Rosenblatt, 1962; Winnicott, 1953) and interpersonal (Sullivan, 1953; Horney, 1950) models of mind have joined the structural model as important descriptive and explanatory constructs in psychodynamics; an increasingly important component of such models is self-representation. With the advent of these newer models, the explanation of anxious states of mind has undergone revision.

The purpose of this chapter is twofold. First, we follow the theoretical trail connecting current models of anxiety that utilize self-representations, with the earliest models in psychoanalytic thought that do not, but that nevertheless provided the groundwork for the later developments. We begin with Freud's two models and continue with a discussion of Sullivan and Horney, both of whom placed anxiety at the core of their interpersonal theories and also posited mental representations of self as descriptive concepts. Moving on to object relational and self psychology views of anxiety, we next focus on the theories of Klein, Fairbairn, Kernberg, and Kohut. The second purpose is to outline a preliminary "person schemas" theory of anxiety, one that builds on its predecessors in psychodynamic theory and also draws constructs from cognitive science.

FREUD'S TWO THEORIES OF ANXIETY

Freud had two theories of anxiety: an early "toxic" theory, or what we will call the *wine-to-vinegar* theory, and a later *signal anxiety* theory. It is primarily in the second that self-representation plays a role, if only an approximating and adumbrative one.

Wine to Vinegar

Freud's first view of neurotic anxiety—that is, anxiety not resulting from realistic concerns about one's environment—predominated in his thought, at least from 1894 when he first explicitly addressed the topic of anxiety, until the publication of "Inhibitions, Symptoms, and Anxiety" in 1926. Although it took different forms through the years, Freud held to the view that neurotic anxiety was the consequence of transformed sexual drive energy. This is summed up in a footnote to his "Three Essays on the Theory of Sexuality" (1905/1953):

> One of the most important results of psychoanalytic research is this discovery that neurotic anxiety arises out of libido, that it is the product of a transformation of it, and that is thus related to it in the same kind of way as vinegar is to wine. (p. 224)

The wine-to-vinegar formulation initially took a purely physiological form, but this was soon rejected in favor of a predominantly psychical form.

The physical model posited no mental apparatus at all. The view was that anxiety is generated by a physical factor in an individual's sexual life, typically a woman's fear of becoming pregnant, a man's fear "that his device might not succeed" (Freud, 1954, p. 88), and a couple's practice of *coitus interruptus*. Freud summed up the physical theory in the phrase: "Where there is an accumulation of *physical* sexual tension, we find anxiety neurosis" (1954, p. 90). The mechanism Freud suggested is consistent with his lifelong adherence to the tension-reduction model; it assumes the gradual buildup of physical sexual tension, which normally would pass a threshold and become an idea. Anxiety occurs when this transformation does not occur, or occurs insufficiently, and instead the physical tension is transformed into anxiety.

Freud (1894/1962) soon abandoned the physical version of the wine-to-vinegar theory in favor of a psychical version that emphasized ideogenesis and the role of unconscious processes, particularly repression. The principle of conversion of libido to anxiety remained unaltered, but the mechanism became psychic processes. He now proposed that internal or external forces lead to a buildup of libidinal energy; but, instead of a physical conversion to anxiety, Freud assumed that an idea or wish is attached to the libido from the outset, and at a certain point becomes detached from the libido (which, in his view, is identical to affect) and is repressed. The "unattached" energy is then converted into anxiety. Thus, the model posits a sequential set of events: incompatible idea leads to repression, which leads to anxiety. After the publication of "The Ego and the Id" in 1923, Freud attempted to translate the wine-to-vinegar theory into structural terms. The new formulation was that a "person represses libidinal cathexes made by the id via anticathexes put up by the ego and superego, and then in time this combined libido is transformed (converted) into an anxiety dream or a symptom of neurosis" (Rychlak, 1981, p. 89).

Freud became increasingly unhappy with the wine-to-vinegar theory. It posed theoretical difficulties relating to the mechanism by which the libido generated and maintained anxiety. The notion that repression leads to anxiety also created difficulties because it assumes, at least in part, that repression is an intentional act, that an individual generates a "will to forget." An additional problem was the occurrence of "war neuroses" in World War I veterans. Soldiers' repetitive dreams and intrusive images of the battlefield did not seem well explained by the notion of transformed libido. The weight of these problems, and the impetus provided by Rank's (1924/1929) treatise that anxiety is the prime motivator of neurosis, led Freud to formulate his signal anxiety model in 1926.

Signal Anxiety

The signal anxiety theory represents a significant remodeling and partial reversal of Freud's earlier views. The belief that libidinal forces contribute significantly to anxiety was not completely rejected, but played a far less important role in the new theory. Anxiety was no longer simply transformed libido, but was governed by ego processes. Freud (1926/1959) now posited that the ego produces anxiety in response to a threat "with the unmistakable purpose of restricting that distressing experience to a mere indication, a signal" (p. 162). This "signal" then triggers the processes of repression. In this respect the anxiety serves as an "inoculation, submitting [the ego] to a slight attack of the illness in order to escape its full strength"

(p. 162). Freud defined the threat that leads to the ego's issuance of a signal as a "danger-situation" or a "recognized, remembered, expected situation of helplessness" (p. 166).

The specific threat that induces anxiety depends in part on one's developmental level. The developmental sequence Freud posited is the birth experience itself, the loss of a caretaker, the loss of the caretaker's love, castration anxiety in boys, and breaches of moral conduct. What all of these have in common is that they threaten to render the individual helpless. As we show later, our view of anxiety as representing a "taste" of a dreaded role-relationship model is analogous to Freud's formulation of anxiety representing an "inoculation."

Self-representation in Freud's Model of Anxiety

With each advance in Freud's notion of anxiety, a role for self-representation was increasingly approximated, although Freud never actually used the term. Some authors have pointed out, however, that he used the term "ego" in two ways: sometimes to mean a structure that mediates demands of the id and of reality, and sometimes to mean the "self" (Hartmann, 1964; see, e.g., Freud, 1919/1955, p. 209). In the physiological version of the wine-to-vinegar theory, no mental function was invoked. In the psychical version, Freud originally held that an incompatible idea led to anxiety by becoming detached from libido, which, in turn, was transformed into anxiety. No self was posited, but he moved from the physical to the psychic world. In a later version of this theory, he postulated similar processes, but within the framework of separable ego functions and id drives.

With the signal anxiety theory, we have Freud's closest approximation to a concept of self-representation. The ego is now empowered as the "seat of anxiety" (1926/1959, p. 162). Its powers in relation to the id, as originally set forth in "The Ego and the Id," are clarified, and we see that it is not entirely at the mercy of the id, but possesses the capacity to ward off a danger situation by inoculating itself and initiating repression of the feared idea, wish, or impulse that is connected with the danger situation.

An advantage to this later model is that by positing the ego as the seat of anxiety, Freud was able to classify anxiety into a typology that better fit the variety of experiences that generate it. For example, as mentioned, one inadequacy of the wine-to-vinegar theory was that it did not sufficiently account for anxiety related to previous war experience. Similarly, anxiety that seemed to be a healthy and adaptive response to a genuine and immediate threat was not well accounted for. The new model led Freud to classify anxiety as either realistic, neurotic, or moralistic, depending on whether the ego was viewed as in conflict with reality, the id, or the superego. In this manner, internal and external sources of anxiety were incorporated into a single model.

A second advantage of the signal anxiety model is that, as Schafer (1983) noted, it casts the processes of forming anxious states into more cognitive terms. This is indicated by the definition of a danger situation as one that is "recognized, remembered and expected" (p. 97). By viewing anxiety in more cognitive terms, Freud moved closer to self-representations. The notion of a danger situation suggests a reflected-upon self-entity that stands in relation to a threat.

LATER PSYCHODYNAMIC THEORIES OF ANXIETY

Harry Stack Sullivan and Karen Horney focused on anxiety in an interpersonal context but still utilized self-representational language. In contrast, the three subsequent theorists discussed in this section—M. Klein, Fairbairn, and Kernberg—gave anxiety a less central role in their theories but placed great emphasis on internal mental representations. The final theorist discussed here, Kohut, emphasized both anxiety and internal mental representations.

Harry Stack Sullivan

Perhaps more than any other theorist, Sullivan (1953) placed anxiety at the core of his theory of personality and psychopathology. Although his focus was primarily on the dynamics, or process, of interpersonal exchange, self-structures also play a role in his theory. According to Sullivan, most of our experience is organized and regulated by the "self system." The purpose of the self-system is to minimize anxiety and maintain a feeling of security, even at the cost of distorting one's view of self and other. The self-system includes structures that Sullivan termed the "good me," the "bad me," and the "not me." These arise out of an individual's childhood interpersonal experiences and reflect the first form of mental differentiation, that between anxious and nonanxious states.

The "good me" represents an internalization of the child's experiences with the "good mother," that is, all experiences with a caretaker that promote non-anxious states of mind such as well-being, security, self-confidence, and calm. It is reflected in the individual's conscious self-concept of pleasing self-attributes.

Conversely, the "bad me" is an organization of experiences that are associated with the "bad mother." These reflect behaviors of the child that make the caretaker increasingly tense, which the child is attuned to, and which, in turn, give rise to anxious states of mind in the child. The "bad me" reflects those aspects of an individual's self-concept that he/she is aware of but disapproves and tries to disguise or conceal.

Whereas the "good me" and "bad me" form a large part of conscious experience, the "not me" is only rarely experienced, and then in a relatively primitive and unintegrated manner. It is originally associated with states of intense anxiety in the mother, which overwhelm the infant and seem to have no connection to cause and effect. In later life, the "not me" is reflected in the "uncanny emotions" of dread, wonder, terror, loathing, disorientation, and awe. The most common example of a "not me" experience is that of awaking in a disoriented state from a nightmare.

As mentioned earlier, Sullivan asserted that each of these self-structures arises out of interpersonal experience. In his view, the infant is closely attuned to the experiences of its caretakers; this is particularly crucial in the experience of anxiety, and the connection is a direct one: "the tension of anxiety, when present in the mothering one, induces anxiety in the infant" (Sullivan, 1953, p. 259). Through the process of "prehension," a rudimentary form of perception, the child responds sensitively to subtle signs exhibited by the caretaker—for example, a frown, postural tension, or a sudden movement—and adjusts its behavior so as to avoid eliciting anxiety-arousing behavior in its caretakers. These are the beginnings of what later develop into more complex "security operations."

Like the self-system, security operations involve configurations of self-structures. The development of "me–you patterns" is a primary means by which an individual redirects her/his experience away from feared situations. For example, an individual who fears authority figures may develop an inflated or exaggerated sense of self as powerful in relation to others, who are viewed as potentially critical and demanding. Competent observers may agree, however, that the individual is avoiding the anxiety-arousing view of self as weak and ineffectual, and that the authority figure involved actually behaves benignly. Me–you patterns anticipate what we call role-relationship models.

Sullivan's view of anxiety can be seen as an extension and redirection of Freud's signal theory. Anxiety is the consequence of anticipating a more dreaded, or "uncanny" state. It is "a sign of *foreseen* lowering of self-esteem" (1954, p. 207) or an "anticipated unfavorable appraisal of one's current activity by someone whose opinion is significant" (1953, p. 113). Thus, it is not so much an internal danger situation that provides the impetus for anxiety, but an external, interpersonally significant, feared situation that is anticipated. Although he made use of terms suggesting mental structures, he did so cautiously because he viewed personality primarily as a pattern of activity rather than a structural organization. This is illustrated by his choice of the terms "dynamism" and "self system" rather than "entity" and "self structure." Sullivan's use of structural entities are better viewed as tools to describe mental experience than as concepts to explain it.

Karen Horney

Like Sullivan, Horney (1937, 1945, 1950) focused on anxiety and an individual's attempts to minimize it as the key to understanding personality development, particularly neurotic development. As Horney developed her theory, she gave increasing importance to the concept of self. In her early writings, she focused on "neurotic trends" (1937); later she concentrated on interpersonal patterns that characterize neurotic interaction (1945). It was not until the final formulation of her theory (1950) that the self came to the forefront of her thinking. Self-representation took the form of three entities: the "real self," the "glorified self," and the "despised 'real' self." The "real self" is "that central inner force, common to all human beings and yet unique in each, which is the deep source of growth" (1950, p. 17). The "glorified self" and "despised 'real' self" are consequences of the individual's efforts to manage anxiety; along with the "real self," they constitute what Horney called "the pride system."

In Horney's system, "basic anxiety" arises when a child is caught between feelings of hostility and dependency toward inconsistent, neglectful, or otherwise abusive caretakers. The unstable "solution" of repressing the hostility leads to the feeling of basic anxiety, directed not just toward the caretaker but toward the world at large. She defined it as "the feeling of being isolated and helpless in a world conceived of as potentially hostile" (1950, p. 18). Through imagination, the individual attempts to minimize basic anxiety and its crippling loss of self-esteem by forming an idealized or "glorified" self-image. Eventually, he/she identifies with the "glorified self" and seeks to actualize it. The energy previously directed toward the actualization of the "real self" becomes redirected toward the "glorified self." This goal is impossible, however, because the "glorified self" is an anxiety-induced, rigid, perfectionistic, and unrealistic construction of the individual. From the perspective of the "glorified self," the "real self" is distorted and hated by the individual. Horney calls the self that develops from these distortions the "despised 'real' self."

Like Sullivan, Horney was primarily a clinical pragmatist; theory construction was secondary. She never articulated the composition of the various "selves" she proposed, and seems to have used them principally as tools for formulating her thoughts rather than proposing them as actual mental structures.

Melanie Klein

The loci of anxiety in Klein's (1948/1975) model are "bad" internalized objects, or introjects, which may be "part" (e.g., the mother's breast) or "whole" (i.e., person) representations. Such objects are created primarily through the workings of the life and death instincts, and secondarily as the consequence of caretaker behavior. The mind "splits" (a term introduced by Klein) the object of these instinctual wishes into "good" and "bad" components—the "good" representing gratifying experiences with the external object and the projection onto it of the life instinct, the "bad" reflecting frustrating experiences and the projection onto it of destructive impulses originating in the death instinct. "Persecutory anxiety" arises as a result of conflict between the ego—which all infants are endowed with at birth, according to Klein—and the "bad" object, which seeks to destroy the ego. "Depressive anxiety" arises when an individual realizes she/he has both feelings of destructiveness and love toward a single object.

Klein's theory of anxiety incorporated Freud's wine-to-vinegar and signal anxiety theories. As in Freud's earlier model, anxiety is based in instinctual forces, although for Klein, the death instinct takes precedence over the life instinct. Klein altered Freud's theory by positing introjected objects that "contain" the aggressive impulses. It is the "bad" objects, rather than the ego, that appear primarily responsible for anxiety. She also differed from Freud by placing a greater emphasis on the role of projection. Like Freud, Klein did not posit the construct of a self-representation, but used the term "ego" in ways that suggest a self.

W. R. D. Fairbairn

Fairbairn agreed with Klein that the primary form of anxiety is the threat of ego dissolution, although he emphasized this in an interpersonal context (Rinsley, 1979). In outlining his model, he made considerable use of her concepts of internalized objects and splitting, but applied them in a different framework. Unlike Klein, Fairbairn categorically rejected Freud's instinct model of motivation and replaced it with a motivational system based entirely on object relations. He asserted that libido is primarily object seeking, not pleasure seeking—that is, there is no fundamental need for instinctual release, but only for human contact. Fairbairn also disagreed with Klein by claiming that "bad" objects are entirely compensatory, that there would be no motivation to construct internal objects if the ideal amount of contact were provided to an infant. In Fairbairn's system, there is no death instinct to provide such motivation.

According to Fairbairn, anxiety, and indeed all psychopathology, whether neurotic or psychotic, can be traced to problems of infantile dependence. The basic conflict is between a regressive wish to remain completely dependent upon others and a progressive wish to be maturely dependent on the other. As Eagle and Wolitzky (1988) explained, acquiescing to the regressive wish

> carries the threats of engulfment and loss of identity. . . . On the other hand, pursuing the progressive urge toward separation and renunciation of infantile

dependence generates anxiety over feeling isolated, alone, and unsupported. One, then, is impelled to retreat back to the relative safety of home base.... This step, however, while it reduces the immediate intense anxiety, does not constitute a stable solution. For, after the immediate relief, the individual will often begin to feel imprisoned and engulfed and will attempt another foray to the outside world, thereby beginning the process all over again. (p. 262)

As suggested by his object relations approach to motivation, self and other representations play a major role in Fairbairn's view of anxiety. Without going into the complex details of his theory, we will comment only that he made great use of the splitting defense to ward off anxious or dreaded states of mind, that he agreed with Freud that the ego is the seat of anxiety, and that he differed with Freud in emphasizing relationships between the split-off aspects of the ego and corresponding internalized objects, rather than instinctual forces, as the primary source of anxiety. In sum, Fairbairn's theory marked a significant shift toward a self-representational view of anxiety.

Otto Kernberg

Kernberg's model of personality, including his thoughts about anxiety, is similar in key ways to Fairbairn's, but also owes much to the work of Hartmann (1964) and Jacobson (1964). As a number of writers have pointed out (e.g., Greenberg & Mitchell, 1983; Klein & Tribich, 1981), Kernberg speaks the language of Freud's instinct model, but reorganizes it in significant ways toward a more self and object relational perspective. For example, Kernberg's theory of affect retains the notions of libidinal and aggressive drives, but conceptualizes drives as built up from internalized self and other representations, thus effectively shifting objects to a primary, explanatory role, and instincts to a subordinate role. In Kernberg's (1984) words,

> Libido and aggression in turn become hierarchically supraordinate motivational systems which express themselves in a multitude of differentiated affect dispositions under different circumstances. Affects, in short, are the building blocks, or constituents, of drives; affects eventually acquire a signal function for the activation of drives. (p. 236)

An additional contribution of Kernberg's is his restriction of the term "object" to refer only to persons. "Part" objects, which play a major role in the models of Klein and Fairbairn, have no place in Kernberg's system (Greenberg & Mitchell, 1983, p. 328). Instead, Kernberg substitutes diverse and contradictory ego states and objects.

Kernberg based his theory, including his thoughts about anxiety, on his observation of characteristic transference reactions in his severely disturbed patients. These reactions include splitting, projection, projective identification, primitive idealization, and devaluation. Particularly when they emerge intensely and early in psychotherapy, Kernberg sees these reactions as indicators of characteristic relationship patterns that have become internalized. When Kernberg pointed out these contradictory ego states to patients, they became highly vulnerable to anxiety states. In his view, this reflected conflict associated with these internalized relationship patterns, or "relational configurations."

Relational configurations have three components: a self-representation, an object representation, and an affective tone linking the two. An individual is highly susceptible to anxiety when such configurations are highly charged affectively and are poorly differentiated. For example, an individual may have a configuration made up of a self-representation of him/herself as weak and vulnerable, an object representation characterized by ruthless domination, and a violent affective tone. When this configuration is activated in psychotherapy, the patient may become highly anxious and resort to one of the characteristic transference reactions in an attempt to reduce anxiety.

Kernberg hypothesizes that these psychic structures occur prior to the development of an integrated ego, which is capable of repression and other higher level defense mechanisms that characterize well-adapted individuals. As we will point out in more detail later, Kernberg's concept of relational configurations contributed to our notion of role-relationship model configurations.

Heinz Kohut

Kohut (1971, 1977, 1984) accepted Freud's theory of signal anxiety, but added to it a description of "disintegration anxiety," which he originally theorized is experienced by individuals with a narcissistic personality organization, but later extended to people generally. Whereas signal anxiety implies a coherent mental representation of the self that fears a specific danger situation, disintegration anxiety reflects a threat to the self-organization. Kohut models this type of anxiety in self and other representational terms, specifically, the "archaic grandiose self" and the "idealized parent imago." Developmentally, these are postulated to develop very early in childhood, prior to the setting in place of the Freudian tripartite structures.

Inevitably, shortcomings in parental child-rearing behavior disturb a child's "primary narcissism," or sense of perfection. To compensate for this loss, the child develops an unrealistic, grandiose, and exhibitionistic mental representation of him/herself, the "archaic grandiose self." He/she also develops a mental representation of the parents, the "idealized parent imago," to make up for their perceived shortcomings. These mental representations are termed "selfobjects" by Kohut. They are "archaic" because they develop early in life and are not experienced as separate and independent from the self. Mature forms of selfobjects may also develop in life, but for the narcissistic individual they are typically disturbed by the influence of corresponding archaic forms. In the normal course of development, these mental representations coalesce into the ego and superego, respectively, and become part of the mature adult personality. Such a person would not be highly vulnerable to disintegration anxiety.

When the parents consistently fail to provide adequately for the child's primary narcissistic needs, the archaic grandiose self and the idealized parent imago may become hardened and may not integrate into the developmentally subsequent structures. They continue to exist in a substratum of the individual's psychic organization and cause disturbances and distortions in the individual's view of self and relationships with others. The person fails to experience others as separate individuals with their own minds and feelings, but instead projects his/her own inadequately differentiated mental representations of self and others onto those on whom he/she is dependent. The individual becomes highly vulnerable to rapid and extreme fluctuations of self-esteem, and often experiences lassitude, emptiness, work inhibition, and a vague sense of discomfort. Kohut (1971, p. 17) explains these experiences as resulting from the ego's walling off of the unrealistic, and at times godlike, claims of the archaic grandiose self, and powerful longings for infusions of self-esteem from others. To compensate for these deficiencies and needs, the person attempts to dominate and control important others. This is one way of assuring that a ready supply of self-esteem remains available, the individual not possessing the psychic structure to obtain this in mature, reciprocal, adult relationships. In his later writings, Kohut (1984) made clear his belief that fulfilling interpersonal relationships are essential to successfully warding off anxiety.

Kohut's model of anxiety differs from Freud's in its emphasis on structural rather than drive features. For Freud, drive strength plays an important role: Either it is so strong that it is converted into anxiety, or it overwhelms the ego. In Kohut's model—as in Fairbairn's—it is psychic structures themselves, in the form of self and other representations, that play the primary role in the experience of anxiety. This is clearly the case for disintegration anxiety, but even in signal anxiety, Kohut (1977) holds to the view that the primary threat is to the cohesiveness of mental structure.

PERSON SCHEMAS AND ANXIETY

Our model of maladaptively anxious states of mind is an extension and elaboration of the work just reviewed. It reflects a synthesis of these views and an attempt to utilize knowledge from cognitive science. In this section, we briefly define terms, present our model, suggest how it may be used to model a variety of specific anxiety disorders, and, finally, address research issues.

Terminology and General View of Theory

The notion of multiple schemas of self and other is central to our model. These exist as *person schemas* (either of self or other) and as *role-relationship models* (RRMs). Horowitz (1991) defines a person schema as an enduring codification and structure of meaning that is not experienced, but can, when activated, influence the formation of a self-concept. Person schemas may be combined into a more complex schema of self-in-relationship-with-other, or what we call a role-relationship model. An RRM may be defined as an enduring template that can, when activated, affect the formation of a role-relationship concept, as well as serve in organizing the actual patterns of interpersonal transaction (Horowitz, 1991). In an RRM, self and other are linked in scriptlike sequences comprising interactional patterns that influence an individual's relationships with others. They involve wishes, expectations, and appraisals one person has toward another. For example, an individual may wish love from another, but expect rejection and thus withdraw.

A role-relationship-model configuration (RRMC) incorporates a repertoire of RRMs to depict a set of maladaptive interpersonal behavior patterns or a set of wishes, fears, and defenses in relation to a specific theme. Strong wishes can be represented in a *desired* RRM, fears in a *dreaded* RRM, and the derivatives of defensive operations as either *adaptive compromise* or *problematic compromise* RRMs. Both compromise RRMs represent the relative attenuation of affect; that is, when active as organizers of information, they are unlikely to lead either to highly enjoyable states of mind or to intensely anxious ones. An adaptive RRM represents a compromise that has no maladaptive signs or symptoms; it enables an individual to achieve a portion of what was wished for, but a limited portion. A problematic RRM comprises negative affects or maladaptive traits, but at a more manageable level of intensity than a dreaded RRM. RRMCs may also depict supraordinate sets of strong and weak self-schemas.

To understand an RRMC, it is useful to begin with the desired RRM. Enactment of a desired RRM may be frustrated by the threat of entry into a state of mind organized by a dreaded RRM. The individual may then seek a compromise or attenuated "solution" to the desired wish and thus activate an adaptive compromise RRM. Although this provides partial gratification of a wish, it may not be enough; thus, the individual may express his/her wish more strongly, moving him/her into a problematic RRM, one that produces symptoms, but not disabling ones. Once the individual is in a state of compromise—adaptive or problematic—he/she may have enough restoration of self-esteem to once again attempt to activate the desired RRM. Thus, an RRMC may represent an "obligatory" linkage between RRMs in the sense that a mental state organized by one RRM, such as a desired RRM, can trigger a subsequent state organized by another RRM, such as a dreaded RRM. The pattern just explained is only one of several that may describe how an individual manages a frustrated wish.

The mechanism of change in this model is informationally and affectively driven; it does not depend upon Freudian instinct theory. We think that parallel distributed processing (PDP) theory offers an attractive account of the mental architecture that may underlie the larger order schematic processing just described. The PDP model presupposes large numbers of relatively simple and slow processing units that, like neurons, assume inhibitory or excitatory states. Large-scale networks of such units exhibit distinctive, dynamic, activation patterns. Cognitive processes such as remembering, planning, sensing, perceiving, problem solving, and emoting may reflect different activation patterns. These activation patterns may also give rise to complex, emergent information structures such as person schemas and RRMs. For a fuller discussion of the relation between PDP models of cognition and person schemas, see Stinson and Palmer (1991).

Person Schematic Modeling of Anxiety

How can the person schemas model be applied specifically to anxiety? In general, we propose that anxiety arises out of a mismatch between schemas and incoming information. This can occur in two distinct ways: anxiety as anticipation of a dreaded schema, and anxiety as a brief "taste," or instantiation, of a dreaded schema.

Anxiety as Anticipation of a Dreaded RRM

Earlier, we stated that one link in an obligatory linkage between RRMs may be movement from a desired RRM to a compromise RRM due to a threat posed by entering a dreaded state of mind. For example, an individual may have a strong desire to be loved and appreciated by a powerful other who can provide guidance, but because this RRM is linked to a dreaded RRM in which the powerful other becomes exploitive, the individual shifts to the compromise of keeping the powerful other distantly present, or of passively resisting his/her efforts to provide guidance. This can happen when incoming information—that is, genuinely benign behavior by the helping other—is misinterpreted by the individual as threatening.

When mental processes such as these occur in the course of an individual's interactions in the interpersonal world, the threat must register quickly if the dreaded outcome is to be avoided. This registration is what we experience as anxiety. It is a "felt process," in Bowlby's (1969) terms, that is, a mental process that reaches awareness. It may occur over an extended period of time as intrusive phenomena (e.g., distorted ideas about the intent of the powerful other), accompanied by physiological arousal, or in an extremely brief period of time, which quickly leads to a restabilization of mood. Intensification of control processes to ward off the onset of a dreaded schema may lead to omissive phenomena, such as an individual failing to recall the threatening person's name. In any case, the specific content of the dreaded RRM does not come clearly into awareness.

The "dreaded outcomes" that we propose are organized by dreaded RRMs and are not typically events in the external world, or at least not merely events in the external world. When only external events are at issue—for example, when we are in physical danger—we are more likely to call our feeling "fear." By and large, the dreaded outcomes in anxiety are mental representations and states of mind experienced as unpleasant and out of control. More specifically, anxiety is the experienced anticipation that a dreaded RRM (or the dreaded part of another RRM) will become the working model of the current situation. In this sense, the dreaded RRM is a mismatch to the incoming information, which may be innocuous to most individuals. Note the similarity of this view of anxiety to Freud's signal anxiety model.

PDP theory provides a model of the above relationships among RRMs. The associations among working models—that is, the currently instantiated RRM and others, such as dreaded RRMs—can be understood as the tendency for a certain activation state (the instantiation of an RRM), to be followed by the activation of a specific alternate state (instantiation of another RRM). Just as RRM activation states can rapidly—and at times inaccurately—fill in missing details, so too can activation states shift in meaningful, chained sequences that can be viewed as purposive. The sequence leading to a dreaded RRM is a consequence of this higher order association. Personal experience of these transitions, and perhaps an inner monitoring of the approaching changes (Pribram, 1970), leads to the anticipation, which is felt as anxiety.

Anxiety as a Brief Instantiation of a Dreaded RRM

Anxiety may also be generated when a mismatch between incoming information and schemas leads to the brief "taste," or instantiation, of a dreaded RRM. From this perspective, RRMs not only provoke feelings such as anxiety, they also *are* the mental representations of feelings or emotions. Emotions are thus viewed as complex structures involving views of self and other, interactions among them, and interpretations of sensations of arousal. While the RRM *is* the affect, in the sense just described, the critical locus is the script elements that link person schemas, implying an interpersonal context for emotion. (This is similar to Kernberg's focus on affective tone as the linking element in relational configurations.) This view of emotion helps explain their complexity, including the important influence that situation and context have upon them.

This second type of anxiety can be illustrated by a patient who had recently lost her husband, whom she loved, in a sudden death and who soon fell in love with another man, whom she viewed as more exciting and charismatic than her husband. The woman became suddenly anxious on the rare occasions that she allowed herself to think that she might love the new man more than her deceased husband. This experience might be explained by the brief instantiation of an RRM in which she sees herself as an unfaithful wife who humiliates her dependable but unexciting husband. See Horowitz, Fridhandler, and Stinson (1991) for further elaboration of this view of emotion.

Application to Specific Anxiety Disorders

Our person schematic theory of anxiety can be used to model specific anxiety disorders. We will illustrate this with Social Phobia, Post-traumatic Stress Disorder, and Generalized Anxiety Disorder.

Social Phobia

In Social Phobia, social situations threaten to instantiate a dreaded scenario of humiliation. This condition is particularly intractable when there are obligatory links from a desired RRM to a dreaded RRM and thence to compromise RRMs. For example, some social phobics see themselves as secretly superior to the people before whom they act submissively. This suggests a link between a compromise RRM of being a peer among equals, and a desired RRM of dominating and triumphing over others. This, in turn, may be linked to a dreaded RRM in which the self is vindictively shamed by those over whom the individual has secretly triumphed, but who now appear powerful and threatening.

Thus, for example, when a social phobic is about to engage in a performance before observers, the individual may secretly feel superior and desire recognition and acclaim but may be so incapacitated by anticipatory anxiety as a consequence of the dreaded humiliation scenario, that a poor performance is intentionally given. This behavior, and face-saving claims such as "I wasn't really trying," "I didn't care," or "I could have performed well if I had really wanted to" reflect the individual's entry into a state organized by a compromise RRM. The act of sabotage has the effect of bringing under control what otherwise seemed to be an uncontrollable situation. It thus restores at least a modicum of self-esteem, but eliminates the possibility of achieving the desired goal of shining before others. Note that the audience's reaction may, in fact, have been receptive and supportive, as reflected by applause or a warm introduction. Were this the case, the social phobic's responses would reflect a mismatch between enduring schemas, in which derision is expected, and incoming information. Both the anticipatory and brief instantiation models of anxiety can be applied in this example. Anxiety may be seen as the anticipation of dreaded representations and also as brief experiences of humiliation—that is, brief instantiations of the dreaded RRMs.

Post-traumatic Stress Disorder

Individuals with Post-traumatic Stress Disorder (PTSD) have experienced unusually threatening or damaging events that are vividly encoded into memory, but are not integrated into the individual's prior, enduring schema of the self as invulnerable. When the traumatic experiences are not integrated into such a schema, they are subject to repeated activation into conscious representation, as incoming information is misinterpreted to be relevant to the traumatic experiences. Incoming information may also threaten to instantiate a dreaded RRM in which the self is weak, assaulted, and overwhelmed, or in which others who are vital to the self are harmed or killed, and the self, in turn, feels guilty for having survived. To avoid this dreaded RRM and the concomitant anxiety, the individual may enter compromise states of denial, depersonalization, restricted affect, or hypervigilance. As with social phobia, the anticipatory and the brief instantiation model of anxiety may be applied here. The person schemas model of PTSD is described in more detail elsewhere (Horowitz, 1986, 1988).

Generalized Anxiety Disorder

In Generalized Anxiety Disorder (GAD), anxiety is present much of the time. The individual is virtually always in a state of apprehension and hypervigilance, ruminating or worrying that some unspecified foreboding event may harm him/her or others. In addition, the individual's autonomic nervous system is overaroused and he/she is motorically tense.

In person schematic terms, the individual with GAD can be viewed as unable to escape the dreaded contents of RRMs. This may reflect one or a combination of two "internal situations": either the inability to achieve a stable state in which a dreaded RRM is successfully warded off and a compromise state is entered, which does not have anxiety as a feature, or the inability to avoid a compromise or desired RRM, which itself contains dreaded components.

Consider a clerical worker experiencing virtually constant anxiety in the office. Such an individual may have a dreaded RRM in which the self is viewed as incompetent, blundering, and stupid, faced with punishing mentors who may fire him/her for the slightest indiscretion. The anxiety persists because the person is unable to successfully ward off this dreaded scenario, experiencing, instead, multiple instantiations of it. When he/she does ward off the dreaded RRM, however, it may be through entering a state organized by a compromise RRM that contains a dreaded component. For example, the individual withdraws from others, working silently at his/her desk and avoiding all social chit-chat. This alleviates the intense anxiety mobilized by the dreaded RRM, but contains a component in which the individual anticipates harsh judgments of coworkers who may view him/her as cold, aloof, strange, and "not a team player." This may trigger the anxiety anew and cast the individual back into the more anxious state organized by the dreaded RRM.

The brief instantiation model of anxiety seems more descriptive of GAD, although the anticipatory model is also relevant. The former is reflected in the individual's experience of multiple instantiations of the dreaded RRM, the latter to the extent that the individual withdraws from others to avoid the more intense anxiety organized by the dreaded RRM.

Research Issues

The person schemas approach to anxiety is amenable to empirical research. A key issue is achieving reliability in determining RRMs and RRMCs for particular cases. Results from the one reliability study that has been conducted on the RRMC method of case formulation (Horowitz & Eells, in press) have been encouraging. The method, based on the theory advanced earlier in this chapter, involves listing roles, characteristics, and traits of the self and others; these are then linked according to wish–fear dilemmas and assembled into RRMCs (Horowitz et al., 1991). Horowitz and Eells had clinical judges rate the goodness-of-fit between a set of RRMCs and videotaped psychotherapy sessions. The judges were able to match the "correct" RRMC to the patient in every case and achieved high levels of agreement on the ratings. Although these patients suffered from grief disorders, similar results would likely be obtained with patients suffering from anxiety disorders.

A more detailed method of achieving reliability is currently under development by the first two authors of this chapter, and others. It involves elaborating, condensing, and paraphrasing psychotherapy dialogue. This is done in a sequence of steps that eventually leads to a set of RRMs or RRMCs for a particular case. One advantage of this method is that it allows the investigator to trace all inferences contained in an RRMC to the dialogue upon which it is based.

Validity is also a key issue in research on person schemas theory. Evidence for convergent validity of clinical inferences was obtained by Horowitz, Luborsky, and Popp (1991). These researchers compared two case formulations for a social phobic. One was developed according to the RRMC method and the other according to the Core Conflictual Relationship Theme (CCRT) (Luborsky & Crits-Christoph, 1990) approach. Qualitative and quantitative analyses showed considerable overlap in the formulations. The average inter-rater reliability coefficient for comparing the formulations was .88.

Further support for a multiple self-representational view of anxiety is provided by Tunis, Fridhandler, and Horowitz (1990). These researchers had a social phobic rate a set of self-generated descriptors in the context of nine views of herself (e.g., actual self, undesired self, self with husband, self at center of attention.) Hierarchical cluster analysis, validated by the INTREX short form (Benjamin, 1988), suggested that this subject had four key self-schemas. These selves may be interpreted as corresponding to an obligatory script involving desired, dreaded, adaptive compromise, and dreaded compromise RRMs. Similar results in cases of grief disorder were found by Merluzzi (1991) and Eells (1992).

Each of the validity studies just cited utilized single-subject methodologies. For at least four reasons, this may be an important avenue for empirical research about self-representations and emotional disorders.

1. Many anxiety disorders are modeled in a developmental framework. The processes involved in developing an emotional disorder may be such that summing and averaging them across subjects, as is typically done in group studies, distorts the shape and meaningful variability of the processes. In the context of learning theory, for example, Sidman (1952) demonstrated that the shape of learning curves based on group data is usually different from that based on individuals.

2. The content and perhaps the form of schematic representations in anxiety and other emotional disorders are unique for each individual. By aggregating across individuals, the findings may apply to the "average" individual, but not to any specific individual in the study.

3. Self-representation in emotional disorders may be reflected in multiple variables that interact in complex ways. These variables include nonverbal signs of defensiveness (e.g., eye gaze, posture, facial expression), speech patterns (e.g., dysfluencies, topic shifts, idiosyncratic vocabulary, discourse markers), physiological measures, and sensitivity to the interpersonal context of a situation. Modeling the interaction of these variables can only be done in single-subject research.

4. Group methodologies that base inferences on the results of statistical hypothesis testing have many epistemological limitations. This is particularly the case in "soft" psychology, as argued, for example, by Bakan (1967) and Meehl (1978, 1986). These limitations make drawing inferences about individual psychological function extremely problematic (Thorngate, 1986; Valsiner, 1986). A research strategy of sequential single-case studies may provide insights precluded by the limitations of group studies (Russell & Trull, 1986). Conducting multiple single-subject studies allows us to

stand on firmer ground when making cause-and-effect inferences and when generalizing to others. The importance of assessing individual schematic representations, even if not in the context of a single-subject study, has been noted by Fiske and Linville (1980), Higgins (1987), and Kihlstrom and Cunningham (1991).

COMPARISON OF MODELS

In this section, we highlight salient similarities and differences in the models of anxiety discussed in this chapter. Note, first, that all but Freud's wine-to-vinegar theory involve some mental representation of self providing the conditions for anxiety. Second, the role of self-representation becomes more explicit as Freud's signal anxiety model is built upon by others. Third, most theories posit multiple self-representations, not a single, monolithic self-representation. Fourth, the notion of anticipatory anxiety is common to many models. This is explicit in Freud's signal anxiety model, in Sullivan, Fairbairn, and Kohut, and in the person schemas model.

A final similarity is that, just as the role of self-representations become more explicit in later models, so too does the role of representations of others. The importance of how others influence anxious as well as nonanxious states is illustrated by Fairbairn's rejection of Freud's instinct theory as a primary motivation, in favor of his theory that the primary human drive is human relationships. Sullivan's me–you patterns, Kernberg's relational configurations, and our RRMs all illustrate the increased role given to introjections of interpersonal experiences. Note, however, that while me–you patterns and RRMs have in common a model of self-in-relation-to-other, the former is used entirely for defensive purposes, whereas the latter can represent adaptive relationships as well. Relational configurations and RRMs are very similar, although Kernberg emphasizes affective tone and we emphasize affect as well as a cognitive component in the form of a schematized script.

The theories differ in the mechanism of anxiety. Freud's signal anxiety theory posits the ego as both emitting and receiving anxiety to ward off a danger situation. In Sullivan's theory, an interpersonal context—specifically, the anticipated unfavorable appraisal by a significant other—produces anxiety. For Horney, anxiety is triggered in the context of an individual's attempts to actualize an idealized self. In the theories of Klein and Fairbairn, bad objects threaten ego integration, which, in turn, precipitates anxiety. Kernberg's model posits certain internalized relationship configurations that leave one vulnerable to anxiety states. In Kohut's model, disintegration anxiety occurs when an individual's selfobjects fail to supply self-esteem needs adequately. Finally, the person schemas model posits anxiety as the consequence of anticipated or briefly experienced RRMs.

A further difference among the models relates to risks posed to the ego, or self. In Freud's signal model the ego is viewed as intact, but subject to being rendered helpless. The models of Klein, Fairbairn, Kernberg, and Kohut give ego, or self-dissolution, a more prominent role in anxiety. (One explanation may be their focus on more severe personality disorders than those focused on by Freud.) The person schemas model posits a set of self-states represented in RRMs, some of which are far more threatening and destructive than others. A dreaded RRM may involve potential dissolution of self.

A final difference has to do with the availability to awareness of a self-representation. Sullivan, Horney, and Kernberg appear to suggest that the self-structures in their models are available to consciousness. Sullivan's good-me, bad-me, and not-me are all part of an individual's self-concept, although the not-me is the least well-integrated of the three. Similarly, Horney's glorified self and despised real self reflect an individual's self-concept; reidentification with the real self becomes the primary goal of psychotherapy. Kernberg also postulates that the self-representations are available to the subjective awareness of the individual. In contrast to Sullivan, Horney, and Kernberg, we view self and other representations as unconscious organizers of subjective experience, but not directly experienced themselves.

CONCLUSIONS

In this chapter, we have described the role that self and other representations have played in psychodynamic models of anxiety states and have tried to show the links between our person schemas model of anxiety and earlier models. Although self-representation has played a more central theoretical role in psychodynamic models over time, few of the theories described have been subjected to formal scientific investigation. Such scrutiny would enable one to assess empirically the relative advantages and disadvantages of the models, and to evaluate what one gains, if anything, by positing self-representation as a key to understanding anxiety. New methods that are adequate to clinical data and the demands of science are required.

ACKNOWLEDGMENT

This research is supported by the Program on Conscious and Unconscious Mental Processes of the John D. and Catherine T. MacArthur Foundation.

REFERENCES

Bakan, D. (1967). *On method: Toward a reconstruction of psychological investigation*. San Francisco: Jossey-Bass.

Benjamin, L. (1988). *SASB short form user's manual*. Salt Lake City, UT: INTREX Interpersonal Institute.

Bowlby, J. (1969). *Attachment and loss: Vol. 1. Attachment*. New York: Basic Books.

Eagle, M., & Wolitzky, D. L. (1988). Psychodynamics. In C. G. Last & Michel Hersen (Eds.), *Handbook of anxiety disorders* (pp. 251–277). Elmsford, NY: Pergamon Press.

Eells, T. D. (1992). *Role reversal: A convergence of clinical and quantitative evidence*. Unpublished manuscript.

Fairbairn, W. R. D. (1941). A revised psychopathology of the psychoses and psychoneuroses. *International Journal of Psycho-Analysis, 22*, 250–279.

Fiske, S. T., & Linville, P. W. (1980). What does the schema concept buy us? *Personality and Social Psychology Bulletin, 6*, 543–557.

Freud, S. (1953). Three essays on the theory of sexuality. In J. Strachey (Ed. and Trans.), *The standard edition of the complete psychological works of Sigmund Freud* (Vol. 7, pp. 125–245). London: Hogarth Press. (Original work published 1905)

Freud, S. (1954). *The origins of psycho-analysis: Letters to Wilhelm Fliess, drafts and notes: 1887–1902*. New York: Basic Books.

Freud, S. (1955). Psychoanalysis and the war neuroses: An introduction. In J. Strachey (Ed. and Trans.), *The standard edition of the complete psychological works of Sigmund Freud* (Vol. 17, pp. 205–215). London: Hogarth Press. (Original work published 1919)

Freud, S. (1959). Inhibitions, symptoms, and anxiety. In J. Strachey (Ed. and Trans.), *The standard edition of the complete psychological works of Sigmund Freud* (Vol. 20, pp. 87–174). London: Hogarth Press. (Original work pubished 1926)

Freud, S. (1961). The ego and the id. In J. Strachey (Ed. and Trans.), *The standard edition of the complete psychological works of Sigmund Freud* (Vol 19, pp. 3–66). London: Hogarth Press. (Original work published 1923)

Freud, S. (1962). The neuro-psychoses of defence. In J. Strachey (Ed. and Trans.), *The standard edition of the complete psychological works of Sigmund Freud* (Vol. 3, pp 45–61). London: Hogarth Press. (Original work published 1894)

Greenberg, J. R., & Mitchell, S. A. (1983). *Object relations in psychoanalytic theory*. Cambridge, MA: Harvard University Press.

Hartmann, H. (1964). *Essays on ego psychology: Selected problems in psychoanalytic theory*. New York: International Universities Press.

Higgins, E. T. (1987). Self-discrepancy: A theory relating self and affect. *Psychological Review, 94*, 319–340.

Horney, K. (1937). *The neurotic personality of our time*. New York: W. W. Norton.

Horney, K. (1945). *Our inner conflicts, a constructive theory of neurosis*. New York: W. W. Norton.

Horney, K. (1950). *Neurosis and human growth: The struggle toward self-realization*. New York: W. W. Norton.

Horowitz, M. J. (1986). *Stress response syndromes*. Northvale, NJ: Jason Aronson.

Horowitz, M. J. (1988). *Introduction to psychodynamics: A new synthesis*. New York: Basic Books.

Horowitz, M. J. (1991). Person schemas. In M. J. Horowitz (Ed.), *Person schemas and maladaptive interpersonal patterns* (pp. 13–31). Chicago: University of Chicago Press.

Horowitz, M. J. & Eells, T. D. (in press). Case formulations using role-relationship model configurations: A reliability study. *Journal of Psychotherapy Research*.

Horowitz, M. J., Fridhandler, B., & Stinson, C. D. (1991). Person schemas and emotion. *Journal of the American Psychoanalytic Association*, *39*, 173–208.

Horowitz, M. J., Luborsky, L., & Popp, C. (1991). A comparison of the role-relationship models configuration and the core conflictual relationship theme. In M. J. Horowitz (Ed.), *Person schemas and maladaptive interpersonal patterns* (pp. 213–219). Chicago: University of Chicago Press.

Horowitz, M. J., Merluzzi, T. V., Ewert, M., Ghannam, J. H., Hartley, D., & Stinson, C. H. (1991). Role-relationship models configuration. In M. J. Horowitz (Ed.), *Person schemas and maladaptive interpersonal patterns* (pp. 115–154). Chicago: University of Chicago Press.

Jacobson, E. (1964). *The self and object world*. New York: International Universities Press.

Kernberg, O. (1984). *Severe personality disorders*. New Haven, CT: Yale University Press.

Kihlstrom, J. F., & Cunningham, R. L. (1991). Mapping interpersonal space. In M. J. Horowitz (Ed.), *Person schemas and maladaptive interpersonal patterns* (pp. 311–336). Chicago: University of Chicago Press.

Klein, M. (1975). On the theory of anxiety and guilt. In *Envy and gratitude and other works: 1946–1963* (pp. 25–42). London: Hogarth Press. (Original work published 1948)

Klein, M., & Tribich, D. (1981). Kernberg's object-relations theory: A critical evaluation. *International Journal of Psycho-Analysis*, *62*, 27–43.

Kohut, H. (1971). *Analysis of the self*. New York: International Universities Press.

Kohut, H. (1977). *Restoration of the self*. New York: International Universities Press.

Kohut, H. (1984). *How analysis cures*. New York: International Universities Press.

Luborsky, L., & Crits-Christoph (1990). *Understanding transference: The core conflictual relationship theme method*. New York: Basic Books.

Meehl, P. E. (1978). Theoretical risks and tabular asterisks: Sir Karl, Sir Ronald, and the slow progress of soft psychology. *Journal of Consulting and Clinical Psychology*, *46*, 806–834.

Meehl, P. E. (1986). What social scientists don't know. In D. Fiske & R. Schweder (Eds.), *Metatheory in social science* (pp. 315–338). Chicago: University of Chicago Press.

Merluzzi, T. V. (1991). Representation of information about self and other: A multidimensional scaling analysis. In M. J. Horowitz (Ed.), *Person schemas and maladaptive interpersonal patterns* (pp. 155–166). Chicago: University of Chicago Press.

Pribram, K. H. (1970). Feelings as monitors. In M. A. Arnold (Ed.), *Feelings and emotions* (pp. 41–53). New York: Academic Press.

Rank, O. (1929). *The trauma of birth*. New York: Harcourt Brace. (Original work published 1924)

Rinsley, D. (1979). Fairbairn's object-relations theory. *Bulletin of the Menninger Clinic*, *43*, 489–514.

Russell, R. L., & Trull, T. J. (1986). Sequential analysis of language variables in psychotherapy process research. *Journal of Consulting and Clinical Psychology*, *54*, 16–21.

Rychlak, J. F. (1981). *Introduction to personality and psychotherapy: A theory-construction approach* (2nd ed.). Boston: Houghton Mifflin.

Sandler, J., & Rosenblatt, B. (1962). The concept of the representational world. *Psychoanalytic Study of the Child*, 17, 128–145.

Schafer, R. (1983). *The analytic attitude*. New York: Basic Books.

Sidman, M. (1952). A note on functional relations obtained from group data, *Psychological Bulletin*, *49*, 263–269.

Stinson, C. H., & Palmer, S. E. (1991). Parallel distributed processing models of person schemas and psychopathologies. In M. J. Horowitz (Ed.), *Person schemas and maladaptive interpersonal patterns* (pp. 339–377). Chicago: University of Chicago Press.

Sullivan, H. S. (1953). *The interpersonal theory of psychiatry*. New York: W. W. Norton.

Sullivan, H. S. (1954). *The psychiatric interview*. New York: W. W. Norton.

Thorngate, W. (1986). The production, detection, and explanation of behavioral patterns. In J. Valsiner (Ed.), *The individual subject and scientific psychology* (pp. 71–93). New York: Plenum Press.

Tunis, S., Fridhandler, B., & Horowitz, M. J. (1990). Identifying schematized views of self with significant others: Convergence of quantitative and clinical methods, *Journal of Personality and Social Psychology*, *59*, 1279–1286.

Valsiner, J. (1986). Different perspectives on individual-based generalizations in psychology. In J. Valsiner (Ed.), *The individual subject and scientific psychology* (pp. 391–404). New York: Plenum Press.

Winnicott, D. W. (1953). Transitional objects and transitional phenomena. *International Journal of Psycho-Analysis*, *34*, 89–97.

Commentary

RICHARD J. MCNALLY
Harvard University

IN THIS COMMENTARY on Eells, Horowitz, Stinson, and Fridhandler's chapter, I shall first comment on general issues concerning psychoanalytic thinking on self-representation and anxiety, and discuss several salient points of contact between the psychodynamic and cognitive perspectives. I shall then comment directly on their person-schematic psychodynamic model.

PSYCHOANALYSIS, SELF-REPRESENTATION, AND ANXIETY

It is obvious from Eells et al.'s excellent review of the literature that psychodynamic theorists have devoted far more attention to self-representation and anxiety than have their cognitive–behavioral counterparts.[1] But most of this theorizing has been done by clinicians who have not endeavored to test their conjectures empirically. Accordingly, the evidential basis of these theories is often unclear. For example, Melanie Klein asserts that the infant forms representations of the mother's breast and the father's penis. How does she know this? What evidence does she have that infants do, in fact, develop such representations? How might we test such notions to determine their validity? Although these questions are not a call for the exhumation of operationism, verificationism, and other long-abandoned relics of logical positivism (e.g., Leahey, 1980; Meehl, 1986), controlled observations and testable hypotheses, for example, ought to strengthen the psychoanalytic program by stimulating the interplay between data and theory. In the absence of data, we can only appeal to the authority of our favorite theorists and their clinical observations and insights.

As Eells and colleagues point out, traditional psychoanalysis emphasized an internal, instinctual origin of threat in anxiety disorders. Freud, it seems, acknowledged the possibility of an external origin of threat only when confronted with cases of combat-related PTSD. By contrast, traditional behavioral theorists emphasized the external origin of anxiety disorders, as established through Pavlovian conditioning (Wolpe & Rachman, 1960).

However, several contemporary cognitive–behavioral theories depart from the traditional emphasis on external feared stimuli as the primary locus of pathological anxiety. In their influential reanalysis of agoraphobia, Goldstein and Chambless (1978) emphasized that agoraphobia is not so much a fear of open or public places as it is a "fear of fear." Similarly, Clark (1986) suggested that panic attacks result from the catastrophic misinterpretation of certain bodily sensations (e.g., a skipped heartbeat as a sign of an impending heart attack). Despite their focus on internal fear cues, these theories are still distinguishable from Freud's in that they do not postulate instinctual drives as etiological factors in anxiety disorders.

Another apparent similarity between cognitive and psychoanalytic theories of anxiety is an emphasis on the unconscious determinants of behavior (e.g., Mathews, 1990; Williams, Watts, MacLeod, & Mathews, 1988). Cognitive theories emphasize pathological memory organization (Foa & Kozak, 1986), involuntary semantic activation of threat concepts (McNally, Riemann, & Kim, 1990), and processing of threat cues without awareness (Mathews & MacLeod, 1986) as responsible for the maintenance and perhaps the etiology of anxiety disorders. The unconscious of cognitive psychology comprises structures and processes that operate outside of awareness and subserve relatively automatic, "unintelligent" functions. The unconscious is not a repository of creative thinking or incubation (Weisberg, 1986), nor does it possess intentional attributes (e.g., wishes). In contrast, as Lang (1978) noted, the Freudian unconscious possesses most of the properties of the conscious mind (e.g., feelings, wishes)—except consciousness itself. Thus, the similarities between the cognitive and psychodynamic perspectives on the unconscious are more apparent than real.

THE PERSON-SCHEMATIC PSYCHODYNAMIC MODEL

The development of psychoanalysis has been stimulated more by the insights of the consulting room than by the discoveries of the laboratory.

Accordingly, I was surprised to find references to parallel distributed processing (PDP) architecture, neural nets, and the like, in a chapter on the psychodynamics of anxiety. On the one hand, Eells et al. are a step ahead of their cognitive experimental psychopathology counterparts who have yet to explore the relevance of connectionism for understanding the anxiety disorders. On the other hand, it remains to be seen how psychoanalysis, an exemplary symbol-processing paradigm, can be integrated with connectionism—a paradigm that dispenses with symbol processing.

It is unclear whether Eells et al. regard connectionism as a radically new approach to the mind wholly distinct from the physical symbol-system approach of traditional artificial intelligence (Simon, 1981), or whether they view connectionism as merely an implementational strategy for instantiating the concepts of psychoanalysis (Fodor & Pylyshyn, 1988). Given that they retain the explanatory apparatus of psychoanalysis, Eells et al. appear to subscribe to the implementational construal of connectionism.

Self-schemas and role-relationship models (RRMs) play a prominent role in Eells et al.'s theorizing. They suggest that anxiety results from one's anticipating or experiencing a "dreaded self-concept." That is, anxious individuals worry that a dreaded RRM will become the current working model of the immediate situation. They also conceptualize anxiety as an objectless fear, a signal that some unknown threat is about to materialize.

There are several potential problems with this perspective. First, it is unclear whether activation of a dreaded self-concept fits all cases of pathological anxiety. Fear of a dreaded self-concept appears to apply to some anxiety disorders (e.g., social phobia) much better than to others (e.g., snake phobia). For example, in what sense does a snake phobic fear the activation of a dreaded self-concept versus simply fearing the snake?

Second, although Eells et al. view anxiety as objectless fear, several studies suggest that Generalized Anxiety Disorder (GAD) patients are quite capable of specifying what worries them (e.g., Craske, Rapee, Jackel, & Barlow, 1989; Hibbert, 1984). The object of these worries varies widely from finances and family matters to illness and nuclear war.

Third, Eells et al.'s model seems to limit anxiety to species capable of self-representation. If anxiety is the consequence of experiencing a dreaded self-concept, infrahuman species incapable of developing self-concepts should be incapable of experiencing anxiety—a conclusion inconsistent with fear-conditioning research in animals (Mineka, 1985). Either animals have self-concepts and therefore experience anxiety, or the anxiety experienced by human beings is qualitatively distinct from that experienced by infrahumans. At issue, then, is the phylogenetic continuity of emotion.

Relevant to this issue is the ingenious research conducted by comparative psychologists that establishes that at least some infrahuman species can develop self-representations, and by implication, experience anxiety as Eells et al. define it (for a review, see Gallup, 1985). In the first systematic demonstration of this phenomenon, Gallup (1970) exposed chimpanzees to full-length mirrors, and found that they acted as if they were viewing an unfamiliar chimpanzee only for the first 3 days. During the next 10 days, they used the mirror to inspect and groom parts of their bodies that were otherwise visually inaccessible. To demonstrate conclusively the existence of self-representations, Gallup anesthetized the chimpanzees, removed them from their cages, and applied a bright red, nonirritating dye to regions of their faces that were visually inaccessible without a mirror. When they returned to their cages, they used the mirror to inspect the reddened regions, whereas a second group of chimpanzees that had not received any previous mirror exposure did not inspect the red marks on their faces. Unlike the chimpanzees who had received previous mirror exposure, they acted toward their image as if it were another chimpanzee. These findings indicate that the mirror-exposed subjects learned that the image in the mirror was a reflection of themselves, thus implying the existence of a cognitive self-representation. Using this paradigm, comparative psychologists have determined that chimpanzees and orangutans, but not gorillas, are capable of self-recognition (Gallup, 1985). Taken together, these findings indicate that at least some species can develop self-representations.

Eells et al. postulate control processes that counteract anxious states of mind. This hypothesis has its roots in Freud's concepts of suppression and repression, and in Sullivan's concept of unconscious selective inattention to threat cues. Experimental research on attentional bias in anxiety disorders is relevant to this hypothesis. Consistent with Eells et al.'s hypothesis of control processes, nonanxious individuals seem characterized by an automatic bias for diverting attention away from threat. Anxiety-disordered patients, however, are characterized by a bias for directing attention toward threat cues, thus exhibiting a breakdown in a control process that otherwise counteracts anxious states of mind (Mathews, 1990).

In the clearest demonstration of this phenomenon, MacLeod, Mathews, and Tata (1986) devised an attentional deployment task to study the processing of threatening information. They presented anxious, depressed, and normal subjects with pairs of words on a computer screen. On each trial, the subject had to name the top word of the pair. On other trials, a faint dot appeared where one of the words had been, and when this happened, subjects had to push a button as quickly as possible. On some trials, one of the words had a threatening meaning. Anxious subjects responded faster when the dot replaced a threat word at the top (when a neutral word was at the bottom) than when it replaced a neutral word at the top, and were slow to respond when the dot replaced a neutral word at the top (when a threat word appeared at the bottom). Control subjects exhibited the opposite pattern. Taken together, these results suggest that anxious patients exhibit selective attention for threat material, whereas normal control subjects (and depressed patients) exhibit selective avoidance of threat. Cast in the terminology of Eells et al., nonanxious people do, indeed, exhibit rapid, unconscious control processes that curtail anxious states of mind, whereas GAD subjects exhibit a failure of such control, and accordingly are plagued by anxious states of mind.

CONCLUSIONS

Are cognitive and psychodynamic views on self-representation and anxiety ripe for integration? Certainly Eells et al. have embarked on such an endeavor; their model is as much cognitive as psychoanalytic. Their approach is exciting because it promises to strengthen the empirical basis of psychoanalysis while introducing affective and psychopathological themes into connectionist cognitive science.

It is too soon to tell whether psychoanalysis and cognitive psychology *must* be integrated to capture the relevant generalizations about self-representation and anxiety. Certainly, increased communication between these two traditions ought to be heuristically valuable. Perhaps the wisest strategy is to promote a proliferation of diverse perspectives, and to subject them to as much conceptual and empirical scrutiny as possible.

NOTE

1. Bandura's (1977) cognitive–behavioral theory of self-efficacy constitutes an important exception to this generalization. Because this theory has uncertain ramifications for PTSD, I did not address it in my target chapter.

ACKNOWLEDGEMENT

Preparation of this chapter was supported in part by National Institute of Mental Health Grant #MH43809 awarded to the author.

REFERENCES

Bandura, A. (1977). Self-efficacy: Toward a unifying theory of behavioral change. *Psychological Review*, *84*, 191–215.

Clark, D. M. (1986). A cognitive approach to panic. *Behaviour Research and Therapy*, *24*, 461–470.

Craske, M. G., Rapee, R. M., Jackel, L., & Barlow, D. M. (1989). Qualitative dimensions of worry in DSM-III-R generalized anxiety disorder subjects and nonanxious controls. *Behaviour Research and Therapy*, *27*, 397–402.

Fodor, J. A., & Pylyshyn, Z. W. (1988). Connectionism and cognitive architecture: A critical analysis. *Cognition*, *28*, 3–71.

Foa, E. B., & Kozak, M. J. (1986). Emotional processing of fear: Exposure to corrective information. *Psychological Bulletin*, *99*, 20–35.

Gallup, Jr., G. G. (1970). Chimpanzees: Self-recognition. *Science*, *167*, 86–87.

Gallup, Jr., G. G. (1985). Do minds exist in species other than our own? *Neuroscience and Biobehavioral Reviews*, *9*, 631–641.

Goldstein, A. J., & Chambless, D. L. (1978). A reanalysis of agoraphobia. *Behavior Therapy*, *9*, 47–59.

Hibbert, G. A. (1984). Ideational components of anxiety: Their origin and content. *British Journal of Psychiatry*, *144*, 618–624.

Lang, P. J. (1978) Anxiety: Toward a psychophysiological definition. In H. S. Akiskal & W. L. Webb (Eds.), *Psychiatric diagnosis*: *Explorations of biological predictors* (pp. 365–389). New York: Spectrum.

Leahey, T. H. (1980). The myth of operationism. *Journal of Mind and Behavior*, *1*, 127–143.

MacLeod, C., Mathews, A., & Tata, P. (1986). Attentional bias in emotional disorders. *Journal of Abnormal Psychology*, *95*, 15–20.

Mathews, A. (1990). Why worry? The cognitive function of anxiety. *Behaviour Research and Therapy*, *28*, 455–468.

Mathews, A., & MacLeod, C. (1986). Discrimination of threat cues without awareness in anxiety states. *Journal of Abnormal Psychology*, *95*, 131–138.

McNally, R. J., Riemann, B. C., & Kim, E. (1990). Selective processing of threat cues in panic disorder. *Behaviour Research and Therapy*, *28*, 407–412.

Meehl, P. E. (1986). Diagnostic taxa as open concepts: Metatheoretical and statistical questions about reliability and construct validity in the grand strategy of nosological revision. In T. Millon & G. L. Klerman (Eds.), *Contemporary directions in psychopathology*: *Toward DSM-IV* (pp. 215–231). New York: Guilford Press.

Mineka, S. (1985). Animal models of anxiety-based disorders: Their usefulness and limitations. In A. H. Tuma & J. D. Maser (Eds.), *Anxiety and the anxiety disorders* (pp. 199–244). Hillsdale, NJ: Lawrence Erlbaum.

Simon, H. A. (1981). *The sciences of the artificial* (2nd ed.). Cambridge, MA: MIT Press.

Weisberg, R. W. (1986). *Creativity*: *Genius and other myths*. New York: W. H. Freeman.

Williams, J. M. G., Watts, F. N., MacLeod, C., & Mathews, A. (1988). *Cognitive psychology and emotional disorders*. Chichester, UK: Wiley.

Wolpe, J., & Rachman, S. (1960). Psychoanalytic "evidence": A critique based on Freud's case of Little Hans. *Journal of Nervous and Mental Disease*, *131*, 135–148.

III

Depression

5

A Cognitive Perspective on Self-representation in Depression

ZINDEL V. SEGAL
Clarke Institute of Psychiatry,
University of Toronto

J. CHRISTOPHER MURAN
Beth Israel Medical Center,
Mount Sinai School of Medicine

THE SYNDROME OF depression currently ranks among the most prevalent mental health complaints of North Americans (Myers et al., 1984). The risk of developing the disorder within one's lifetime has been estimated as 12% for men and 20% for women (Sturt, Kumakura & Der, 1984). The occurrence of depression is associated with an increased risk for the condition to become chronic, since anywhere from 15% to 39% of cases may still meet the diagnostic criteria for depression up to 1 year after symptom onset (Berti Ceroni, Neri, & Pezzoli, 1984; Van Valkenburg, Akiskal, Puzantian, & Rosenthal, 1984), and in 22% of cases may continue to do so up to 2 years later (Keller, Lavori, Lewis, & Klerman, 1983). In recognition of the pervasive nature of this disorder, there has been a concerted effort over the past 25 years to develop effective treatment modalities, which has met with some success (Beckham, 1990). This must be considered as only a partial solution to the problem, because there is good evidence to suggest that single episodes of Major Depressive Disorder are relatively rare, and if the time of observation is extended beyond 15 years, they are practically never observed (Keller, Lavori, Endicott, Coryell, & Klerman, 1983). It seems as if patients who recover from their first episode of depression are at a pivotal point in charting the future course of their disorder, since they have a higher probability of relapse; should this occur, they have an approxiamtely 20% chance of remaining chronically depressed (Belsher & Costello, 1988; Keller, Lavori, Lewis & Klerman, 1983; Segal & Dobson, 1992).

Current diagnostic convention as spelled out in DSM-lll-R (American Psychiatric Association, 1987) emphasizes that the syndrome of depression can be discerned on the basis of the occurrence of 5 out of 9 cardinal symptoms, which reflect affective, cognitive, and somatic complaints, as well as the ruling out of competing conditions that would explain these features. As Arieti and Bemporad (1980) remind us, however, the affects of sorrow and sadness have a currency that is much wider than that recognized by nosological schemes and reflect a variety of meanings descriptive of both normal and pathological emotional states. The import of this for self-representation is that aspects of a view of the self or a manner of personal regard, which may dominate during a full-blown depression, may be exhibited, if only partially, in normal, everyday moods. This, in fact, is one of the premises behind a good deal of research examining the role of personality factors in depression (Hirschfeld, Klerman, Clayton, & Keller, 1983). Although it is generally accepted that a worsening of depressed mood is accompanied by changes in other spheres, such as bodily complaints, physiological disturbances, motivation, and behavioral routines, this chapter focuses primarily on the cognitive aspects of depression and on those phenomena that illuminate the model of self subscribed to by depressed individuals.

THE COGNITIVE SIDE OF DEPRESSION

Cognitive theories of depression were spawned at a time when a more general shift within psychology toward the adoption of models stressing cognitive mediation was occurring. Beck's (1967) cognitive model, Seligman's (1975) learned helplessness model and its reformulated incarnation as the hopelessness theory (Abramson, Metalsky, & Alloy, 1989), and Rehm's (1977) self-control model subscribe to a number of common assumptions regarding (1) the ability of cognitive activity to affect behavior, (2) the potential for such activity to be monitored and altered, and (3) the possibility of arriving at change in behavior through prior cognitive change (Segal & Dobson, 1992). Since, in our view, the latter two models are less than explicit in elaborating the implications of their premises for the representation of the self in depression, they will only be mentioned briefly.

Cognitive theories of depression that emphasize the role of attributions were originally based on the observation that when humans expect that they cannot control events in their lives they manifest certain changes consistent with depression (e.g., negative expectations, loss of incentive).

Of specific relevance seemed to be the nature of the individual's explanations for this uncontrollability. Three dimensions were identified as descriptive of a depressive attributional style: internal versus external, stable versus unstable, and global versus specific. Depression was predicted to result from internal, stable, and global attributions for negative events, a feature that most clinicians would recognize as a tendency toward self-blame. Two vignettes may help to clarify the role of this type of meaning that makes for self-representation in depression.

In the first scenario, two friends (Greg and Tom) are out for a morning jog. In their usual discussion, the topic of politics arises, and Greg makes a number of inflammatory statements against women, leftists, and the poor, which he does not really believe, but which he knows will sound outrageous and provocative. Flushed as he is with the emotion of denouncing some of the favorite causes of his running partner, he fails to notice a pothole on the trail and twists his ankle. This, fairly rapidly, changes the mood of the moment, with concern and sympathy replacing debate. In trying to explain how or why the sprain came about, Greg says that he is being punished for being insulting and profane; he could have avoided the injury if he had not been so immature and childish. He views the injury as both a retaliation and a warning. He hobbles back to the gym, and Tom finishes his run. When Tom returns, Greg is icing his ankle and in response to Tom's inquiries about his state of mind, Greg jokingly admits that he will vote for the socialists in the next election. Greg also acknowledges that choosing to jog down that particular winding muddy trail 1 hour after it had rained was a poor choice, especially since his ankle had been tender from a previous pull 2 weeks before. His explanation now seems more focused on the risks that the slippery trail could present to any runner, and he is thinking about other ways of exercising while staying off his ankle.

In the second case, Carla, a depressed patient receiving cognitive therapy, describes being informed by the president of her firm that the contract position for which she was initially hired will expire in a month. The president goes on to tell Carla that the firm was very pleased with her work and will keep her in mind for future consulting opportunities. In recounting this incident during therapy, Carla recalls her automatic thoughts at the moment as being, "She is firing me," "Once again this means I have failed," "If I were more competent she would have found a way to keep me on," and "The only reason she is saying those things about my performance is because she pities me." Even though the patient knew at the time of hiring that the position was time limited, and that "rationally, I know that they have not misled me," she continues to feel as if this outcome confirms a deeper sense of things not working out in her life. She remains convinced of her responsibility for negative occurrences and, at some inchoate level feels that the fates have not chosen her as someone who is destined to live a happy life.

We would suggest that the pertinence of these vignettes to the question of self-representation is that, while self-blame was evident in both instances, there was a difference in the extent to which these explanations of cause could be spontaneously controverted by the individual and an alternative perspective considered. Could it be that one reason for this difference is that depressive attributions may arise as part of the activation of a more general depressive self-organization, of which attributions are only one element? Unfortunately, attribution-based models of depression are relatively silent with respect to issues of cognitive organization.

The model developed by Beck (1967, 1976), on the other hand, is more explicit about this possibility and places great emphasis on the content of an individual's self-view as determining vulnerability to depression in the face of social adversity. Depressive symptoms are explained in terms of the operation of three cognitive concepts: the cognitive triad, cognitive distortions, and schemas. The cognitive triad describes negative thinking patterns about the person's view of the world, future, and self, whereas cognitive distortions represent faulty information processing, systematic errors in logic, or misinterpretations of objective events such that the conclusions drawn by depressed individuals confirm their previously held negative expectations. Schemas are the underlying cognitive structures that generate these cognitive patterns and errors; they are abstract representations of a domain of self-knowledge that is presumed to be largely negative and punitive in nature (Segal, 1988). A complete account of the conditions under which these schemas are formed and what is actually represented has been lacking in the theory. Beck, however, suggested that painful childhood experiences, such as those of loss, deprivation, and death of a significant other, provide the basis for the formation of negative self-schemas (1967), and that these schemas may be latent or hypovalent, but can be activated by specific circumstances analogous to those experiences initially responsible for embedding the structure (Kovacs & Beck, 1978).

According to the particulars of Beck's conceptualization, a negative self-schema is activated, in turn, when a negative life event impinges on a dysfunctional attitude. Dysfunctional attitudes are excessively rigid, absolute rules for interpreting the meaning of certain situations or occurrences and may be related to the underlying view of the self which the person holds. The attitudes that have received the greatest attention are those that are stated as self-worth contingencies or conditional statements—"If I succeed at all tasks important to me, then I am worthwhile" (Kuiper & Olinger, 1986)—and those that are cast as noncontingent or unconditional statements of self-worth—"I am a failure" (Beck, 1976). Measures of dysfunctional attitudes and have been shown to correlate significantly with depression (e.g., Eaves & Rush, 1984; Segal & Shaw, 1986).

The activation of the negative self-schema subsequently results in an increasing flow of negative views that emerge rapidly, without any apparent antecedent reflection, and are so-called automatic thoughts. In other words, these automatic thoughts are the cognitive products of the negative self-schema, reflective of the cognitive triad and the faulty information processing characteristic of depression. Several studies have documented an increase in negative automatic thoughts in depression, with a corresponding return to normal levels when the depression remits (e.g., Dobson & Shaw, 1986; Eaves & Rush, 1984; Hollon, Kendall, & Lumry, 1986). Automatic thoughts operate out of awareness but can be accessed through attention. It is through attending to a constellation of automatic thoughts that one can infer the nature of the dysfunctional attitude implicit to the schematic structure. For example, Richard, a male patient who had been self-employed as a businessman in the community decides to go to a meeting at a downtown hotel to learn about new franchise opportunities in the city. He is currently in treatment for depression resulting from his being released from his firm for having a management style that his coworkers found to be aggressive and competitive. In describing the experience at the hotel, Richard explains to the therapist that he noticed his mood shift when he entered the hotel suite in which the presentations were being made, and he recalls the following automatic thoughts: "This room is for winners only, which rules me out since being fired shows I am a loser," "I can tell from how these guys are dressed that they are all more successful than I am," "I just don't belong," "If they knew my story, they would tell me to get lost," "I'm now the type of guy that I used to look down on when I was still working." A therapist intent on abstracting a particular self-worth contingency from these thoughts may want to explore with the patient such possibilities as "If I fail at what I choose to do, then I am worthless," or "If I cannot compete and win, then I am weak and useless."

SELF-SCHEMAS

Beck (1967) borrowed the schema construct from contemporary cognitive psychology, particularly from the work of Bartlett (1932), who used the construct to account for the influence of old knowledge on the perception of, and memory for, new information. Bartlett considered a schema to be a generic cognitive representation that the mind extracts in the course of exposure to particular instances of a phenomenon. Piaget (1954) also used the schema construct to describe the cognitive development of the child. Specifically, he described a process of interaction between schemas and the environment, which consists of assimilation and accommodation as the basic mechanisms producing increasingly complex knowledge domains in the child.

Since Bartlett and Piaget, there has been a notable proliferation of use of the schema construct (Bobrow & Norman, 1975; Neisser, 1976; Rumelhart, 1975; Schank & Abelson, 1977), resulting in a great many definitions and a good deal of conceptual confusion (Segal, 1988). In fact, it is generally accepted that the construct has no single, fixed definition (Brewer & Treyens, 1981; Taylor & Crocker, 1981). As a result, there have been recent efforts to rigorously conceptualize schema. For example, Williams, Watts, MacLeod, and Matthews (1988) have established a set of criteria for determining schematic operation: (1) a schema is a stored body of knowledge that interacts with the selection of new information, the abstraction of meaning from the information, the interpretation of the meaning according to a preexisting schema, the integration of the meaning with previously acquired information, and the reconstruction of memories (Alba & Hasher, 1983); (2) a schema has a consistent internal structure that is imposed on the organization of new information; (3) the knowledge contained within a schema is generic in nature, comprising abstract prototypical representations of environmental regularities; and (4) the format in which this information is represented is akin to a package, or module, of generic information, such that activation of any one part will tend to produce activation of the whole (pp. 154–155).

Social cognition has also contributed in important ways to the evolving definition of the self-schema construct, and in this case the work of Markus (1977) is especially relevant. According to her, self-schemas are defined as "cognitive generalizations about the self, derived from past experience, that organize and guide the processing of self-related information contained in an individual social experience (p. 64). Markus and Nurius (1986) broadened this definition of self-schema to include the idea of "possible selves," which are defined as an individual's ideas of what he/she might become, would like to become, and is afraid of becoming. This theoretical expansion establishes a rationale for the investigation of self-knowledge in terms of rules, standards, or strategies that individuals use to evaluate, guide, and control their own behavior. Such a conceptualization of self-schema is more compatible with the use of self-schema in the cognitive therapy tradition, where it is used to account for self-worth maintenance.

More recently, Markus (1990) has described the self as a multidimensional set of structures, or a collection of self-schemas, that plays a critical role in organizing all aspects of behavior. In her emerging view of the self, she conceptualizes each person as holding multiple representations of the self:

> the good me, the bad me, the not me, the actual me, the ideal me, the ought me, the possible me, the undesired me, the hoped-for me, the expected me, the feared me, and the shared me (i.e., me-in-relation-to my mother; me-in-relation-to-my spouse, etc.). Of this universe of self-representations, only some will become focal for the individual and receive a high degree of cognitive,

> affective, or somatic elaboration. Those representations that, for whatever reasons, become the target of such intensive elaboration are the self-schemas. And it is the self-schemas that will dominate consciousness, and perhaps unconsciousness, and that can be considered the "core" self. (p. 242)

This most recent conceptualization highlights two important aspects that are receiving more attention in self-schema theory: the role of affect and behavior and the role of the other in the self-system.

In terms of affect and behavior, self-schemas have come to be conceptualized as structures that include affective and motoric as well as cognitive components (Cantor, 1990; Muran, 1991; Safran & Segal, 1990; Segal, 1988). This is consistent with Leventhal's (1984) notion of emotional schemas, which are representations in memory of specific perceptions, expressive motor (instrumental and autonomic) reactions, and situationally specific stimuli. Both Bower (1981) and Lang (1985) have proposed similar models of the processing of emotion information. Subsequently, what distinguishes the depressogenic schemas from those of other emotional disorders is only the content of the self-schemas; in other words, the cognitive component would include devaluation, the affective component would include sadness, and the motoric component would include avoidance and withdrawal from activities of normal functioning.

As for the role of the other, Markus's (1990) idea of "shared me" introduces the interpersonal nature of the self into the self-system and is echoed in Neisser's (1988) inclusion of "the interpersonal self" in his most recent exposition on self-knowledge. In a related vein, Safran (1990) introduced the construct of the "interpersonal schema" to represent beliefs and expectations of others, as well as assumptions about how an individual must act in order to maintain relatedness to others.

What is most significant about addressing the interpersonal nature of the self is that it sheds light on the development of the self and the etiology of depressogenic self-schemas. As noted previously, a somewhat murky picture has been painted regarding this issue. At best, self-schemas are simply attributed to learning from early painful experiences (Beck, Rush, Shaw & Emery, 1979). It is still unclear what types of "past experiences" may be pivotal to this developmental process. As Harter (1990) reminded us, the significant role of the other in the development of one's self-schemas is something that children become increasingly sensitized to with age. In time, they learn to use these views to verify and refine their own self-representations. Bowlby (1969) also suggested that finely tuned, contingent responding from those in one's social environment may be a key to the development of viable self-schemas. As these authors would argue, a clearer picture regarding what exactly is represented in the self-schemas is obtained when the role of the other is addressed.

WHAT IS REPRESENTED IN DEPRESSIVE SELF-SCHEMAS?

This section is perhaps best started with a caveat that the answer to the question in the heading is not definitively known. In its place, all we can offer is speculation informed by research and clinical experience (at this point the reader may surmise the operation of a "do not promise more than you can deliver" self-worth contingency).

It seems to be generally accepted that during an episode of depression, most patients go through a transition from a healthy to a corrosive self-regard. As Segal and Vella (1990) pointed out, markers of such a process might include

> not only self-disparaging comments, low expectations of personal efficacy, or harsh judgments arising from strict and often unrealistic standards, but, perhaps more telling, a tendency to process information in a fashion which minimizes positive and maximizes negative appraisals, in effect enshrining a continuing view of self as fundamentally inadequate or worthless (Beck, 1967, 1976). (p. 162)

This suggests that depressed patients' self-views are not monolithic, but rather contain different aspects that may dominate at a particular point in time. The information reflected in the elements, which combine to fashion a unitary sense of self, probably varies along a number of dimensions (e.g., valence, salience, temporality). To understand fully how such features may come to be organized, we must consider what is known about social knowledge representation in general.

Social-cognitive accounts of the interactions between people have stressed the importance of understanding the meaning of social events, as conveyed through the different personal constructs employed by individuals (Higgins & Bargh, 1987; Wyer & Srull, 1986). The basic units of social perception are thought to be those constructs or categories utilized by people to contain their social experience and render it interpretable within preexisting conceptual frameworks. For example, a serious dieter may categorize food-related social situations in terms of those that present risks for overeating or a danger of violating caloric intake limits, whereas someone who values social manners and etiquette may categorize the same situations as requiring restraint simply because overindulgence would be seen as unacceptable behavior. The same situation would thus elicit identical responses from both parties, but they would come about through the operation of largely unrelated social constructs (Bruner, 1957; Kelly, 1955). Furthermore, research has shown that of the those constructs a person has stored in his/her memory (referred to as "available constructs") certain categories will come to mind more easily than others (referred to as "accessible constructs") (Higgins & King, 1981; Higgins & Bargh, 1987). Construct accessibility has been shown to vary as a function of the recency of previous activation of the construct, expectations, motivation, salience, and affect.

The relevance of this for the study of self-processes in depression is that the self can be thought of as a construct whose activation follows the same principles enunciated above for other social categories (Kihlstrom & Cantor, 1984; Markus, 1990). There seem to be credible parallels between what is meant by the activation of the self construct and clinical accounts of the dominance of negative constructs in depression (e.g., about the world, the future, the self; Beck, 1967) to the exclusion of other information. At the level of phenomenology, what is experienced is the sudden coming to mind of various self-descriptors in response to some internal or external cue (Auerbach, 1985; Dunn, 1985). The next question concerns how the features of the depressed person's self construct (i.e., the self-descriptors) are organized and how this differs from the self constructs of individuals who are not depressed.

Two possibilities are suggested by an accessibility/availability account. In the first case, depressed individuals may have different features stored in memory so that activation of the self would lead to constructs related to failure, worthlessness, or rejection coming to mind, rather than confidence, desirability, or efficacy. This suggests that self-representation is determined through the availability of constructs and that depressed and nondepressed persons draw upon different content during self-instantiation. A second possibility is that both depressed and nondepressed individuals have similar self constructs stored in memory, but that the accessibility of features descriptive of failure, worthlessness, or rejection is greater for one group than the other. This suggests that self-representation is determined through those constructs most accessible at any given time, within the limits of what is available to a person (Higgins & King, 1981; Higgins, King, & Mavin, 1982; Riskind & Rholes, 1984).

Given the strong evidence in favor of a relation between affect and accessibility (Blaney, 1986; Bower & Cohen, 1982; Isen, 1984), an accessibility account seems more tenable. Since, by definition, depressed individuals are in a chronic state of negative mood activation, negative self constructs will come to mind more easily than will positive or neutral alternatives, even though they may be available in memory. More frequent activation of these negative constructs makes it easier for them to be activated in future instances and thus to continue their potential domination over fresh or disconfirming information in the person's mind (Bower, 1981; Teasdale & Russell, 1983). This process can be altered by effort on the part of the subject to recall other stored constructs, but such work usually requires paying less attention to the content of the information recalled most immediately. It is interesting to note that instituting such a "moment of reflection" is an explicit goal of cognitive therapy for depession and is probably achieved by different means in other effective interventions.

In theory, at least, the self-representations of depressed individuals are composed of negative constructs or exemplars of negative evaluation, which come to mind more easily than more positive or neutral features. It is also likely that activation of one negative element will increase the chances of similar elements coming to mind. Whether this occurs as a result of negative elements within the self being interconnected, such that the activation of one will cause activation to spread to neighboring elements (see Bower, 1981, for a fuller description of a network theory of associative memory), is still an open question. If it were to be the case, it might explain why thinking about one setback brings to mind other instances of failure or remorse, even in the absence of a congruent mood state.

RESEARCH ON SELF-SCHEMAS IN DEPRESSION

Using these models as its starting point, a large empirical literature has investigated the content of depressed persons' self-representations, and it is to this work that we now turn. The dimension of depressed individuals' self-representations most frequently investigated has been that of valence, that is, the extent of positivity or negativity in self-based productions. At least three hypotheses have been proposed and tested. The first suggests that nondepressed individuals are characterized by an asymmetry of positive over negative constructs (Matlin & Stang, 1978), whereas the second suggests that they have a balance of both types in contrast to depressives' negative asymmetry (Kuiper & Derry, 1982). A third possibility is that the content of a self-structure is less important than the complexity of its organization, so that depressive mood states are associated with less complex self-organizations (Linville, 1987).

Although self-report inventories are of limited utility in shedding light on the nature of depressed persons' self-representations (Segal, 1988), they do represent some of the initial methodologies employed to address this query. The Dysfunctional Attitude Scale (DAS) (Weissman, 1979) was purposely designed to measure depressogenic schemas and contains 40 items describing contingencies between behavior and feelings of self-worth that subjects are asked to endorse. This scale has correlated positively with measures of cognitive distortions assessed during the depressive episode, and depressed patients generally score higher than normal or psychiatric controls (Giles & Rush, 1983; Hollon, Kendall, & Lumry, 1986). What can be culled from endorsement patterns of this sort is a description of clusters of beliefs or attitudes, but one cannot surmise that they are directly tied to a self construct. In addition, the poor specificity of the DAS in comparisons between depressed and schizophrenic subjects suggests that rather than reflecting a proceess of self-worth maintenance, which is unique to depression, scores on this measure may simply tap a general distress or devaluation factor associated with psychiatric disorder.

Perhaps in response to the ambiguity entailed in relying on self-report measures of depressogenic schemas, a number of investigators have chosen instead to examine on-line processing of information relevant to self-description. The work of Kuiper and his colleagues is perhaps most representative in this regard (Derry & Kuiper, 1981; Kuiper & McDonald, 1983; Kuiper & Olinger, 1983). This group modified the self-referent encoding task (SRET), a method originally developed by cognitive psychologists to examine the relation between depth of processing and memory (Craik & Tulving, 1975) for the purpose of studying how negative and positive information about the self is processed (Rogers, Kuiper, & Kirker, 1977). Subjects are typically presented with a number of personal adjectives and asked to make a yes–no decision about whether the adjective is self-descriptive. The amount of time required to make the judgment, the number of words endorsed as self-descriptive, and an incidental recall test are all measures afforded by this task.

This body of work supports the notion that the self-schemas of depressed individuals contain mostly negative information, through findings such as higher recall of negative adjectives following the SRET by depressed subjects, and higher recall of positive adjectives by nondepressed controls. Depressed subjects tend to rate negative adjectives as being self-descriptive, whereas nondepressed controls rate more positive adjectives as describing them. Finally, when the time taken to arrive at these ratings is examined, nondepressed subjects are quicker in their decisions about whether positive adjectives describe them (schema congruent) than they are about negative adjectives (schema incongruent), but the opposite pattern is evident for clinically depressed subjects. The SRET has made an important contribution to the field by operationalizing schematic processing in a testable fashion and beginning the process of describing possible content differences between depressed and nondepressed individuals.

There is a problem with this paradigm, however, concerning the reliability of its findings with respect to supporting the existence of an organized cognitive structure for negative or positive information. Two difficulties arise in this context that need to be considered. Although the observed differences between the groups is not being debated, the processes underlying their existence is, since such findings may be obtained through the operation of factors that are not necessarily reflective of cognitive organization for the material being studied. One possibility is that the differences are obtained as a result of enhanced accessibility for information that is mood congruent, in which case depressed persons should show a processing advantage for negative information, and nondepressed persons should show the same for positive material. The operation of an accessibility heuristic is certainly consistent with the existence of an underlying cognitive structure, but it is equally possible that the interrelation for negative or positive information is due to the influence of mood alone. In fact, when we examine the typical stimulus items presented to subjects in this paradigm, many of the personal adjectives actually describe a dysphoric mood (e.g., bleak, weary, dismal, depressed, upset, unhappy). In this instance, depressed patients' superior recall of these items, or their tendency to choose them as descriptive of self, may be due more to the match between the content of the word and the individual's mood state than to the activation of an organized self-structure. More apropriate stimuli may have been adjectives that capture qualities of self-esteem while avoiding affective connotations (e.g., unattractive, clumsy, inferior).

Yet another programmatic approach to the study of self-schema in depression has been undertaken by Hammen and colleagues (Hammen, 1985, 1991; Hammen, Marks, Mayol, & DeMayo, 1985), whose use of longitudinal designs and the study of developmental/familial factors in depressive self-representation sets a challenging standard for investigators in the field. The measures of schematicity used in this work are similar to those reported above, but were obtained through slightly different procedures (e.g., the incidental recall of previously rated personal adjectives, the time required to decide whether an adjective is self-descriptive, and the retrieval from memory of behavioral exemplars of times when a subject felt sad or self-critical). Although evidence in favor of a negative self-view for both depressed adults and children is presented (Hammen, 1991), the same questions regarding the implications of these findings for the organization of this material in the form of a cognitive structure apply. In fact, Hammen suggests that these measures tap processes that are more reflective of dysphoria, since they covary strongly with the depressed episode: "[S]tudies of the incidental recall task of self-schema for adults . . . have strongly suggested that these measures capture current depression, rather than underlying vulnerability" (p. 102).

It thus appears that the research reviewed up to this point has answered some questions, while leaving others unresolved. Differences in content between depressed and nondepressed subjects have been demonstrated in adults as well as in children as young as 8 to 10 years old. The main finding is that negative information or self-description is more characteristic of depressed groups, and positive self-views are descriptive of the nondepressed ones. It should also be emphasized that this is by no means a dichotomous relationship, since depressed individuals are still capable of endorsing a good deal of positive information as being self-relevant (e.g., 70% of personal adejctives chosen by depressed patients in two separate studies were positive; Segal, Hood, Shaw, & Higgins, 1988; Segal & Vella,

1990). The differences emerge when comparisons with nondepressed persons are performed (5% of personal adjectives chosen by nondepressed persons were negative). Whether such content differences reflect the operation of an organized self-structure needs to be determined in a more forceful manner, since the measures that have produced these findings do not address the interpretive alternatives proposed by an accessiblity account, which capitalizes on the effects of mood as an organizing principle, rather than the interrelation among the elements in the self-structure.

In an attempt to achieve this resolution, investigators have begun to turn to experimental tasks that emphasize less effortful and more automatic aspects of depressed patients' information processing and that have been used to tap cognitive structure in other knowledge domains.

DEPRESSOGENIC SELF-SCHEMAS AS COGNITIVE STRUCTURES

Since most investigators would agree that a depressive self-schema ought to exert an automatic influence over social perception, it seems reasonable, then, to suggest that using measures capable of demonstrating automatic or uncontrolled (Shiffrin & Schneider, 1977) information processing in depression might be valuable in addressing some of the difficulties outlined above. Tasks that operate at a level of attention or awareness over which the subject has little intentional control can serve to bypass possible response strategies or response styles aimed at faciliating performance (e.g., Ferguson, Rule, & Carlson, 1983). Requirements of this type make it easier to rule out extraneous influences, such as mood, on schema-driven responding. This is important because the effects of mood may mimic the effects of an organized cognitive structure, thereby confounding efforts to evaluate the contributions of each of these variables separately.

One measure capable of meeting the requirements for the assessment of cognitive structure at a relatively automatic level is the Stroop Color-Word Interference Naming Test (Stroop, 1935), in which subjects are asked to name the color of ink in which a stimulus word is printed while attempting to ignore the word itself. Although the exact mechanism behind this effect is still a matter of debate (MacLeod, 1991), it is generally agreed that word meaning is automatically activated and interferes with the subject's task of color-naming. Its value for addressing the accessibility versus cognitive structure issue is that the goal of color-naming conflicts with predictions of structural relatedness among elements in a schema. It is, therefore, more difficult for response sets or strategies to confound the measures from which structure is inferred, because the effects produced by the activation of the cognitive structure (i.e., more of the word's meaning gaining awareness) go in the opposite direction of the subject's response goal (i.e., suppression of the word's meaning in order to facilitate color-naming).

In spite of its proclaimed virtues, it is still possible for tasks that measure more automatic information processing to fall prey to the same difficulties that were associated with the SRET. An early pair of studies (Gotlib & McCann, 1984; Gotlib & Cane, 1987) conducted with the Stroop test reported that depressed subjects took longer to color-name depressed content words than nondepressed content words. Because the words presented to subjects were descriptive of depressed mood, manic mood, and neutral mood, all we can conclude from this work is that subjects take longer to color-name words that describe how they are feeling at the time than they do to color-name words that describe an opposite or unrelated feeling state. As original as this work is—and the testing of patients in both the depressed and remitted states is a laudable feature of the second study—it tells us very little about whether highly descriptive personal traits are represented within a self-structure.

A more powerful design for attacking the issue is one that tests the organization of traits assumed to be related, and contrasts this with traits considered to be unrelated (Higgins, Van Hook, & Dorfman, 1988; Segal, 1988; Strauman & Higgins, Chapter 1, this volume). Segal et al. (1988) and Segal and Vella (1990) examined the responses of depressed patients, anxious patients, and normal controls to a modified version of the Stroop test, which incorporated a priming component and was based on Posner and Warren's (1972) investigation of the cogntive organization of natural categories. In these two studies, subjects were primed by the presentation of a word that was either related or unrelated to the target that was to be color-named. For example, a subject's stimuli set would include words previously chosen as being descriptive of his/her dominant self-view (let's assume these are "inferior," "clumsy," and "awkward"), along with words that were not self-descriptive (let's assume these are "stingy," "critical," and "nosey"). Subjects were shown either a pair of self-descriptive words (i.e., "inferior" as the prime, presented in black and white, followed by "clumsy," printed in blue ink) or a non-self-descriptive prime (i.e., "nosey") followed by a self-descriptive target (i.e., "clumsy," printed in blue ink). With this approach, cognitive structure is inferred from vocal reaction time differences for color-naming produced by comparing latencies for related versus unrelated pairs of self-descriptors.

According to the operationalization afforded by this paradigm, cognitive structure refers to an organization among the descriptors stored in memory, such that activation of one element will result in subthreshold activation of its neighbors. In the absence of any interrelation, elements would tend to be represented in a random fashion throughout semantic memory and differences between related and unrelated pairs of personal adjectives would not be expected. In the two studies we conducted to test the hypothesis that self-descriptive traits form a cognitive structure similar to that underlying semantic memory, our results provided tentative support for this notion (Segal et al., 1988; Segal & Vella, 1990). As illustrated in Table 5.1, depressed subjects took longer to color-name a personal adjective when it was primed by an equally self-descriptive adjective than when it was primed by an adjective that was not self-descriptive. Although these data are intriguing, the specific question of whether individuals who are depressed have negative or depressogenic self-schemas still needs to be considered. According to the findings from these two studies, depressed individuals do not have a global negative view of self that does not permit any positively tinged material to be represented. Recalling that all subjects endorsed more positive than negative adjectives as being self-descriptive, the Stroop interference latencies would argue that any self-structure would contain both types of material. The critical question is whether there is an interrelation among the negative personal adjectives so that activating the self-structure would make it more likely that the negative content would come to mind. In fact, Strauman and Higgins (Chapter 1, this volume) make a similar suggestion when they report their failure to find evidence of structural interrelatedness for self-concept attributes. They do not believe that this argues against the possibility of such interconnectedness existing, but rather, suggest that it may only exist for attributes that are "problematic" (i.e., "mismatches," in the language of self-discrepancy theory) such that they evoke awareness of a discrepancy concerning who the person thinks he/she is, would like to be, or ought to be.

Another possibile configuration of elements in the self-schemas of depressed individuals comes from the finding that adjectives rated as extremely nondescriptive also show some evidence of structural interconnectedness (Segal & Vella, 1990). An example of this might be the case of a nun endorsing the adjective "pious" as extremely descriptive, but "promiscuous" as extremely nondescriptive (or a judge endorsing "fairminded"

TABLE 5.1. Response Latency Means and Standard Deviations across Conditions

	Group					
	Depressed (n=14)		Normals (n=14)		Anxious (n=9)	
Type	X	(SD)	X	(SD)	X	(SD)
Adjectives						
Related	1,137.68	(415.93)	935.89	(189.87)	950.14	(147.24)
Unrelated	1,021.81	(285.56)	912.33	(161.80)	948.37	(115.29)
Nouns						
Related	1,074.50	(313.76)	920.78	(138.40)	967.47	(116.32)
Unrelated	974.93	(222.92)	878.52	(124.54)	877.97	(127.82)

and "dishonest"). In both instances the person's stated identity is incompatible with these traits, but the descriptors may, nonetheless, play a role by forming a sort of negative boundary condition against which the construction of an identity can begin. As might be expected, depressed patients showed a tendency ($p < .08$) to choose more positive adjectives as being extremely nondescriptive of their self-view. Lamiell (1981) argued that a dialectical process of this type may be better suited to describing the formation of personal identity. By putting forth the possibility that self-representations may be structured in terms of polarities of possessed and avoided characteristics, Lamiell's (1981) work forces us to reconsider the notion of a structure composed of unitary elements.

In stepping back from this body of work and trying to reach some conclusions, it seems that there is some support for the notion of a self-structure that is composed of self-attributes, at least some of which may be interconnected, so that activating one will give rise to subthreshold activation of neighboring elements. It is also probable that the content of the schema is not composed of entirely negative information and may indeed contain predominantly positive material. What seems to be important in this context is the possibility of interrelation among negative elements, even within such a structure, and the conditions under which this suborganization may override ongoing information processing. There is also the suggestion that extremely nondescriptive self-relevant information may be structurally organized, but the full implications of this have yet to be fully explored.

THE IMPORTANCE OF PRIMING IN CONSTRUCT ACTIVATION

The operation of depressive self-schemas has always been described within the context of a stress-diathesis model in which an environmental trigger is required to activate the cognitive structure in such a way that the schema becomes an increasingly powerful influence on subsequent information processing (Beck, 1967; Kovacs & Beck, 1978). Implicit in this formulation is the notion of a type of priming of the self-system which may "unlock" or "unfreeze" elements of a self-representation, which, in the absence of particular adversity, have remained relatively unaccessed. Unfortunately, priming manipulations or an effort to activate the construct one is interested in measuring before testing for its effects have rarely been a feature of work in this area (Riskind & Rholes, 1984; Segal, 1988; Uleman & Bargh, 1989). There are some indications, however, that the value of primimg-based models of construct activation is gaining influence, and the results of studies using this conception are particularly informative of the nature of self-representation in depression.

The first group of studies to be described consists of laboratory-based inquiries of self-description by individuals who have recovered from an episode of depression and are tested while in a mildly dysphoric mood. Teasdale and Dent (1987), for example, reported that women who had recovered from a major depression showed better recall of negative self-descriptive adjectives, during a depressed mood induction, than did women with no history of the disorder. Miranda, Persons, and Byers (1990) demonstrated that reports of dysfunctional attitudes varied as a function of patients' mood state and stage of recovery. Following a depressed mood induction, higher endorsements of dyfunctional beliefs were obtained for patients who had a history of depression than for subjects who had never been depressed, but there were no differences between the groups when they were tested in normal mood. Although still preliminary in scope, these findings suggest that some aspects of depressive self-representation may emerge, if properly primed. Furthermore, the content of such representation seems to be concordant with clinical accounts of a negative and deprecatory view of self (Arieti, 1977; Beck, 1967; Bibring, 1953).

A more intriguing possibility is that a representation of this kind may follow from experience with an episode of major depression and that this work is descriptive of a type of "scar" found in individuals who have recovered from the disorder. The work of Lewinsohn has been important in outlining some possible tests of this hypothesis (Lewinsohn, Steinmetz, Larson, & Franklin, 1981; Rohde, Lewinsohn, & Seeley, 1990). Assessements of the psychological functioning of recovered patients (in these studies) have generally yielded few traces of characteristics that are not state dependent, suggesting a low likelihood of residual deficits that would characterize persons at risk for becoming depressed again. The important caveat to bear in mind seems to be that the measures utilized failed to incorporate priming conditons before testing patients, and the functions assessed did not focus on particular self constructs. Social skills, general health, life satisfaction, and emotional reliance were more descriptive of the variables of interest. Although the work on mood priming discussed above is not sufficient to controvert these findings completely, it certainly suggests that asking the same questions with a conceptualization of "scarring," which includes a priming condition as well as measures capable of detecting the organization of self-referent material, is worthy of further empirical scrutiny.

ARE COGNITIVE STRUCTURES ACTIVATED WHEN SOCIAL ADVERSITY MATCHES PERSONAL VULNERABILITY?

A departure from the use of laboratory-based measures of self-representation in depression can be found in the literature on congruency between life stress and personal vulnerability. Hammen's work in this area is exemplary and provides a good deal of support for the notion that when patients who have high needs for affiliation or achievement experience life-stress-related losses in these domains, they are more likely to become depressed than patients who experience noncongruent life stress of equal severity (Hammen, 1991). This effect seems robust enough to have been replicated by a number of investigators (e.g., Zuroff & Mongrain, 1987), studied in both student and clinical populations (Hammen, Marks, Mayol, & DeMayo, 1985; Hammen, Ellicott, Gitlin, & Jamison, 1989), in children (Hammen, & Goodman-Brown, 1990), and shown to be related to depressive relapse (Segal, Shaw, Vella, & Katz, 1992).

This work has drawn liberally from clinical descriptions of depressed patients' presentations, especially those that have emphasized dependent and self-critical themes (Arieti & Bemporad, 1980; Beck, 1983; Blatt, Quinlan, Chevron, McDonald, & Zuroff, 1982). Although the intent of much of this work has not been the explicit investigation of self-representational processes, its findings are nonetheless relevant. When considered from a priming perspective, the probability of activating self-structures can be enhanced by choosing subjects who possess personality characteristics, such as dependency or self criticism, and testing for schematic operation once certain risk situations have been encountered, such as rejection or failure. Naturally occurring events can thus serve as primes, and the contribution of environmental variables to self-construct activation can be evaluated in a more ecologically valid fashion (Safran, Segal, Hill, & Whiffen, 1990).

The general picture to emerge from this work is that the power of congruency to predict depression is greater than noncongruency (Blaney & Kutcher, 1991; Nietzel & Harris, 1990). The exact configuration of matches, however, is still somewhat variable, with some studies supporting the pairing of achievement stress in self-critical individuals, while others have reported stronger effects for interpersonal stress in dependent subjects (see Hammen, 1991; Nietzel & Harris, 1990, for a review). The important point for the purposes of this chapter is that one mechanism by which these effects have been proposed to operate is that certain types of adversity eventuate in depression for some people through the activation of a cognitive structure (Segal, Shaw, Vella, & Katz, 1992). The toxicity of the match between stress and this cognitive predisposition, then, may lie in the event's potential for confirming or supporting the content of this cognitive structure over others that may also be self-relevant, but less depressogenic.

At this point, such proposals are clearly speculative, but they have the value of suggesting links between the organization of information about the self and environmental experience, which can either strengthen or weaken the relations between the elements. The congruency findings seem robust enough to suggest that they say something meaningful about the prediction of depression, but whether the disorder comes about through the specific pathway described above or through some other route, not necessarily predicated on the operation of a self-structure, awaits testing. There have been no studies, to date, in which measures capable of detecting cognitive structure have been used in a longitudinal design for the purposes of assessing changes in self-representation associated with either the onset of a new episode of the disorder or the return of symptoms following recovery.

A NARRATIVE-BASED MEASURE OF SELF-REPRESENTATION

The notion that self-representation develops out of the stories or vignettes people tell themselves and others is an approach to identity formation that draws a great deal from symbolic interactionist theory and defies the division of self-attributes into discrete units, as is often the case in experimental or cognitive studies of self (Alexander, 1988; Gergen & Gergen, 1988; Rosenberg, 1988). The study of stories generated by subjects in response to probes for self-description has revealed a number of intriguing rules and structures that have served to illuminate the subject's relationship to him/herself and to others. For example, Gergen and Gergen (1988) have identified the following components as essential to the construction of a narrative: the establishment of a valued endpoint, the selection of events relevant to the goal state, the ordering of events, the establishment of causal linkages, and the inclusion of points of demarcation. If the contention that we know who we are through the stories we tell ourselves and others is true, then studying these descriptions may be informative of the processes underlying how one's view of self changes as a result of experiencing clinical depression.

This rationale has not been lost on researchers studying self-schemas in clinical disorders, who have questioned the construct validity of paper-and-pencil measures of cognitive structure and the representativeness of cognitive-psychology-based tasks for reflecting events both clinically meaningful and phenomenologically veridical. Although the final verdict on the value of the types of measures described has yet to be delivered (and will probably be more damaging for questionnaires than laboratory-based measures), the existence of diversity in approaches and conception in the field is a salutary development. We are still some time away from a consensus on which measures are best suited to reflect cognitive organization in depression.

Script theory (Abelson, 1981; Schank & Abelson, 1977), for example, may offer a clue to the development of a narrative-based assessment of self-schemas in depression. Scripts are considered procedural schemas that are less abstract and tied more specifically to a class of situations. They represent fixed sequences of behavior that are formed through repeated exposure to well-structured events, allowing the creation of what has been referred to as "standardized generalized episodes" (Schank & Abelson, 1977) or "generalized event representations" (Nelson & Greundel, 1981). Script theory has drawn the attention of a number of theorists and researchers (e.g., Carlson, 1981; Teller & Dahl, 1986; Tompkins, 1987) to describe what Tompkins has coined as a "nuclear scene," which represents a core pathological pattern or schema. This notion of a generalized event representation or nuclear scene is very much related to the use of psychobiography (see Alexander, 1988) and case formulations (see Luborsky & Crits-Christoph, 1990) to describe the central life themes operative for any individual.

An approach that attempts to represent this nuclear scene would be a step in the direction of construct and ecological validity, since it could provide a picture of how an individual reacts to and interacts with his/her environment. In line with the priming notion, we would argue in favor of representing schematic activity in the face of those stimulus situations that potentially activate it. Furthermore, since schematic activity seems to influence and reflect how an individual thinks, feels, and behaves in a particular set of circumstances, a nuclear scene that represents the cognitive, affective, and motoric components constituting schematic structure would provide a more complete picture of this activity.

SELF-SCENARIOS

One assessment approach that attempts to capture self-schemas in terms of nuclear scenes is called self-scenarios (Muran & Segal, in press; Muran, Segal, & Samstag, 1991). They entail extended vignettes of highly distressing events that are idiographically constructed for each patient and are assessed along several signficant parameters. Each scenario depicts a particular patient's recurrent cognitive, affective, and motoric patterns of responding to a particular stimulus situation, which are derived from information observed in assessment interviews. The content of each scenario, therefore, establishes a highly self-referent context for the patient, making it an extremely salient discriminative stimulus, which should prime the patient's recognition of his/her schematically driven or habitual ways of responding. Self-scenarios differ most prominently from inventory-based and adjective-based schematic assessment measures in that they allow the patient to have substantial input in the generation of assessment stimuli, they present a broader picture of schematic activity, and they measure this activity on multiple parameters.

Self-scenarios are idiographically constructed from a standardized procedure. Each scenario consists of four components and is structured according to the paradigm of stimulus situation, affective response, motoric response, and representations of emotionally evocative circumstances of conditions, such as "When I am in social situations. . . . " Affective responses involve statements that reflect the patient's affective lexicon and state, such as "I become very anxious and nervous." Motoric responses include descriptions of instrumental or somatic predispositions, such as "I tend to act in a quiet and inhibited manner." Cognitive responses consist of a statement regarding automatic thinking, such as "I'm always wondering what people think of me," as well as a conditional statement of self-worth, self-protection, or interpersonal relatedness, such as "If I do not succeed at all things important to me, then I am worthless," "I must take great precautions in order to feel safe and secure," or "I must be strong in front of others in order to gain their acceptance and approval." Thus, a scenario complete with all its components may read as follows:

> When I think about my past accomplishments, I become very sad and depressed. I tend to withdraw and hide. I typically wallow in self-pity and think, "What have I done? I hate my past! I hate myself!" Because of my lack of great success, I believe I am a complete failure.

From two assessment interviews designed to evaluate suitability for short-term cognitive therapy (Safran & Segal, 1990), a third-party observer constructs one to three scenarios that he/she considers to be clinically relevant and representative of the patient's presenting problems. These scenarios are combined with others that are considered to be less relevant in order to total five scenarios altogether. The other scenarios are extracted from other patients who were previous subjects or participants in a pilot study and also presented with similar problems. They are incorporated in order to establish through a process of discrimination the clinical relevance of the scenarios.

The 5 scenarios are then broken down into their respective components, a procedure adapted from one devised by the Mount Zion Group for case formulations (Curtis, Silberchatz, Weiss, Sampson, & Rosenberg, 1988). Each component is separated into a single sentence or statement. Only the stem "I have great difficulty . . . " is added as a constant to the dependent clauses representing the stimulus situations in order to complete the sentences, as, for example, "*I have great difficulty* when I am in social situations." This breakdown of 5 scenarios into their respective 4 components results in 20 items that are randomly distributed and subsequently rated in terms of clinical relevance on a 9-point Likert-type scale by the therapist, the patient, and the third-party observer. Reliability estimates of the self-scenarios are analysed. Adequate interrater reliability has been previously reported with average coefficients ranging from .80 to .93 for each of the components (Muran & Segal, in press; Muran, Segal, & Samstag, 1991).

With the establishment of adequate reliability, the 5 scenarios are reconstructed into their original form and presented to the patient to rate on 8 questions scaled in a 9-point Likert-type format that correspond to the following 8 parameters: Frequency ("How often has such a scenario occurred recently?"), Preoccupation ("How concerned have you been about this happening recently?"), Accessibility ("How easily can you imagine such a scenario?"), Alternatives, ("How easily can you imagine alternatives to this scenario?"), Self-efficacy ("How confident are you about your ability to act on these alternatives?"), Self-view ("How well does this scenario describe you?"), Interpersonal view ("How well does this scenario describe your relationships with others?"), and Chronicity ("How far back in your life can you recall this scenario occurring?"). These ratings are used to further discriminate the most clinically relevant scenarios from the other ones.

SOME RESEARCH FINDINGS WITH SELF-SCENARIOS

At this point, we would like to present some data collected as a result of administering self-scenarios to four depressed outpatients (two males and two females) who received 20 treatment sessions of cognitive-interpersonal therapy. Their ages ranged from 32 to 41. The female patients were diagnosed as dysthymic; the male patients were diagnosed as having double depression. At intake, they completed the Social Desirability Scale (SDS) (Crowne & Marlowe, 1960), on which they scored a mean of 6.0 (SD = 2.5), which suggested no contaminating response sets. They also completed the Symptom Checklist-90 (SCL-90) (Derogatis, 1977) at intake, termination, and a 3-month follow-up. In short, results examining reliable change (RC) (Jacobson & Truax, 1991) on the Global Severity Index (GSI) of the SCL-90 indicated that there were some insignficant gains on average from intake to termination (RC = 1.06, p = .29), and that there was, on average, some significant movement toward relapse by follow-up (RC = 1.41, p = .16).

All the patients completed the 20-item rating form pertaining to their self-scenarios after the 1st session, and the ratings on all 5 of their scenarios after the 2nd session, from which the clinically relevant scenarios were discriminated. From the 3rd to the 20th and at follow-up, they received only the clinically relevant scenarios and completed the corresponding ratings after each session. The mean number of clinically relevant scenarios per patient was 2.5 (SD = .5). These scenarios were rated on the items for all the parameters, except Chronicity, which only required a single rating and received a mean rating of 7.8 (*SD* = .6). The therpists who conducted the assessment interviews and the third-party observers completed the 20-item rating form within one week of the 2nd and final interview session.

Interrater reliability was calculated immediately after the first therapy session, when all three participants in each case had completed the 20-item ratings. Adequate reliability was established with the four cases, with ratings between interviewer and patient averaging .83 (*SD* = .11) for stimulus situation, .83 (*SD* = .10) for affective component, .86 (*SD* = .08) for motoric, and .86 (*SD* = .09) for cognitive; ratings among interviewer, patient, and observer averaged .91 (*SD* = .04) for stimulus situation, .92 (*SD* = .03) for affective component, .94 (*SD* = .03) for motoric, and .92 (*SD* = .04) for cognitive.

The results regarding the parameters of the self-scenarios as rated across treatment are presented in Figures 5.1 through 5.7. The figures represent ratings averaged across the four patients and collapsed into 4-session segments, which translates into session quintets, or 5 data points per parameter (e.g., the first session quintet equaled 1 through 4). Accordingly, the patients experienced fewer occurrences of their problematic scenarios across treatment and through follow-up (Figure 5.1). Similarly, they reported less preoccupation with the possible occurrence of these scenarios (Figure 5.2). Their ability to access or imagine such scenarios, though, remained fairly high and constant throughout (Figure 5.3). As for their ability to generate alternatives (Figure 5.4) and their confidence in enacting these alternatives (Figure 5.5), both demonstrated substantial improvement that continued through follow-up. Their sense of self-efficacy (Figure 5.5), however, never reached more than a modest rating level.

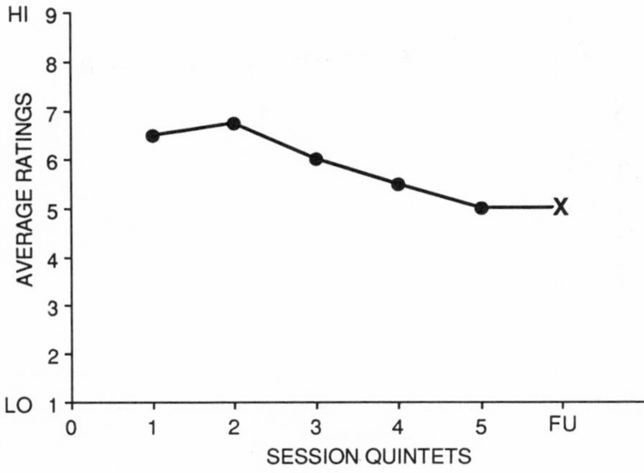

FIGURE 5.1. Frequency.

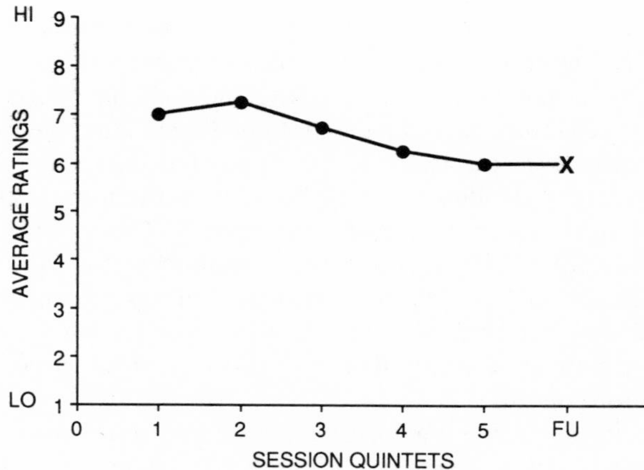

FIGURE 5.2. Preoccupation.

As for how representative these scenarios were of themselves (Figure 5.6) and their relations with others (Figure 5.7), modest movement was evidenced, and the problematic scenarios remained highly representative even at follow-up.

The final three figures (Figures 5.5–5.7) probably best account for the marginal indications of change and relapse. Considering the chronic nature of the depression reported by all the patients, and the short-term nature of the treatment itself, it seems hardly unusual to see such dis-

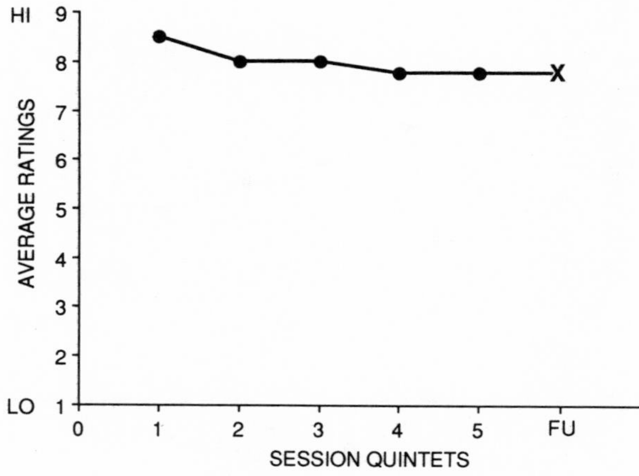

FIGURE 5.3. Accessibility.

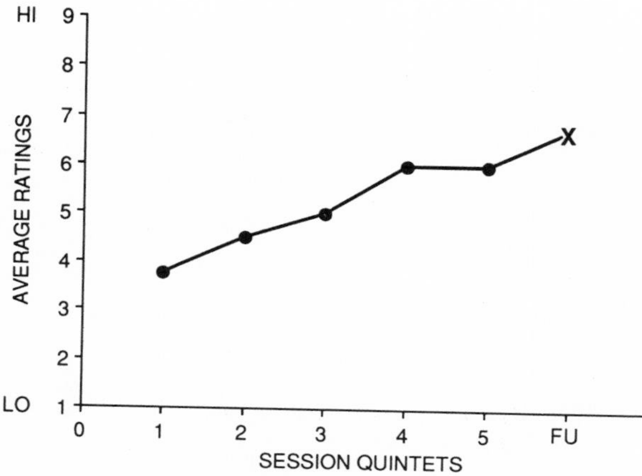

FIGURE 5.4. Alternatives.

appointing outcome results. As for evaluating the sensitivity of self-scenarios as a schematic measure, ratings on the parameters of Self-efficacy, Self-view, and Interpersonal view seem to reflect the lack of significant gains and to predict the trend toward relapse. Of course, these findings are preliminary and in need of further replication, but they are promising and suggest the value of using idiographic vignettes and exploring multiple scaling parameters in order to capture the complicated nature of schematic activity.

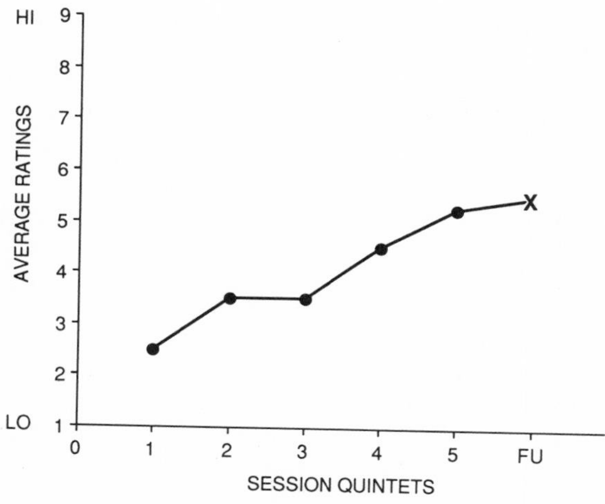

FIGURE 5.5. Self-efficacy.

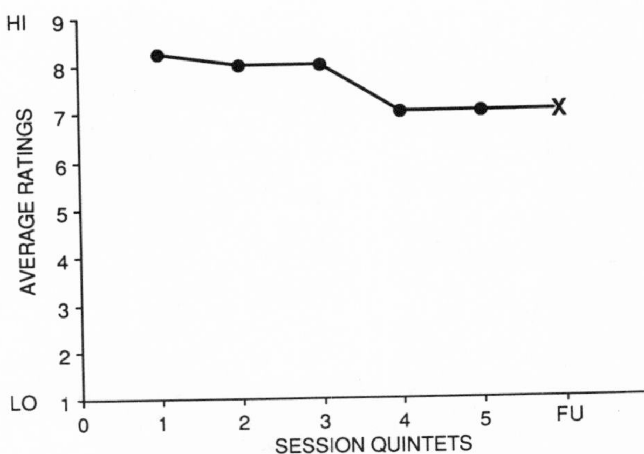

FIGURE 5.6. Self-view

SUMMARY

The idea that the self-view of depressed patients offers them little more than a devalued and consistently inferior sense of who they are is a compelling clinical feature of this disorder. Only recently have cognitive theories of depression begun to acknowledge that this may be a fruitful staring point for interventions aimed at alleviating the suffering caused by depression, as well as modeling the process by which people either become depressed or

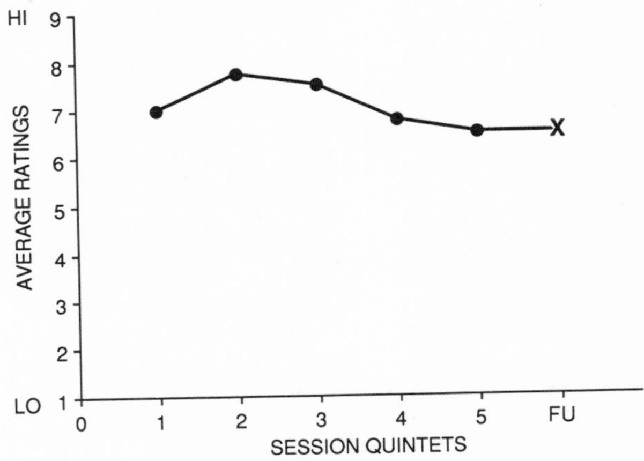

FIGURE 5.7. Interpersonal view.

experience depression following recovery (Segal & Dobson, 1992). The variety of measures developed to tap into self-representation have been closely allied to conceptions of the self in social and cognitive psychologies and have provided some evidence of a possible organization for attributes that are both self-relevant and problematic. The continuing challenge in this area will be to refine our understanding of the nature of the material represented, determine whether the content is specifically depressogneic, explain the interaction of environmental adversity and cognitive structures to produce depression, and give greater consideration to priming the constructs we are interested in testing.

At this point we can admit to having supported some of the more durable aspects of clinical descriptions of depressive self-representation, but better maps of the terrain in front of us are required if we are to try to work toward changing the landscape in favor of one that is less inclined toward depressive experience.

REFERENCES

Abelson, R. P. (1981). Psychological status of a script concept. *American Psychologist, 36*, 715–729.

Abramson, L. Y., Metalsky, G. I., & Alloy, L. B. (1989). The hopelessness theory of depression: A metatheoretical analysis with implications for psychopathology research. *Psychological Review, 96*, 358–372.

Alba, J. W., & Hasher, L. (1983). Is memory schematic? *Psychological Bulletin, 93*, 207–231.

Alexander, I. E. (1988). Personality, psychological assessment, and psychobiography. *Journal of Personality, 56*, 265–294.

American Psychiatric Association. (1987). *Diagnostic and statistical manual of mental disorders* (3rd ed. rev.). Washington, DC: Author.

Arieti, S. (1977). Psychotherapy of severe depression. *American Journal of Psychiatry, 134*, 397–406.

Arieti, S., & Bemporad, J. (1980). The psychological organization of depression. *American Journal of Psychiatry, 137*, 1360–1365.

Auerbach, C. (1985). What is a self? A constructivist theory. *Psychotherapy, 22*, 743–746.

Bartlett, F. C. (1932). *Remembering.* London: Cambridge University Press.

Beck, A. T. (1967). Depression: Clinical, experimental and theoretical aspects. New York: Harper & Row.

Beck, A. T. (1976). Cognitive therapy and the emotional disorders. New York: International Universities Press.

Beck, A. T. (1983). Cognitive therapy of depression: New perspectives. In P. J. Clayton & J. E. Barrett (Eds.), *Treatment of depression: Old controversies and new developments* (pp. 265–290). New York: Raven Press.

Beck, A. T., Rush, A. J., Shaw, B. F., & Emery, G. (1979). *Cognitive therapy of depression:* New York: Guilford Press.

Beckham, E. E. (1990). Psychotherapy of depression research at crossroads: Direction for the 1990's. *Clinical Psychological Review, 10*, 207–228.

Belsher, G., & Costello, C. G. (1988). Relapse after recovery from unipolar depression: A critical review. *Psychological Bulletin, 104*, 84–96.

Berti Ceroni, G., Neri, C., & Pezzoli, A. (1984) Chronicity in major depression: A naturalistic prospective study. *Journal of Affective Disorders, 7*, 123–132.

Bibring, E. (1953). The mechanism of depression. In P. Greenacre (Ed.), *Affective disorders* (pp. 13–48). New York: International Universities Press.

Blaney, P. H. (1986). Affect and memory: A review. *Psychological Bulletin, 99*, 229–246.

Blaney, P. H., & Kutcher, G. S. (1991). Measures of depressive dimensions: Are they interchangeable? *Journal of Personality Assessment*, *56*, 502–512.

Blatt, S., Quinlan, D., Chevron, E., McDonald, C., & Zuroff, D. (1982). Dependency and self-criticism: Psychological dimensions for depression. *Journal of Consulting and Clinical Psychology*, *50*, 113–124.

Bobrow, D. G., & Norman, D. A. (1975). Some principles of memory schemata. In D. G. Bobrow & N. Collins (Eds.), *Representation and understanding: Studies in cognitive science* (pp. 131–149). New York: Academic Press.

Bower, G. H. (1981). Mood and memory. *American Psychologist*, *36*, 129–148.

Bower, G. H., & Cohen, P. R. (1982). Emotional influences in memory and thinking: Data and theory. In M. S. Clark & S. T. Fiske (Eds.), *Affect and cognition* (pp. 241–331). Hillsdale, NJ: Lawrence Erlbaum.

Bowlby, J. (1969). *Attachment and loss: Vol. 1. Attachment*. New York: Basic Books.

Brewer, W. F., & Treyens, J. C. (1981). Role of schemata in memory for places. *Cognitive Psychology*, *13*, 207–230.

Bruner, J. S. (1957). On perceptual readiness. *Psychological Review*, *64*, 123–152.

Cantor, N. (1990). From thought to behavior: "Having" and "doing" in the study of personality and cognition. *American Psychologist*, *45*, 735–750.

Carlson, R. (1981). Studies in script theory: Adult analogs of a childhood nuclear scene. *Journal of Personality and Social Psychology*, *40*, 501–510.

Craik, F. I. M., & Tulving, E. (1975). Depths of processing and the retention of words in episodic memory. *Journal of Experimental Psychology: General*, *104*, 268–294.

Crowne, D., & Marlowe, D. (1960). A new scale of social desirability independent of psychopathology. *Journal of Consulting Psychology, 24*, 349–354.

Curtis, J. T., Silberchatz, G., Weiss, J., Sampson, H., & Rosenberg, S. E. (1988). Developing reliable psychodynamic case formulations: An illustration of the plan diagnosis method. *Psychotherapy*, *25*, 256–265.

Derogatis, L. (1977). *The SCL-90 manual: Scoring and administrative procedures.* Baltimore: Clinical Psychometric Research.

Derry, P. A., & Kuiper, N. A. (1981). Schematic processing and self-reference in clinical depression. *Journal of Abnormal Psychology*, *90*, 286–297.

Dobson, K. S., & Shaw, B. F. (1986). Cognitive assessment with major depressive disorders. *Cognitive Therapy and Research, 10*, 13–29.

Dunn, R. J. (1985). Issues of self-concept deficit in psychotherapy. *Psychotherapy*, *22*, 747–751.

Eaves, G., & Rush, A. J. (1984). Cognitive patterns in symptomatic and remitted unipolar major depression. *Journal of Abnormal Psychology, 93*, 31–40.

Ferguson, T., Rule, B., & Carlson, D. (1983). Memory for persistently relevant information. *Journal of Personality and Social Psychology, 44*, 251–261.

Gergen, K. J., & Gergen, M. M. (1988). Narrative and the self as relationship. In L. Berkowitz (Ed.), *Advances in experimental social psychology* (Vol. 21, 176). New York: Academic Press.

Giles, D. E., & Rush, A. J. (1983). Cognitions, schemas, and depressive symptomatology. In M. Rosenbaum, C. M. Franks, & Y. Jaffe (Eds.), *Perspectives on behavior therapy* (pp. 184–199). New York: Springer-Verlag.

Gotlib, I. H., & Cane, D. B. (1987). Construct accessibility and clinical depression: A longitudinal investigation. *Journal of Abnormal Psychology, 96*, 199–204.

Gotlib, I. H., & McCann, C. D. (1984). Construct accessibility and depression: An examination of cognitive and affective factors. *Journal of Personality and Social Psychology, 47*, 427–439.

Hammen, C. L. (1985). Predicting depression: A cognitive- behavioral perspective. In P. C. Kendall (Ed.), *Advances in cognitive-behavioral research and therapy* (Vol. 4, pp. 30–74) New York: Academic Press.

Hammen, C. (1991). *Depression runs in families.* New York: Springer-Verlag.

Hammen, C., Ellicott, A., Gitlin, M., & Jamison, K. R. (1989). Sociotropy/autonomy and vulnerability to specific life events in unipolar and bipolar patients. *Journal of Abnormal Psychology, 98*, 154–160.

Hammen, C., & Goodman-Brown, T. (1990). Self-schemas and vulnerability to specific life stress in children at risk for depression. *Cognitive Therapy and Research, 14*(2), 215–227.

Hammen, C., Marks, T., Mayol, A., & deMayo, R. (1985). Depressive self-schemas, life stress, and vulnerability to depression: *Journal of Abnormal Psychology, 94*, 308–319.

Harter, S. (1990). Developmental differences in the nature of self-representations: Implications for the understanding, assessment, and treatment of maladaptive behavior. *Cognitive Therapy and Research, 14*, 113–142.

Higgins, E. T., & Bargh, J. A. (1987). Social cognition and social perception. *Annual Review of Psychology, 38*, 369–425.

Higgins, E. T., & King, G. A. (1981). Accessibility of social constructs: Information-processing consequences of individual and contextual variability. In N. Cantor & J. F. Kihlstrom (Eds.), *Personality, cognition, and social interaction* (pp. 69–121). Hillsdale, NJ: Lawrence Erlbaum.

Higgins, E. T., King, G. A., & Mavin, G. H. (1982). Individual construct accessibility and subjective impressions and recall. *Journal of Personality and Social Psychology, 43*, 35–47.

Higgins, E. T., Van Hook, E., & Dorfman, D. (1988). Do self-attributes form a cognitive structure? *Social Cognition, 6*, 177–207.

Hirschfeld, R. M. A., Klerman, G. L., Clayton, P. J., & Keller, M. B. (1983). Personality and depression: Empirical findings. *Archives of General Psychiatry, 40*, 993–998.

Hollon, S. D., Kendall, P. C., & Lumry, A. (1986). Specificity of depressotypic cognitions in clinical depression. *Journal of Abnormal Psychology, 95*, 29–52.

Isen, A. M. (1984). Affect, cognition and social behavior. In R. S. Wyer & T. R. Srull (Eds.), *Handbook of social cognition* (Vol. 3, pp. 179–236). Hillsdale, NJ: Lawrence Erlbaum.

Jacobson, N. S., & Truax, P. (1991). Clinical significance: A statistical approach to defining meaningful change in psychotherapy research. *Journal of Consulting and Clinical Psychology, 59,* 12–19.

Keller, M. B., Lavori, P. W., Endicott, J., Coryell, W., & Klerman, G. L. (1983). "Double Depression": A two-year follow-up. *American Journal of Psychiatry, 148,* 689–694.

Keller, M. B., Lavori, P. W., Lewis, C. E., & Klerman, G. L. (1983). Predictors of relapse in major depressive disorder. *Journal of the American Medical Association, 250,* 3299–3304.

Kelly, G. A. (1955). *The psychology of personal constructs: A theory of personality* (2 vols.). New York: Norton.

Kihlstrom, J. F., & Cantor, N. (1984). Mental representations of the self. In L. Berkowitz (Ed.), *Advances in experimental social psychology* (Vol. 15, pp. 1–47). New York: Academic Press.

Kovacs, M., Beck, A. T. (1978). Maladaptive cognitive structures in depression. *American Journal of Psychiatry, 135,* 525–533.

Kuiper, N. A., & Derry, P. A. (1982). Depressed and nondepressed content self-reference in mild depressives. *Journal of Personality, 50,* 67–80.

Kuiper, N. A., & MacDonald, M. R. (1983). Self and other perception in mild depressives. *Social Cognition, 1,* 223–239.

Kuiper, N. A., & Olinger, L. J. (1986). Dysfunctional attitudes and a self-worth contingency model of depression. In P. C. Kendall (Ed.), *Advances in cognitive-behavioral research and therapy* (pp. 115–142). Orlando, FL: Academic Press.

Lamiell, J. T. (1981). Toward an idiothetic psychology of personality. *American Psychologist, 36,* 276–289.

Lang, P. (1985). The congitive psychopathology of emotion, fear and anxiety. In A. Tuma & J. Maser (Eds.), *Anxiety and anxiety disorders* (pp. 131–170). Hillsdale, NJ: Lawrence Erlbaum.

Leventhal, H. (1984). A perceptual-motor theory of emotion. In L. Berkowitz (Ed.), *Advances in experimental social psychology* (Vol. 17, pp. 117–182). New York: Academic Press.

Lewinsohn, P. M., Steinmetz, J. L., Larson, D. W., & Franklin, J. (1981). Depression-related cognitions: Antecedent or consequence? *Journal of Abnormal Psychology, 90,* 213–219.

Luborsky, L., & Crits-Christoph, P. (1990). *Understanding transference: The CCRT method.* New York: Basic Books.

MacLeod, C. M. (1991). Half a century of research on the Stroop effect: An integrative review. *Psychological Bulletin, 109,* 163–203.

Markus, H. (1977). Self-schemata and processing information about the self. *Journal of Personality and Social Psychology, 35,* 63–67.

Markus, H. (1990). Unresolved issues of self-representation. *Cognitive Therapy and Research, 14,* 241–253.

Markus, H., & Nurius, P. (1986). Possible selves. *American Psychologist, 41,* 954–969.

Matlin, M. W., & Stang, D. J. (1978). *The Pollyanna principle: Selectivity in language, memory and thought*. Cambridge, MA: Schenkman.

Miranda, J., Persons, J. B., & Byers, C. N. (1990). Endorsement of dysfunctional beliefs depends on current mood state. *Journal of Abnormal Psychology, 99,* 237–241.

Muran, J. C. (1991). A reformulation of the ABC model: Implications for assessment and treatment. *Clinical Psychology Review, 11,* 399–418.

Muran, J. C., & Segal, Z. V. (in press). The development of an idiographic measure of self-schemas: An illustration of the construction and use of self-scenarios. *Psychotherapy*.

Muran, J. C., Segal, Z. V., & Samstag, W. (1991). *The use of self-scenarios as an idiographic measure of self-schemas.* Paper presented at the Society for Psychotherapy Research, Lyon, France.

Myers, J. K., Weissman, M. M., Tischler, C. E., Holzer, C. E., Orvaschel, H, Anthony, J. C., Boyd, J. H., Burke, J. D., Kramer, M., & Stoltzman, R. (1984). Six-month prevalence of psychiatric disorders in three communities. *Archives of General Psychiatry*, *41*, 959–967.

Neisser, U. (1976). *Cognition and reality: Principles and implications of cognitive psychology*. San Francisco: Freeman.

Neisser, U. (1988). Five kinds of self-knowledge. *Philosophical Psychology*, *1*, 35–59.

Nelson, K., & Greundel, J. M. (1981). Generalized event representations: Basic building blocks of cognitive development. In M. E. Lamb & A. L. Brown (Eds.), *Advances in developmental psychology* (Vol. 1). Hillsdale, NJ: Lawrence Erlbaum.

Nietzel, M. T, & Harris, M. J. (1990). Relationship of dependency and achievement/autonomy to depression. *Clinical Psychology Review*, *10*, 279–297.

Piaget, J. (1954). *The construction of reality in the child*. New York: Basic Books.

Posner, M. I., & Warren, R. E. (1972). Traces, concepts and conscious contructions. In A. W. Melton & E. Martin (Eds.), *Coding processes in human memory* (pp. 25–43). Washington, DC: Winston.

Rehm, L. P. (1977). A self control model of depression. *Behavior Therapy, 8,* 787–804.

Riskind, J.H., & Rholes, W. S. (1984). Cognitive accessibility and the capacity of cognitions to predict future depression: A theoretical note. *Cognitive Therapy and Research*, *8*, 1–12.

Rogers, T. B., Kuiper, N. A., & Kirker, W. S. (1977). Self-reference and the coding of personal information. *Journal of Personality and Social Psychology*, *35*, 677–688.

Rosenberg, S. (1988). Self and others: Studies in social personality and autobiography. In L. Berkowitz (Ed.), *Advances in experimental social psychology* (Vol. 21, pp. 57–95). New York: Academic Press.

Rohde, P., Lewinsohn, P. M., & Seeley, J. R. (1990). Are people changed by the experience of having an episode of depression: A further test of the scar hypothesis. *Journal of Abnormal Psychology*, *99*, 264–271.

Rumelhart, D. E. (1975). Notes on a schema for stories. In D. G. Bobrow & A. M. Collins (Eds.), *Representation and understanding* (pp. 211–236). New York: Academic Press.

Safran, J. D. (1990). Towards a refinement of cognitive therapy in light of interpersonal theory: Theory. *Clinical Psychology Review, 10*, 87–105.

Safran, J. D., & Segal, Z. V. (1990). *Interpersonal process in cognitive therapy*. New York: Basic Books.

Safran, J. D., Segal, Z. V., Hill, C., & Whiffen, V. (1990). Refining strategies for research on self-representations in emotional diorders. *Cognitive Therapy and Research, 14*, 143–160.

Schank, R., & Abelson, R. (1977). *Scripts, plans, goals and understanding: An inquiry into human knowledge structures*. Hillsdale, NJ: Lawrence Erlbaum.

Segal, Z. V. (1988). Appraisal of the self-schema construct in cognitive models of depression. *Psychological Bulletin, 103*, 147–162.

Segal, Z. S., & Dobson, K. S. (1992). Cognitive models of depression: Report from a consensus development conference. *Psychological Inquiry, 3*, 219–224.

Segal, Z. V., Hood, J. E., Shaw, B. F., & Higgins, E. T. (1988). A structural analysis of the self-schema construct in major depression. *Cognitive Therapy and Research, 12*, 471–485.

Segal, Z. V., & Shaw, B. F. (1986). Cognition in depression: A reappraisal of Coyne and Gotlib's critique. *Cognitive Therapy and Research, 10*, 671–693.

Segal, Z. V., Shaw, B. F., Vella, D. D., & Katz, R. (1992). Cognitive and life stress predictors of relapse in remitted unipolar depressed patients: A test of the congruency hypothesis. *Journal of Abnormal Psychology, 101*, 26–36.

Segal, Z. V., & Vella, D. D. (1990). Self-schema in major depression: Replication and extension of a priming methodology. *Cognitive Therapy and Research, 14*, 161–176.

Seligman, M. E. P. (1975). *Helplessness*. San Francisco: W. H. Freeman.

Shiffrin, R. M., & Schneider, W. (1977). Controlled and automatic human information processing: 2. Perceptual learning, automatic attending, and a general theory. *Psychological Review, 84*, 127–190.

Stroop, J. R. (1935). Studies of interference in serial verbal reactions. *Journal of Experimental Psychology, 18*, 643–662.

Sturt, E., Kumakura, N., & Der, G. (1984). How depressing life is: Life morbidity risk for depressive disorder in the general population. *Journal of Affective Disorders, 7*, 104–122.

Taylor, S. E., & Crocker, J. (1981). Schematic bases of social information processing. In E. T. Higgins, M. P. Herman, & M. P. Zanna (Eds.), *The Ontario Symposium in Personality and Social Psychology* (Vol. 1, pp. 89–134). Hillsdale, NJ: Lawrence Erlbaum.

Teasdale, J. D., & Dent, J. (1987). Cognitive vulnerability to depression: An investigation of two hypotheses. *British Journal of Clinical Psychology, 26*, 113–126.

Teasdale, J. D., & Russell, M. L. (1983). Differential effects of induced mood and the recall of positive, negative and neutral words. *British Journal of Clinical Psychology, 22*, 162–172.

Teller, V., & Dahl, H. (1986). The microstructure of free association. *Journal of the American Psychiatric Association, 34*, 763–798.

Tompkins, S. (1987). Script theory. In V. Aronoff, A. A. Rabin, & R. Zucker (Eds.), *The emergence of personality* (pp. 147–216). New York: Springer-Verlag.

Uleman, J. A., & Bargh, J. A. (Eds.) (1989). *Unintended thought*. New York: Guilford Press.

Van Valkenburg, C., Akiskal, H. W., Puzantian, V., & Rosenthal, T. (1984). Anxious depression: Clinical family history and naturalistic outcome. Comparisons with panic and major depressive disorders. *Journal of Affective Disorders, 6*, 67–82.

Weissman, A. N. (1979). The Dysfunctional Attitude Scale: A validation study (Doctoral dissertation, University of Pennsylvania, 1978). *Dissertation Abstracts International, 40*, 1389B–1390B.

Williams, J. M. G., Watts, F. N., MacLeod, C., & Mathews, A. (1988). *Cognitive psychology and emotional disorders*. New York: Wiley.

Wyer, R. S., & Srull, T. K. (1986). Human cognition in its social context. *Psychological Review, 93*, 322–359.

Zuroff, D. C., & Mongrain, M. (1987). Dependency and self-criticism: Vulnerability factors for depressive affective states. *Journal of Abnormal Psychology, 96*, 14–22.

Commentary

SIDNEY J. BLATT
SUSAN A. BERS
Yale University

IN OUR DISCUSSION of the provocative chapter by Segal and Muran on self-representation in depression, we will consider both the divergences and convergences of their formulations from a cognitive–behavioral orientation with more psychodynamic approaches in the hope of facilitating an integration of the two perspectives and promoting a fuller understanding of the nature, etiology, and treatment of serious psychological disturbances, especially depression.

Segal and Muran define self-schema as the rules, standards, and strategies that individuals use to evaluate, guide, and control their behavior. Throughout much of their chapter, however, Segal and Muran focus on the content of self-schemas as the composite of specific interrelated words or attributes (adjectives and nouns). They believe that depressogenic schemas can be identified primarily by the verbal content of the self-schema. The authors review a wide range of research that demonstrates how particular negative attributes are linked together in a semantic network in depression and how these attributes can be activated, noting that "extreme nondescriptors" also show some evidence of interconnectedness and structural organization in the self-schema. Segal and Muran view the network of extreme nondescriptors as forming a "negative boundary condition" that contributes to the formation of the self-schema. But they fail to consider the possibility that there may be a close relationship between those terms designated as descriptors and those as extreme nondescriptors. Extreme nondescriptors may be defensively related to the fundamental issues expressed in aspects of the descriptors included in the self-schema. Extreme nondescriptors may be important to consider as a dynamic part of the network of descriptors, since they may reflect dimensions that are being defensively avoided by certain facets of the self-schema. Although much of Segal and Muran's formulations are organized around the analyses of the content of single-word attributes that define the self-schema, they seem to recognize the limitations of this approach in their concern that thus far there is no "complete account of how schemas are formed and what is actually represented." Segal and Muran discuss negative self-schemas as the central construct in depression, but they provide no way of considering how or why these negative self-schemas are established and maintained. Are there developmental and motivational dimensions to these self-schemas? What determines the hierarchy of different dimensions of these negative self-schemas? Which elements become the target of intensive elaborations? In attempting to develop therapeutic methods for revising negative schemas, it might be useful to understand some of the motivational factors that led to their formation and that contribute to their maintenance and current activation. Elucidation of these motivational dimensions could help us not only to understand current experiences of depression, but also to identify a vulnerability to depression.

Although Segal and Muran mention that affects and interpersonal relationships are an important part of self-schemas, much of the research they cite pays little, if any, attention to these dimensions. They are aware of the importance of affective, motoric, and interpersonal dimensions of self-schemas, but they consider only cognitive dimensions—the individual attributes (adjectives or nouns) that they assume to be the essential structure of self-schemas and attributional styles. The role of affect is not only ignored in most cognitive–behavioral considerations of self-schemas, but it is often considered an impediment to the assessment of them. Rather than viewing the self-schema as a cognitive–affective structure, research from a cognitive–behavioral orientation often attempts to eliminate or control current mood as possibly confounding the assessment of schemas. Evidence that depressed patients in remission show little residual deficit that would be characteristic of a vulnerability to depression (e.g., Lewinsohn & Rosenblum, 1987), for example, leads some cognitive-behaviorists to the conclusion that current mood states can often contaminate the expression of cognitive structures, including self-schemas. Segal and Muran, however, question the experimental procedures used in Lewinsohn and Rosenblum's study because of their failure to include a priming procedure in studying the cognitive structures of previously depressed patients. More basic, however, is the importance of including affect as an essential part of cognitive schema, especially self-schema in depression. More vulnerable patients in remission may try to avoid some of the issues related to their difficulties, but other previously depressed individuals, who are more integrated and less vulnerable, may be responsive to issues related to their previous difficulties because these issues no longer pose a serious threat to them. Thus, it may be more productive to include affective dimensions as an integral part of a self-schema—to view schemas as cognitive–affective structures, and to evaluate relationships between the cognitive and affective components of schemas. This position would allow investigators to consider the apparent paradox of a high recidivism rate in depression noted by Segal and Muran along with indications that depressed patients in remission show little evidence of a vulnerability to depression. Both cognition and affect must be considered essential elements of schemas, especially schemas of the self.

Segal and Muran report an increasing interest among cognitive–behavioral investigators in assessing cognitions that are out of awareness, because they assume that these schemas are less influenced by mood. "Automatic thoughts" (thoughts often out of awareness and out of conscious control) are considered to be the product of negative self-schemas and to reveal dysfunctional attitudes implicit in depressogenic self-schemas. We welcome this long overdue recognition by cognitive-behaviorists of the existence of unconscious thought and their beginning appreciation of its importance, even though they still restrict the unconscious to a descriptive unconscious devoid of any motivational components. From a psychodynamic perspective, the unconscious is important because it is likely to be more influenced by affects and to exert more subtle but powerful effects on behavior than more conscious cognitions.

The authors also state that the "interpersonal nature of the self" could shed light on the development and etiology of depressogenic self-schemas, but they present little data or formulations to elaborate this important statement other than to note that self-schemas are "simply" (emphasis added) attributed to learning from early painful experiences. Although Segal and Muran note that appreciating the "role of the other" can help clarify self-schemas, they do not pursue this line of investigation further. We fully agree with their suggestion that there is a need to expand the view of self-schemas to include both affective and interpersonal components, especially those derived from early experiences. This would be very compatible with a psychodynamic perspective.

Segal and Muran express concern that much of the cognitive–behavioral research on self-schemas, especially the research on depressogenic self-schemas, has been seriously hampered by the almost exclusive reliance on self-report inventories. They note that the study of on-line information processing as a methodology could facilitate the study of self-schemas by assessing the latency of response to certain attributes, the number of words endorsed, and the capacity for incidental recall of different types of words. They believe that this methodology has identified important properties of depressive self-schemas, such as the emphasis on negative content and the rapidity with which negative information is processed. Yet Segal and Muran, toward the close of their chapter, report on some of their own recent research in the study of self-schemas in which they have begun to study self-schemas, or self-representations, in terms of narrative structures rather than the processing of discrete words (adjectives and nouns). Based on script theory (e.g., Schank & Abelson, 1977), generalized event representations (e.g., Nelson & Grundel, 1981), nuclear scenes (Tomkins, 1987), and core conflict themes (Luborsky & Crits-Cristoph, 1990), Segal and Muran describe procedures through which they attempt to assess "clinically meaningful and phenomonologically veridical" dimensions by asking subjects for extended vignettes of highly distressful events. In these "self-scenarios," they ask the subjects to describe what people were *thinking, feeling, and doing* (our emphasis) during these distressful events.

It is impressive that in their search for methods for assessing cognitive structures that go beyond pencil-and-paper questionnaires and laboratory tests, Segal and Muran developed a procedure that closely approximates "projective" test procedures, such as the Thematic Apperception Test, in order to study representations of schematic activity in terms of stimulus situations that potentially activate schemas. In so doing, they have moved closer to using unstructured, ambiguous, open-ended stimuli in which the subject (or patient) has substantial input in presenting idiographically constructed schematic activity. In addition, this approach allows the subject to introduce affect (reports of feelings) and relationships with others as part of the schematic activity. Segal and Muran deconstruct and reconstruct these scenarios generated by the patient and then present aspects of these scenarios to the patient, therapist, and an independent judge in order to obtain multiple assessments of the patient's self-schema. In our judgment, this procedure is a welcome, long-overdue, major departure from the more narrow focus that has characterized much of cognitive–behavioral approaches to the study of schemas, one that may have considerable potential for discovering important properties of self-schemas in a wide range of individuals.

Although Segal and Muran report "disappointing outcome results" (e.g., little change) in these scenarios over the course of relatively brief cognitive–behavioral treatment, they quite correctly note the limitations of short-term treatment in treating a chronic condition such as depression. Both in their research to develop more unstructured methods for assessing cognitive structures that are "clinically meaningful and phenomenologically veridical" and in their concern about the limitations of short-term treatment, Segal and Muran have moved to a position in which they now share a great deal with psychodynamic approaches. Another common ground with psychodynamic formulations is the recognition by Segal and Muran that depressive experiences are not determined exclusively by negative life events, but that individual predispositions (e.g., early painful experiences) have an important role in determining an individual's response to contemporary life events. These important developments in the cognition–behavioral position (the recognition of the importance of affects, interpersonal relationships, the unconscious, and early painful life experiences, as well as the limitations of short-term treatment) offer considerable potential for integrating dimensions from both cognitive– behavioral and psychodynamic approaches.

Segal and Muran consider depression to be the consequence of the individual's inability to control events; this failure generates feelings and thoughts of helplessness and hopelessness that become generalized as negative expectations and as a loss of incentive. A person becomes depressed as a consequence of developing an attributional style that contains internal, stable, and global ways of dealing with negative events. These depressive attributes become part of a more generalized depressive self-organization. All individuals, however, occasionally experience negative events over which they feel they have little or no control, yet only a portion of them develops depressive styles in response to such experiences. Segal and Muran give little indication of how or why these depressive schemas develop in only some individuals other than to cite the brief suggestion by Beck (1967) that painful childhood experiences (e.g., loss, deprivation, death of significant other) can lead to these negative self-schemas. Depression occurs when these negative self-schemas are activated by contemporary life events that create circumstances analogous to dimensions central to the depressive schema. The authors note that these negative self-schemas can arise when negative life events "impinge" on rigid, absolute (dysfunctional) attitudes, and lead to a transition from a healthy to a "corrosive" self-regard. But they suggest only a few of the necessary and sufficient conditions that lead to the establishment of these dysfunctional attitudes. Although they are willing to acknowledge that childhood experiences may contribute to the formation of dysfunctional attitudes, Segal and Muran, like many cognitive–behavioral clinicians, seem very reluctant to explore these developmental and motivational dimensions.

Several issues concerning depressive schemas are presented: (1) how these schemas are structured, (2) whether depressive attributes are part of a more general depressive self-organization, and (3) how depressive schemas operate to create experiences of depression. Cognitive–behavioral investigators, while not contributing much to the understanding of how depressive self-schemas are formed, have demonstrated how attributional features of the depressive self-construct contain elements of failure, worthlessness, or rejection, and how these interact with contemporary life events to create and maintain depression. But Segal and Muran raise the important question of whether it is the content of these depressive self-schemas that create a vulnerability to depression or whether vulnerability to depression is a consequence of individuals having greater access to these depressive features. They seem to favor the accessibility hypothesis: that depressive self-representations are composed of negative constructs that come to mind more easily. Self-schemas of depressed patients contain many more negative attributes than those of nondepressed patients and are generally less complex in their organization, but it is the ready access of these depressive elements to consciousness that Segal and Muran consider to be the unique characteristic of the schemas of depressed patients. They make little attempt, however, to understand the specific content of these negative self-schemas and the unique meaning they have for a given individual. Yet, it is these meaning systems that must be the central focus of therapeutic interventions.

Segal and Muran are particularly interested in how these depressive self-representations interact with negative environmental events to create a depressive episode, but they are less concerned with how these depressive self-representations are formed. They accept Beck's (1967) brief statement that painful childhood experiences can lead to negative self-schemas, but like many cognitive–behavioral clinicians, they simply accept the presence of these negative self-schemas as a given, and direct their primary attention to identifying the properties of these schemas, how they are organized, and how they interact with environmental events to create and maintain a depressive experience and a depressive episode. The cognitive content of these depressive self-schemas are primarily negative, and they influence more general information processing by creating a more efficient processing (easier access and quicker identification) of negative information. Segal and Muran conclude that activation of this self-schema by environmental experiences creates a greater likelihood that negative content will come to mind. This conclusion, that the essential feature of a depressive schema is a more efficient and rapid processing system, especially for negative information, is interesting given the evidence that one of the primary indications of depression is motor and ideational inhibition (Miller, 1975).

In summary, a cognitive–behavioral approach has identified some aspects of the cognitive content of depressive self-schemas and how they interact with environmental events, resulting in the depressed patient having more rapid and efficient access to negative ideas than to positive ones. But cognitive–behavioral therapists have not adequately addressed the role of affect and interpersonal relations in this cognitive schema, or how it develops in the first place. Understanding of depression would be greatly facilitated by considering depression not as an isolated clinical entity, but rather as an affect state that can range along a wide continuum from relatively appropriate and transient reactions to painful life events and circumstances to a severe and persistent clinical disorder, which may or may not involve distortions of reality (Blatt, 1974). In such an approach, depressogenic schemas would be considered an integral part of experiences of depression, which may or may not lead to a clinical disorder. In addition to addressing the important question of how these depressogenic schemas activate clinical depression, it would be equally important to ascertain how they are formed. Psychodynamic and cognitive–behavioral approaches agree that life circumstances contribute in important ways to the formation of depressogenic schemas, but they differ in their emphasis on the role of early (as compared to current) life events in both the etiology and treatment of depression. The emphasis placed by Segal and Muran on the important but relatively unexplored role of affect and interpersonal relations in these schemas, at least as studied by cognitive–behavioral investigators, however, provides a potential bridge for the integration of cognitive–behavioral and dynamic approaches that may facilitate our achieving greater understanding of how early and current life experiences both contribute to the creation of depressogenic schemas and depressive experiences. An understanding of the developmental and motivational factors that contribute to the formation and maintenance of depressogenic schemas would enrich, not contradict, the focus of cognitive–behavioral clinicians and investigators on current functioning and the role of contemporary life experiences in depression.

REFERENCES

Beck, A. (1967). *Depression: Clinical, experimental, and theoretical aspects.* New York: Harper & Row.

Blatt, S. J. (1974). Levels of object representation in anaclitic and introjective depression. *Psychoanalytic Study of the Child, 29,* 107–157.

Lewisohn, P. M., & Rosenbaum, M. (1987). Recall of parental behavior by acute depressives, remitted depressives and non-depressives. *Journal of Personality and Social Psychology, 52,* 611–619.

Luborsky, L., & Crits-Christoph, P. (1990). *Understanding transference: The CCRT method.* New York: Basic Books.

Miller, W. R. (1975). Psychological deficit in depression. *Psychological Bulletin, 82,* 238–260.

Nelson, K., & Grundel, J. M. (1981). Generalized event representations: Basic building blocks of cognitive development. In M. E. Lamb & A. L. Brown (Eds.), *Advances in developmental psychology,* (Vol. 1). Hillsdale, NJ: Lawrence Erlbaum.

Shank, R. C., & Abelson, R. (1977). *Scripts, plans, goals and understanding.* Hillsdale, NJ: Lawrence Erlbaum.

Tomkins, S. (1987). Script theory. In V. Aronoff, A. A. Rabin, & R. Zucker (Eds.), *The emergence of personality* (pp. 147–216). New York: Springer-Verlag.

6

The Sense of Self in Depression: A Psychodynamic Perspective

SIDNEY J. BLATT
SUSAN A. BERS
Yale University

THE SELF AND depression are complex and controversial concepts that have multiple definitions, even within a psychodynamic perspective. Consistent with the contemporary emphasis in psychodynamic thought, we approach both the concept of the self and that of depression from a phenomenological perspective.

The sense of self is central to experiences of depression; depression always involves a fundamental distortion of the self. Distortions in the sense of self are often an expression of, or a defense against, depression. Various forms of narcissism, for example, can be a defense against depression (Blatt, 1983).

The relationship between depression and distortions, or impairments, in the sense of self is complex and multidimensional and can occur at different developmental levels. One can articulate at least three developmental levels in the evolution of the sense of self and consider the relationship of the self at each of these levels to different types of depressive experiences. More specifically, we distinguish among a rudimentary, an introjected, and a mature level of self. The quality of the depressed sense of self at the first two levels of self, a rudimentary and an introjected level of self, is often expressed in two types of depressive experiences: feelings of loneliness and abandonment or feelings of self-criticism and a lack of self-worth. We initially approach these issues theoretically, and subsequently present both research and clinical data to indicate how this approach contributes to a fuller understanding of the sense of self in depression. In our research, we first examine the relationship of a sense of self to experiences of depression in a group of normal young adults, then we compare differences in the sense of self between patients and nonpatients, and finally, based on these differences, we consider changes in the sense of self of a young, psychotically depressed, adolescent female inpatient over 1½ years of intensive treatment.

A PHENOMENOLOGICAL APPROACH TO THE SELF

The sense of self is primarily a subjective experience; it is the locus of affective experiences (I feel), the source of a sense of agency (I do), and the basis for a sense of self-awareness and self-reflectivity (I am). The experiences of affect, agency, and reflective self-awareness define the self in ways that are consistent with the experiential aspects of traditional psychoanalytic thought, such as the topographic model with its specification of levels of consciousness and awareness. But a phenomenological conceptualization of the self is inconsistent with a more external (e.g., objective and functional) view of psychological functioning based on concepts from the psychoanalytic structural model of the mind as ego, id, and superego. These two perspectives, the external/objective and the internal/subjective, each provide important independent and complementary insights about mental life. These two perspectives, however, also create a dynamic tension, or a fundamental paradox, about mental life that is dominant throughout much of psychoanalytic theory in its various attempts to create an objective science of subjective experiences.

The self can be considered a structure of the mind—the perceiver of one's own means, the organizer of one's perception, and the intending agent of one's actions. But these attempts to link a phenomenological analysis of self to the structural ego often lead to contradictory formulations. A focus on the functional (adaptive and defensive) dimensions of the mind often obscures the articulation of the subjective or phenomenological dimensions of the self as both agent and object. The shift from an objective study of the mind to the study of the subjective world, a shift from the experientially distant to the experientially near, is now a dominant emphasis in contemporary psychoanalytic thought.

It is difficult to create an objective science of subjective experiences because there is a fundamental indeterminacy to the subjective. We can never observe directly the experiences of another; we have access only to derivative phenomena, to verbal reports or resultant actions that are expressions of subjective experiences. In everyday interactions, as well as in the analytic process, we are largely dependent upon the ability and willingness of others to observe and report their experiences. The major access to the experiences of the other is through participation in a relationship with the other—participation, for example, in the special conversations of a therapeutic relationship. The analyst is brought into the matrix of the individual's internal processes and experiences through the analysand's enactments in the transference. Through empathic participation in the transformations of the transference, the analyst can become an observer of the other's subjective experiences. Transference enactments, along with unconscious dimensions expressed in the complexities of verbalizations, provide the analyst with glimpses of the individual's unconscious intentions and subjective experiences and the opportunity to approximate dimensions of the patient's contemporary as well as earlier experiences.

We come to know the experiential self primarily in the same way it is formed: in a relational context. The emotional dialogue between infant and mother (and between analysand and analyst) leads to the emergence of the sense of the self both as agent and as the object of another's desire. The sense of being an object precedes the emergences of the sense of self as subject, but eventually the individual establishes the self as subject by positing another person, exterior to self, as the other. This other is the object of desire, and the subject begins to define more explicitly the self as subject in the wish to establish an affective relationship with the other. Although the self as subject is transcendent to the self as object, the individual eventually becomes aware that he/she also exists as an object, as a you, for the other. Thus, the self–other polarity enables the individual to construct both an internal reality and an external reality. The recognition that both the self and the other exist simultaneously as subject and object facilitates the distinction between the subjective and the objective, as well as the eventual recognition that this distinction is often arbitrary and elusive. The relationship between oneself and another, the experience of simultaneously being both the subject and the object, is central to the individual's capacity to appreciate the subjective, as well as the limitations of the distinction between internal and external, between subjective and objective.[1]

The self as both subject and object exists only in the context of a relationship. The experience of the self develops a fixed meaning and a continuity, but it also continues to derive meaning from the situations in which it exists. These formulations are congruent with aspects of Modell's (1984) view that self is a stable configuration or structure based on prior internalizations, as well as an "evanescent internal perception" whose very existence is determined by, and dependent on, ongoing environmental nutriments and affective communication; the self "takes form from the immediacy of experience" (Modell, 1985, p. 75).

The self is the essence of the subjective: *I* feel, *I* think, *I* am. The self-reflective sense of self—I am—is based on the other two fundamental dimensions of self: (1) the locus of affective experience and (2) the source of agency and intentionality. The *I* as the locus of all subjective experience is an essential part of the developmental transition of experiencing affect as primarily provocative stimuli for discharge, to affect as signals and signs that convey emotional meanings, affective tones and nuances, and personal values (Blatt, 1983). Tomkins (1963) and Izard (1972), for example, noted that affects are initially the regulators of interpersonal interactions, but with the development of the self, affects also become the basis for communication both within the self and with others. The development of the sense of self is also vital for the development of the sense of agency, for the experience of an intentionality of action and of desire; thus, the sense of self has at least a dual dimensionality, as the locus both of affective experience and of agency and intentionality. The self is also the locus for a sense of being as well as a capacity for doing (Erlich & Blatt, 1985). These two functions of the self—affective experience and regulation as well as agency and intentionality—along with a capacity for self-reflectivity, are major developmental milestones in the progression to emotional and psychological maturity.[2]

Developmental Antecedents of the Self

The Rudimentary Self

A formulation of the self based on the integration of a phenomenological perspective with object relations theory enables us to appreciate more fully the developmental antecedents of the self. The self as the locus of affective experiences and the experience of agency emerges from the parent's willingness and capacity to address the child as a partner and to share affective experiences and verbal expressions. The parent's unwillingness or inability to provide these experiences for the child results in a depleted or impaired sense of self, as found in depressed and disturbed individuals.

The sharing of need gratification and affective communication in a context of attachment (Lichtenstein, 1977) and the development of mastery and competence (e.g, White, 1959) establish emotionally significant memories, which become the essential building blocks for the development of the representational world, the templates of caring relationships, which influence all subsequent relationships and the sense of self within these relationships. The parent, for example, provides a protective context in which the infant can experience his/her own impulses and sensations as personal and as emerging from within (Winnicott, 1960). These experiences form the basis for the infant's awareness of affective experiences and, eventually, of the child's capacity to reflect on these experiences (Schaffer & Blatt, 1990).

Initially, the child experiences him/herself as the object of the parent's response, recognition, and love. The parent recognizes and affirms the existence of the infant by making him/her the object of love and desire. The infant's experience of being desired—of being seen, touched, wanted, and loved in active, affective responses—affirms the child's existence as a central object in the parent's psychological world. As Lichtenstein (1977) noted, the infant's identity is acquired at first through "the imprinting of an identity . . . by the mother." This "released" identity is irreversible and compels "the child to find ways and means to realize this specific identity." Lichtenstein stressed that it is the "early mother–child unit and not its breaking up [that] constitutes the primary condition for identity in man." The "extremeness of the symbiotic relation . . . becomes the very source of the emergence of the human identity" (p. 72). The lack of such affirmation can seriously distort developmental processes.

The parent also enables the infant to experience a sense of separateness, a sense of self in the overall context of relatedness. Recognition of, and appropriate response to, the infant's needs provide a sense of organization and cohesion to the infant's initially undifferentiated and unorganized needs. A sense of self emerges from the coherence provided by the parent's organized response to the infant's spontaneous gestures and expressions (Schaffer & Blatt, 1990). As Lichtenstein (1977) observed, "even as an adult, man cannot ever experience his identity except . . . within the variations of a symbiotically structured *Umwelt*" (p.73).

In addition to providing coherence and meaning for the infant's affective experiences, a caring and responsive parent enables the infant to feel valued psychologically, as the infant's spontaneous gestures and actions are accepted and understood. These gestures and actions are a form of communication that facilitates the infant's development of the capacity to use symbols (Werner & Kaplan, 1963; Winnicott, 1963). Understanding of, and response to, the infant's expressions and gestures as a shareable and perceivable communication becomes part of the infant's awareness that experiences can be shared and that the experiences of the other are related to one's own experiences. These shared affective experiences become increasingly differentiated, integrated, and subtle with development.

Appropriate responses to the infant's needs and gestures also provide the opportunity for the infant to experience a sense of agency through an awareness that his/her acts are efficacious (Schaffer & Blatt, 1990). Sensorimotor, enactive, need-gratifying experiences in the attachment relationship form the basis for the earliest internalizations, which over time become increasingly complex and symbolic. The child, in an attempt to preserve psychologically significant aspects of the gratifying relationship, gradually transforms those functions that the relationship previously provided into his/her own enduring self-generated functions and characteristics (Behrends & Blatt, 1985; Blatt & Behrends, 1987). The internalization of the parent's appropriately caring response, for example, provides the basis for the child's feeling loveable. Erikson (1950) considered the first social achievement to be the capacity to allow the mother to be out of sight because "she has become an inner certainty as well as an external predictability" (p. 247). Assuming responsibility for some of the functions previously provided by the caregiver further facilitates the development of the sense of self as active and effective. The child also develops a sense of agency in adopting the parent's role as initiator by actively desiring and seeking to make the parent the object of his/her affection.

This shared state of desire and communication, the state of being loved and of loving, creates a substrate for the basic experiences of the self as feeling simultaneously both an object and a subject in an affective relationship. Being the object of the parent's affection as well as an agent in the relationship provides the basis for affective experiences and is the source of being an active agent seeking the other. The subjective self thus emerges in a relational dialogue that creates the consciously and unconsciously organized constructions of the sense of self as both object and subject within the affective relationship. These psychological functions emerge as a consequence of the shared bodily and communicative experiences between parent and infant; the infant feels psychically alive and actively seeks affective experiences (Winnicott, 1960; Stern, 1985). These experiences of affect and agency become the basic components of the sense of self. The affective experiences initially formed around shared bodily experiences between infant and parent provide a sense of cohesion and organization for fundamental affective experiences with another. In this reciprocity of shared affect and action, the object of the parent's affection also becomes the self who experiences affects and initiates action. As Loewald (1973) pointed out, it is not the caregiving figure who is internalized in the formation of the child's representational world and psychic structures, but the affects and actions shared in the multifaceted experiences of satisfaction in the mother–child relationship. Prelinguistic, descriptively unconscious experiences of shared affect and action—sensorimotor representations of enactive, affect-laden experiences and the figures sharing in them—eventually become encoded as representations of the qualities of the interpersonal relationship and of the individuals who participated in it. Affective sharing and enactive sensorimotor experiences in caring relationships provide the basis for the emergence of a sense of self; this sense of self and the qualities attached to it provide structure for future subjective experiences and intrapsychic processes. The self becomes the locus of affective experience and the sense of agency, as well as the basis for reflective awareness.

The Introjected Self

Rizzuto (1991), based on Benvineste (1966/1971) and Sharpless (1985), noted that the pronouns "I," "me," and "you" first appear around 22 months of age and become meaningful and stable verbal structures at around 30 months. These linguistic structures, initially imposed on the affective, sensorimotor, enactive experiences of love and affection (or its failures and absences), subsequently begin to have organizing functions of their own, including self-referential and self-reflective activities. The differentiation of the verbal structures of "I" and "you" in the development of language provides a medium through which the child can begin to consider variations and transformations of relationships that go beyond the here and now. The child, through imitation, play, dreams, and fantasy, can begin to envision new types of relationships never experienced directly before (Piaget, 1945/1962). The child can begin to consider multiple relationships within the family system, which eventually assume the triadic configurations of the oedipal phase (Blatt, 1983).

Around 30 to 36 months of age, the emergence and stabilization of the linguistic structures of "me," "I," and "you" indicate that the child has established an articulated and stable representation of self and of the other. The child is now able to differentiate between self and other and to be aware of differences in his/her relationships with various others. Initially, the child has an exaggerated, self-conscious sense of self; there is an acute awareness of self as separate, autonomous, and independent. This exaggerated preoccupation with self can lead to excessive feelings of autonomy and pride or excessive feelings of shame and guilt. It is this exaggerated sense of self, either excessively positive or excessively negative, that we refer to as the introjected self. If the sense of self is essentially realistic and positive, the child can enter into a complex developmental process in which the differentiated conception of self and of other begins to define two fundamental developmental lines: (1) the development of the capacity to establish increasingly mature and satisfying interpersonal relationships; and (2) the development of a consolidated, realistic, essentially positive, increasingly differentiated and integrated self-concept or identity (Blatt, 1991a). These two developmental lines normally evolve throughout the life cycle in a reciprocal or dialectic transaction. An increasingly differentiated, integrated, and mature sense of self is contingent on establishing satisfying interpersonal relationships, and, conversely, the continued development of increasingly mature and satisfying interpersonal relationships is contingent on the development of a more mature sense of self and identity. Throughout the life cycle, meaningful and satisfying relationships contribute to the evolving sense of self, and a new sense of self leads, in turn, to more mature levels of interpersonal relatedness. In normal personality development, these two developmental processes evolve in an interactive, reciprocally balanced, mutually facilitating fashion from birth through senescence (Blatt, 1990; Blatt & Blass, 1990; Blatt & Shichman, 1983).

Freud (1930/1961) also articulated a distinction similar to this emphasis on relatedness and self-definition as two fundamental developmental lines:

"the development of the individual seems . . . to be a product of the interaction between two urges, the urge toward happiness, which we usually call 'egoistic,' and the urge toward union with others in the community, which we call 'altruistic' [p.140]. . . . The man who is predominantly erotic will give first preference to his emotional relationship to other people; the narcissistic man, who inclines to be self-sufficient, will seek his main satisfactions in his internal mental processes" (pp. 83–84). Freud (1914/1957, 1926/1959) also distinguished between object and ego libido, and between libidinal instincts in the service of attachment, and aggressive instincts necessary for autonomy, mastery, and self-definition. Attachment and separation are both basic dimensions of a fundamental developmental process. Attachment or separation are both essential for internalization to occur (Behrends & Blatt, 1985). Attachment is an essential precondition for internalization, but it is only with some disruption of this involvement that internalization takes place. Internalization is an attempt to preserve psychologically significant aspects of a relationship by gradually transforming those functions that the relationship had previously provided into one's own enduring, self-generated functions and characteristics (Behrends & Blatt, 1985; Blatt & Behrends, 1987). Thus, attachment and separation are both essential for psychological development. In the attachment developmental line, the child develops a sense of self as a desirable object; in the separation developmental line, the child develops a sense of autonomy and a capacity for initiative and industry. When these qualities develop in an essentially positive form, the child has a sense of self as agent, which enables the child to eventually develop a sense that he/she has the capacity to contribute actively and constructively in relationships with others. When the content of these internalizations is negative and critical, however, a self-critical sense of self results, as found in seriously depressed individuals.

The Mature Self

The early emotional sharing of bodily experiences and communications (gestures and phrases) in the parent–infant dyad are eventually transformed much later in development into a sense of "we." Shared experiences during infancy and beyond, and the development of a sense of self as the locus of affect and agency, provide the basis for the eventual integration of self-definition with the qualities of interpersonal relatedness in the formation of an identity in late adolescence. Identity formation in adolescence is based on prior identifications, but this identity, or mature self, is more than a simple summation of earlier internalizations. Identity involves an integration of all prior identifications into a new gestalt that transcends any particular set of identifications, and integrates the components of the various internalizations and identifications into an organized and stable identity. Thus, while identification and internalization are the primary mechanisms for the development of psychic structures prior to adolescence, they are replaced by integration as the primary mechanism for the development of psychic structures from adolescence onwards (Blatt & Blass, 1990). This integration of prior identifications into a new gestalt, into an identity, defines the sense of self not only in relation to another, but also involves a reflective self-awareness, a sense of self as unique, with specific qualities that one brings to relationships, some of which are highly congruent with the perceived needs of the other. And conversely, the other is perceived as possessing special qualities that are uniquely congruent with particular needs of the self. This definition of a self-in-relation, this sense of "we," is an extension and an elaboration of the implicit, preverbal togetherness of infancy. But this more mature sense of "we" is very different from the togetherness of infancy in that it now includes a self-reflective awareness of one's unique qualities as contributing to the establishment and maintenance of the relationship. The self and the other each recognize and acknowledge both the independence and interdependence of one and the other (Blatt & Blass, 1992).

The fourth personal pronoun, "we," like the earlier "me," "you," and "I" in the development of an introjected self, is a central aspect of the psychological development of the mature self. Although the "we' has its *anlage* in the unity of the early caring relationship, the full sense of "we" can occur only after the "I" and the "you" are experienced as separate, well-articulated entities and then come together again to establish a mutually meaningful, reciprocal, intimate relationship: the mature sense of "we."

As George Klein (1976) noted: "The terminology of subject and object has contributed to misleading conceptualizations of selfhood and especially to obscuring its We aspect. The traditional view of man as becoming gradually aware of himself as subject confronting others as objects may be applicable *morphologically* but it does not describe the dynamic whole" (pp. 178–179). Klein was particularly interested in the establishment of identity as a "specifically human necessity" that involved two aspects: (1) an autonomous distinction from others as a locus of action and decision (agency), and (2) a "we-ness" as a necessary part of the self that transcends one's autonomous actions. Identity for Klein always has to be defined "as having aspects of both separateness and membership in a more encompassing entity" (p. 177). Thus, Klein saw psychoanalysis as eventually developing a theory of "wego," corresponding to its theory of ego. Such a theory would account for a concept of the "we" as emerging from the dialectic interaction between the sense of self as separate and autonomous as well as related to another. Klein, influenced by Erikson, stressed the sense of continuity, coherence, and integrity in an identity that is defined in terms of "aspects of both separateness and membership in a more encompassing entity . . . reflect[ing] one's role in a relationship with a larger entity" (p. 177).

This sense of belonging, or of "we-ness," has its earliest prototype in the parent–infant unit. From this matrix emerges "a feeling of being part of a larger identity" (Klein, 1976, p. 179). More recent investigation, primarily infant research such as that done by Lichtenstein and by Stern, addressed this dialectic developmental process between separation and relatedness and its creation of schemas not only of self and of other, but of the "self-with-other" (Stern, 1983). Stern took the "being-with" experience in normally developing infants beyond the differentiation of self and other schemas, and established the "self-with-other" experience as a positive human capacity associated with an intact schema of self and other together. Emde (1988), in a discussion of the work of Stern and others who have begun to consider the dialectic between the sense of self and a sense of relatedness, viewed the emergence of this dual emphasis as an important theoretical development: "[W]e are beginning to see a different aspect of psychology, a 'we' psychology in addition to a 'self' psychology. . . . [T]his represents a profound change in our world view" (p. 36). Emde discussed three dynamic aspects of the "we" system: (1) the experience of self; (2) the experience of the other (e.g., the attachment figure); and (3) the experience of the self with the other, or the "we" (Blatt & Blass, 1990).

These formulations of the development of a sense of "we" from a psychoanalytic perspective are consistent with the recent emphasis of feminist theorists (e.g., Chodorow, 1978, 1989; Gilligan, 1982, 1988; Miller, 1984; Surrey, 1984) on the importance of including in formulations of personality development the "self-in-relation." The concept of the "we" is also consistent with Sampson's (1985, 1988) distinction between individualism, or the sense of self, as "self-contained," or "ensembled" (Blatt & Blass, 1992).

The sense of self emerges out of the shared, reciprocal, loving relationship between parent and child during the first 3 years of life; later in development, the processes of self-definition and interpersonal relatedness evolve in a reciprocal, interactive, or dialectic process in which these two fundamental developmental lines are increasingly integrated in more mature and reflective ways. A full integration of these developmental lines occurs in late adolescence, when the consolidation of identity results in a definition of the "self-in-relation" and the capacity to establish enduring, reciprocal, mutually facilitating, satisfying, intimate interpersonal relationships.

PHENOMENOLOGICAL APPROACHES TO DEPRESSION

We also approach the concept of depression primarily from a phenomenological perspective. Numerous attempts have been made to differentiate subtypes of depression based on the manifest expressions of different clusters of symptoms. Because of the remarkable heterogeneity of symptoms in both nonclinical and clinical samples, however, most of these attempts to differentiate subtypes of depression based on objective differences in manifest symptoms have been relatively unsuccessful. Dissatisfaction with these objective classifications of depression based on manifest symptoms has led several independent groups of clinical investigators, from very different theoretical perspectives, to propose differentiating types of depression on the basis of the life experiences or issues that lead individuals to become depressed. In these approaches, depression is considered not just a clinical disorder, but an affect state that ranges from mild and appropriate transient reactions to difficult life events to a profound, sustained, and disabling clinical disorder involving intense and persistent dysphoria, distorted cognition (especially a distorted sense of self), and neurovegetative disturbances such as sleep and weight loss and loss of libido (Blatt, 1974).

Investigators from several different theoretical positions have discussed two major types of experiences that lead to depression: (1) disruptions of gratifying interpersonal relationships (e.g., object loss); and (2) disruptions of an effective, essentially positive, sense of self (e.g., failure and guilt). These two types of depressive experiences have been characterized by several psychoanalytic investigators as anaclitic and introjective (e.g., Blatt, 1974; Blatt & Shichman, 1983), as dependent and self-critical (Blatt, D'Afflitti, & Quinlan, 1976; Blatt, Quinlan, Chevron, McDonald, & Zuroff, 1982), as dominant other and dominant goal (Arieti & Bemporad, 1978, 1980), and as anxiously attached and compulsively self-reliant (Bowlby, 1969, 1973, 1980, 1988). An unusual degree of convergence emerges from these formulations of depression from three different strands of psychoanalytic theory: the contributions of Arieti and Bemporad derive primarily from an interpersonal orientation; Blatt's contributions derive primarily from an integration of psychoanalytic ego psychology with developmental-cognitive theory; and Bowlby's formulations are influenced by ethological theory and are based primarily on extensions of object relations theory. In addition, these psychoanalytic formulations of the phenomenology of depression are consistent with more recent formulations from a cognitive–behavioral perspective in which Beck (1983) has differentiated between a socially dependent (sociotropic) and an autonomous type of depression. These various psychoanalytic and cognitive–behavioral theoretical formulations suggest an impressive degree of agreement about the phenomenology of depression derived from both clinical experience and research findings (Blatt & Maroudas, 1992).

These four theoretical positions on depression (Arieti & Bemporad, Beck, Blatt, and Bowlby) are all based on the belief that a fuller understanding of depression can be gained from a phenomenological analysis of life experiences that lead individuals to become depressed. And all four theoretical positions stress the importance of impaired cognitive structures and distorted early interpersonal relationships in the development of depression. Although the four theoretical groups use different terms and make different basic assumptions about the etiology and treatment of depression, they all describe two major types of depressed patients: (1) those excessively preoccupied with and dependent on interpersonal relationships; and (2) those excessively preoccupied with achievement, self-definition, and self-worth. The former group of patients is typified by disruptions of interpersonal relatedness and by excessive clinging and feelings of loneliness and of being unloved; whereas the latter group emphasizes disruptions of self-definition and is highly self-critical and preoccupied with feelings of worthlessness and failure. Thus, there is considerable congruence, at least on a descriptive level, among these four theoretical positions. They provide important observations that could eventually lead to a more comprehensive formulation of the nature, etiology, and treatment of depression (Blatt & Maroudas, 1992).

Both Beck (1983) and Blatt (Blatt, D'Afflitti, & Quinlan, 1976, 1979) and their colleagues have developed procedures for assessing these two types of depression. The Depressive Experiences Questionnaire (DEQ) (Blatt et al., 1976, 1979), The Sociotropy–Autonomy Scale (SAS) (Beck et al., 1983), and the Dysfunctional Attitude Scale (DAS) (Weissman & Beck, 1978; Cane, Olinger, Gotlib, & Kuiper, 1986) provide methodologies that can be used to investigate systematically these two types or phenomenological dimensions of depression. Although these scales (DEQ, SAS, and DAS) differ in important ways, they all provide methods for assessing these two dimensions of depression, which could be helpful in addressing the wide range of questions raised by the recent approach to depression based on experiential issues.

THE EXPERIENCE OF SELF IN DEPRESSION

From a phenomenological perspective, the various theoretical formulations of depression provide important leads about the experience of self in depression. In our analysis of the phenomenology of the self, we distinguished three essential components of the self: experiences of affect (I feel), of agency (I think and I do), and of self-reflectivity (I am). These components of the self are expressed in very different ways in a dependent (e.g., anaclitic, sociotropic, anxiously attached, dominant other) and a self-critical (e.g., introjective, autonomous, avoidantly attached, dominant goal) type of depression.

As regards affective experiences, individuals with dependent depression are likely to be very labile. The quality of their affective experience varies widely depending on the presence and availability of a need-gratifying other. When interpersonal contact and need gratification are available, these individuals experience feelings of bliss; but this quickly disappears when contact with the other is threatened, discontinued, or lost. Because these individuals have little sense of the future and live very much for the moment, they can be readily soothed. Even momentary contact with another and the brief satisfaction of a need is experienced as boundless; likewise, loss and deprivation is experienced as never-ending. When contact and gratification are lost, dependently depressed individuals quickly begin to feel depleted, alone, and helpless. Profound feelings of joy thus alternate with intense feelings of despair, resulting in a highly variable and labile sense of self, a sense of self that is very much contingent on environmental experiences. Dependently depressed individuals tend to deny difficulties and avoid expressing anger and dissatisfaction with others because they are fearful that others might abandon them. Rather, they rapidly search for substitute satisfactions that serve to postpone or avoid dysphoric experiences and often express their dissatisfactions and unhappiness in feelings of helplessness and somatic complaints, demanding that others take care of them. In addition to clinging to others, they actively search for alternative sources of gratification. They are relatively unreflective, so that dysphoric affect usually results in some form of discharge rather than in a thoughtful evaluation of aspects of themselves, their interpersonal relationships, and their life circumstances. Their affective tone varies from Pollyannaish bliss to feelings of depletion and exhaustion.

Affective experiences in introjectively depressed individuals, in contrast, are much more persistently pessimistic, corresponding to Beck's description of the depressive triad of negative views of one's self, the world, and the future. Because self-critically depressed individuals are more reflective, they express their morbid unhappiness and feelings of hopelessness more directly. They assume blame and responsibility, especially for negative events; every negative event reflects their inadequacy, failure, or guilt, or is their just reward because they deserve to suffer.

The affective experiences of introjective or self-critically depressed individuals are more stable, persistent, and negative, in contrast to the affective lability of dependently depressed individuals, who are overly responsive to momentary positive events. The reluctance of dependently depressed individuals to find fault with themselves or others is in marked contrast to the level of responsibility assumed by self-critical individuals. Dependently depressed individuals deny difficulties and make excuses for negative events, in contrast to self-critical individuals, who all too readily assume responsibility for these negative events as either their fault or their just deserts. Positive events are experienced as happenstance or luck, or as only brief interludes in a gloomy, pessimistic view of themselves and their world. As described by Freud (1917/1957), introjectively depressed individuals can be destroyed by success.

In terms of a sense of agency, dependently depressed individuals feel helpless, weak, and ineffective, and believe that they must rely on others. They are preoccupied with lost and/or unavailable relationships. In contrast, self-critically depressed individuals are plagued by feelings of guilt over sins of commission, by things they believe they have done poorly, incorrectly, or in violation of legal and/or moral code. Dependently depressed individuals are troubled by feelings of shame about how they appear to others, and worried that others may turn away from them. Self-critically depressed individuals feel hopeless about ever doing anything correctly, and feel guilty about errors, mistakes, or transgressions they believe they have committed. A sense of failure and/or guilt is pervasive.

Self-critically depressed individuals are highly self-reflective and constantly scrutinize their actions, words, deeds, and thoughts in the basic belief that they have done something wrong. They assume inordinate responsibility, especially for negative events, and are markedly ambivalent about themselves, constantly striving to prove that they are worthwhile and competent by seeking to make amends and reparation, but always believing that they have failed in these efforts. Dependently depressed individuals, in contrast, tend to be nonreflective. Though hesitant and reluctant to blame or criticize others, they do not assume responsibility for their misfortunes—negative events are simply a consequence of their bad luck and the neglect of others.

Dependently and self-critically depressed individuals differ markedly in self-reflectivity, in access to and awareness of affective experiences, and in their sense of agency. Although the sense of self is impaired and distorted in both types of depression, there is usually much greater internality in self-critical depression. This introjected sense of self represents a developmental progression beyond the rudimentary sense of self usually seen in dependent depression. The beginning of reflectivity and a sense of affect and agency in an introjected sense of self is an important developmental milestone in normal development and may be an important marker in the therapeutic process. So, although from one perspective, experiences of depression may involve distortions in the sense of self, the development of the capacity to experience, bear, and integrate feelings of depression may be an important part of the treatment process, at least in long-term intensive psychotherapy.

The sense of self in dependent and self-critical depression can occur along a continuum from a rudimentary to an introjected to a mature level. There is usually a close correspondence between an introjected sense of self and issues of self-critical depression because of the greater reflectivity involved in self-criticism. But on occasion, an individual with a self-critical depression may have a more rudimentary sense of self, in which the depressive issues are enacted or projected onto others, resulting in limited self-reflectivity, little access to or capacity for integrating affect, and an exaggerated and overstated sense of agency. Likewise, issues of dependent depression most commonly involve a more rudimentary sense of self, in which there is little self-reflectivity, limited access to and awareness of affect, and an impaired sense of agency, with little capacity for delay and intense feelings of helplessness. Dependent depressive issues, however, can also be expressed at a more differentiated introjected level of self; in this case there is often an intense sense of shame, feelings of loss of a relationship with a particular significant person, and a more general feeling of being a failure about specific interpersonal difficulties. Thus, while it is expected that self-critical depression is more frequently associated with an introjected sense of self, and dependent depression is associated with a rudimentary sense of self, there will be notable exceptions to this overall pattern.

Generally, we expect self-critical depression to be associated with a more introjected sense of self: painful feelings of worthlessness, failure, and an impaired capacity to function effectively. We expect experiences of dependent depression to be associated with a more rudimentary sense of self: diminished self-reflectivity, a sense of helplessness, and little capacity to tolerate and integrate affect. We expect normal mature development—a sense of self as effective and competent, and a capacity to establish mutual and reciprocal interpersonal relationships—to be associated with greater and more realistic self-reflectivity, greater capacity to experience and integrate affect, and a fuller sense of agency. We also expect progress in the therapeutic process to result in the development of this more mature sense of self.

INVESTIGATIONS OF THE SENSE OF SELF IN DEPRESSION

Based on the assumption that the self is predominantly a subjective construction, we sought to evaluate the sense of self by asking nonclinical young adults and psychiatric patients in a relatively open-ended manner to "describe yourself." We expected that the semistructured and phenomenological nature of this task would allow a fuller expression of the sense of self than more structured questionnaires. We were interested in comparing the sense of self and its relationship to depression in both a nonclinical and a clinical sample, as well as in tracing changes in the sense of self during intensive long-term treatment of a seriously disturbed patient. We were particularly interested in the relationships among aspects of the self and the two types of depressive experiences—dependent and self-critical—and whether changes in the self-descriptions of a seriously disturbed patient during long-term, intensive, psychoanalytically informed inpatient treatment paralleled the differences noted between the self-descriptions of normal and hospitalized young adults. We were especially interested in noting whether the self-descriptions of this patient moved toward those observed in our normal subjects, and in trying to understand the role that depression played in the patient's self-descriptions and in her therapeutic process.

The Self and Depression in Normal Young Adults

We first studied the spontaneous descriptions of self in 41 male and 46 female college students by adapting procedures initially developed for evaluating qualitative and cognitive aspects of spontaneous descriptions of significant others (Blatt, Wein, Chevron, & Quinlan, 1978, 1979; Blatt, Chevron, Quinlan, Schaffer, & Wein, 1988; Blatt, Bers, & Stein, 1985).[3]

Twelve qualitative characteristics of the self were rated by a judge on 7-point scales: Affectionate, Ambitious, Benevolent, Constructive Involvement with others, Intellectual, Judgmental, Positive self-regard, Nurturant, Punitive, Strong, Successful, and Warm; the judge also noted when it was not possible to rate a particular quality because of a lack of relevant material. The degree of Ambivalence in the self-description was scored on a 3-point scale. An estimate of the Length of the description was used to assess verbal fluency. Conceptual level, a structural or metacognitive variable, was scored on a 9-point scale that reflected a normal developmental progression of the sense of self ranging from global, amorphous descriptions based on action sequences and need gratification, to more differentiated descriptions emphasizing a limited number of attributes presented in a one-sided manner, and finally to highly articulated, integrated, and complex descriptions. Ratings were done by an experienced judge who had previously established acceptable reliability (*r*'s > .65) in rating these scales.

The 12 qualitative self-description scales and the degree of ambivalence about the self were subjected to a principal-components factor analysis with Varimax rotations. When there was a lack of relevant material to rate a particular scale, the subject was assigned a score at the midpoint of the scale. Length of the self-description was also included in the factor analysis. Conceptual level was not included in the factor analysis because it was considered to be a structural, or metacognitive, variable and hence different from the qualitative variables.

Three interpretable factors with eigenvalues greater than 1 emerged from the analysis, and they accounted for 36.6%, 12.4%, and 10.9% of the variance, respectively. These factors were labeled Warm/nurturant, Positive self-regard, and Striving. As indicated in Table 6.1, the Warm/nurturant scale is composed of items concerning the quality of relationships with others, and the Positive self-regard scale is composed of evaluative items. The Striving scale appeared to be less homogeneous because, in addition to

TABLE 6.1. Factors Underlying 13 Qualitative Variables and Length of the Self-descriptions for 87 Subjects

Factor	Item	Factor loading	Eigenvalue
Warm/nurturant to others			5.12
	Warm	.83	
	Construcitve involvement with others	.80	
	Benevolent	.79	
	Nurturant	.77	
	Affectionate	.74	
Positive self-regard			1.74
	Positive self-regard	.85	
	Successful	.81	
	Strong	.76	
	Ambivalence	−.63	
	Punitive	−.58	
	Judgmental	−.47	
Striving			1.53
	Ambitious	.72	
	Length	.66	
	Intellectual	.60	

items related to striving, it included Length, a potentially confounding element, possibly weakening the stability and meaning of this factor scale. In addition, the internal consistency of the Striving factor scale was low, and there was little evidence for its validity. Reliability and validity seemed well established, however, for the Warm/nurturant and Positive self-regard factor scales (Blatt, Bers, & Stein, 1985).

We examined the relationship of aspects of the self-descriptions, (i.e., the 3 factors, the 13 individual scales, conceptual level, and length) to 2 measures of clinical depression (the Beck [1967] and Zung [1973] depression scales) and to the two types of depressive experiences (DEQ; Blatt et al., 1976): (1) dependent experiences focused on concerns about interpersonal issues of loneliness, abandonment, and dependency; and (2) self-critical experiences concerned with issues of self-worth, failure, and guilt. In addition, the DEQ includes an efficacy factor that consists of items reflecting a sense of resourcefulness and well-being.

As seen in Table 6.2, the data consistently suggest that self-critical depression assessed by the second factor of the DEQ, and clinical depression assessed by the Beck and Zung scales, correlated significantly in both men and women with a sense of the self as cold, negative, and nonnurturing, and as poorly related to others. In addition, dependent depression in women was related to a negative view of the self. It seems that the self-concept of women can be adversely affected by concerns about achievement and accomplishment as well as concerns about interpersonal relationships, whereas the self-concept of males is primarily affected only by the former concerns.

In summary, this analysis of spontaneous open-ended self-descriptions, indicates that valuable data can be gleaned from spontaneous self-descriptions. These analyses provided interesting data and intriguing leads even though these initial scoring procedures were derived from procedures originally designed for analyzing descriptions of others. The data suggested

TABLE 6.2a. Correlations of Self-description Factors and Scales with Measures of Depression for Females

	Depression measures				
	Depressive Experiences Questionnaire				
	Dependency (n = 46)	Self-criticism (n = 46)	Efficacy (n = 46)	Zung (n = 44)	Beck (n = 44)
Self-description factors					
Warm/nurturant	−.04	−.57†	.16	−.55†	−.60†
Positive self-regard	−.18	−.62†	.12	−.67†	−.73†
Striving	−.16	−.10	.19	−.17	.11
Self-description scales					
Warm to others	−.06	−.46†	(.26)	−.47†	−.61†
Constructive involvement with others	.01	−.58†	.18	−.63†	−.64†
Benevolent	−.05	−.56†	.04	−.48†	−.51†
Nurturant to others	.18	−.34*	.17	−.38**	−.38**
Affectionate	.04	−.47†	.00	−.35*	−.39**
Positive self-regard	−.36**	−.51†	.23	−.63†	−.66†
Successful	(−.27)	−.47†	(.28)	−.75†	−.65†
Strong	(−.25)	−.45**	.05	−.62†	−.59†
Ambivalence	.15	.46†	−.05	.38**	.55†
Punitive	−.04	.49†	.06	.34*	−.49†
Judgmental	−.08	.46†	−.04	.46**	−.43**
Ambitious	(−.25)	−.05	(.27)	−.24	.08
Intellectual	−.00	−.22	−.03	−.10	−.08
Level	−.21	−.00	−.05	−.06	.11
Length	−.06	.06	.16	−.01	.23

Note. Because of incomplete questionnaires, the number of subjects varies. *$p < .05$. **$p < .01$. †$p < .001$. ( ) = strong trend.

TABLE 6.2b. Correlations of Self-description Factors and Scales with Measures of Depression for Males

	Depression measures				
	Depressive Experiences Questionnaire				
	Dependency (n = 41)	Self-criticism (n = 41)	Efficacy (n = 41)	Zung (n = 37)	Beck (n = 39)
Self-description factors					
Warm/nurturant	.18	−.34*	.08	−.40*	−.38*
Positive self-regard	−.23	(−.30)	−.01	−.23	−.41**
Striving	−.08	−.33*	.14	(−.29)	−.06
Self-description scales					
Warm to others	.15	−.22	.07	−.27	−.10
Constructive involvement with others	.13	−.21	.03	−.43**	−.36*
Benevolent	.08	−.04	.16	−.46**	−.46**
Nurturant to others	(.28)	−.39**	.16	−.27	−.24
Affectionate	.06	−.42**	.07	−.23	−.34*
Positive self-regard	−.18	−.44**	.15	−.22	−.33*
Successful	(−.26)	(−.30)	.17	−.14	(−.29)
Strong	−.24	−.50†	−.08	−.19	−.37*
Ambivalence	.12	.06	−.02	(.28)	.45**
Punitive	.12	.11	.01	.12	.12
Judgmental	.03	.00	.21	−.06	−.00
Ambitious	−.01	−.14	.21	−.09	.09
Intellectual	(−.27)	−.12	.03	−.35*	−.02
Level	.03	.11	.00	−.10	.24
Length	.10	−.41**	.06	−.16	.06

Note. Because of incomplete questionnaires, the number of subjects varies. *$p < .05$. **$p < .01$. †$p < .001$. ( ) = strong trend.

that it would be worthwhile to score self-descriptions with procedures more directly designed to assess dimensions relevant to the sense of self in both clinical and normal subjects.

The Self and Depression in Patients

Based on a review of the clinical and research literature, new scales were developed to capture dimensions of the sense of self that seemed to be omitted in our first attempt to evaluate self-descriptions (Blatt & Bers, 1987) such as a positive attitude about oneself (Kohut, 1971, 1977), the capacity for connectedness and relatedness (Kernberg, 1976, 1989), self-reflectivity (Feffer, 1970; Flavell, 1977; Selman & Byrne, 1974), differentiation (Blatt, 1983; Flavell, 1977; Kegan, 1982), and conceptual capacities (Bannister & Agnew, 1976; Blatt, 1974; Feffer, 1970; Flavell, 1977; Harter, 1982; Katz & Zigler, 1967; Lee & Noam, 1983; Mullener & Laird, 1971). As indicated in Table 6.3, four categories of scales were developed.

The first category of scales was designed to assess aspects of the self as agent, including weak versus strong (ineffective vs. effective), negative versus positive, and striving (or ambitious and successful). The second group of scales was designed to assess the degree of relatedness to others, expressed in descriptions of the self, including the extent of articulation of relationships, the quality of interpersonal involvement, and the perception of others as agents who affect people in either a negative or a positive way. We assumed that omission of these two major content areas of agency and relatedness in a description of oneself was an indication of a constriction in the sense of self, so we noted when aspects of striving (i.e., ambition and success) or of relations with others were omitted from the self-description.

The third group of scales was designed to assess cognitive-affective dimensions of the self-descriptions, including the extent of depression as indicated by sad, apathetic, and dysphoric feelings about the self, others, and life in general; the degree of self-reflectivity; the extent of tolerance of contradictory aspects of the self; and the differentiation and integration of the self (how many different domains or content areas were used to describe the self).

The fourth group of scales included a rating of the conceptual level of the self-description, which assessed the overall quality of the description along a developmental continuum ranging from sensorimotor-preoperational to formal operational thought. In addition, we evaluated the number of different domains (physical/demographic properties, aspects of manifest behavior and functions, personality traits and attributes, and inner feelings, thoughts, and values) that were included in the self-description in order to assess the degree of "substantiality" of the self-description.

Verbal fluency, or the length of the description, was rated on a 7-point scale. Interrater reliabilities of two independent judges were at an acceptable level for all 16 scales, ranging from .62 to .93.

The self-descriptions of 29 adolescent and young adult female psychiatric patients, hospitalized in a long-term facility, were compared to those of 40 female nonpatients of a similar age range (Bers, Blatt, Sayward, & Johnston, 1993). The primary diagnoses of the patients included schizophrenia spectrum disorders, severe personality disorders, and major affective disorders. Most of the patients had several prior hospitalizations; many of them had been taking psychotropic medications prior to admission and continued to do so during this hospitalization. The comparison subjects were 40 students in a large coeducational public high school or in a college introductory psychology course. In addition to comparing the self-descriptions of patients and nonpatients, we also used the same rating process to

TABLE 6.3. Self-description Scales

I. Sense of Agency
   A. *Weak/strong:* the sense of being mild or weak (1) vs. effective, stable, and strong (7)
   B. *Striving*
      1. *Ambitious:* the degree of aspirations or pressure for achievement in instrumental or occupational domains, from unambitious (1) to highly ambitious (7)
      2. *Successful:* the individual's attitudes toward his/her success at achieving his/her own aspirations, from unsucessful (1) to highly successful (7)
   C. *Negative/positive self-regard:* the extent to which the self-view is critical, harshly judgmental, neglectful, and hateful (1) vs. benevolent, caring, and positive (7)

II. Sense of Relatedness
   A. *Articulation of relationships:* the extent to which others are mentioned in the self-description in terms of relationships, from a vague or global mention of others (1) to the depiction of particular relationships with specificity and elaboration (4)
   B. *Cold/warm to others:* impersonal, unemotional, and cold toward others (1) vs. warm, friendly, and engaged with others (7)
   C. *Negative/positive view of others:* perception of others as agents who impact on others in a negative (1) vs. a positive manner (7)

III. Cognitive-Affective Variables
   A. *Depression:* sad, apathetic, and dysphoric feelings about the self, others, and life in general in the past, present, and/or future, from no depression (1) to high depression (7)
   B. *Reflectivity:* a concrete, literal, and minimally reflective (1) vs. an abstract, conceptual, and introspective view of the self (7)
   C. *Tolerance of contradictory aspects:* the extent of contradictory and opposing aspects of the self and the ability to integrate them, from unidimensional (1) to contradictory and integrated (7)
   D. *Differentiation and integration:* ability to view the self across many domains and the degree of integration of different aspects of the self, from few (1) to many well-integrated domains (7)

IV. Use of Dimensions
   A. *Conceptual level:* the highest developmental level (1–9), based on Piaget, Werner, and developmental psychoanalytic theory (see Blatt, 1974, and Blatt et al., 1988)
   B. *Substantiality:* the number of modes (physical and demographic; behavioral; external personality; and inner feelings, thoughts, and values) included and integrated in the self-view; the capacity to maintain a rich and broad self-view with modes at many developmental levels, from 1 mode (1) to 4 modes included and integrated (7)

examine the changes in the self-description of one psychotically depressed patient over the course of long-term, intensive inpatient treatment from intake to discharge.

The self-descriptions of patients and nonpatients were recorded verbatim (those of the patients were obtained as part of the diagnostic evaluation conducted on admission to the hospital). In addition, the self-descriptions of one patient were also obtained at 6-month intervals thereafter until discharge 19 months later.

Table 6.4 presents examples of two subjects' self-descriptions, those of a 14-year-old female nonpatient and a 13-year-old female patient, Patient

TABLE 6.4. Examples of Self-descriptions

Nonpatient Self-description

What I look like? I'm 5′4″. I have brown hair and light green eyes. I go to New Haven High. I'm really shy. I have plenty of friends though. I just moved from __________. I don't know. My best friend's C. I live in a wee house. I get pretty good grades in school. I'm pretty good friends with my parent. My favorite holiday is the 4th of July. My favorite food is pork roast. My favorite TV show is "General Hospital." Madonna is my favorite singer. I like to listen to music and I love to dance. I've been to gymnastics and dance for 4 years. Do we have to fill up the whole thing? You're going to write that down! Lots of times I like to read. I miss the kids back in ______. This week I'm going to Great Adventure. My favorite subject is English. That's about it.

Patient A's Self-descriptions

Admission
Depends on how I'm feeling. Sometimes I'm outgoing but other times I'm withdrawn. [What else?] I don't know. I don't want to describe myself. [?] 'Cause I get upset when I do. [Can you tell me what upsets you?] I'm either too conceited or too modest to answer, something like this.

Six months
I can't describe myself—you describe me. It's hard— no it's easy. Vulnerable. Hurt. Lonely. Sort of happy. Getting more confident—no—please write gaining more confidence. Considerate.

One year
Depressed, suspicious, alone, manipulative, musical, artistic, sensitive, hopeless. Drug abuser, sympathetic. Can be friendly. Opinionated. Withdrawn. Angry. Chain smoker. Can be humorous. That's it.

Discharge (19 months)
Lonely. Insecure. Hiding behind a facade. Has common sense. Abnormal opinions. One of my abnormal opinions is that people who want to kill themselves should be allowed to kill themselves—and I wasn't referring to myself either. Mature—can be mature—haven't really acted it during psych testing—I sort of fooled around. Should have more confidence.

A, whose descriptions were obtained at admission to the hospital, as well as at 6 months, 1 year, and discharge.

Patients versus Nonpatients

Tables 6.5 and 6.6 present group differences between the patients and nonpatients on the self-description scales. The self-descriptions of nonpatients were significantly more positive than those of patients, with little or no expression of depression and a view of the self as fairly strong or effective. The self-descriptions of patients tended to be more negative, with significantly greater feelings of ineffectiveness and depression. Surprisingly, the patients' overall level of depression, although significantly greater than nonpatients, was only at a relatively mild level. It seems that many patients, though clinically depressed, did not include depressive thoughts and feelings in their descriptions of themselves at the time of their admission to a psychiatric hospital.

The two groups showed similar moderate levels of reflectivity in their self-descriptions; yet nonpatients showed significantly more differentiation/integration and tolerance for contradiction than did patients. In contrast to findings with conceptual level in the study of descriptions of

TABLE 6.5. Mean Scores on Self-description Variables for Nonpatients and Patients at Admission

	Nonpatients (n = 40)		Patients (n = 29)		
Variable (range)	*M*	*SD*	*M*	*SD*	$t(67)$
Sense of agency					
Neg./pos. self (1–7)	5.15	(1.03)	3.90	(1.80)	3.66**
Weak/strong (1–7)	4.70	(1.34)	3.59	(1.59)	3.14*
Sense of relatedness					
Articulation of relationships (1–4)	3.28	(1.71)	3.17	(2.49)	.19
Cognitive-affective variables					
Depression (1–7)	1.38	(.77)	2.48	(1.84)	−3.41**
Reflectivity (1–7)	4.95	(1.40)	4.79	(1.57)	.44
Tolerance of contradictions (1–7)	3.85	(1.39)	2.79	(1.57)	2.96*
Differentiation/integration (1–7)	4.23	(1.49)	2.69	(1.42)	4.31**
Dimensional variables					
Conceptual level (1–9)	6.05	(1.06)	5.69	(1.04	1.41
Substantiality (1–7)	4.68	(.89)	3.00	(1.46)	5.90**
Length (1–7)	5.63	(1.37)	2.41	(1.52)	9.16**

*$p < .01$. ** $p < .001$.

TABLE 6.6. Percent of Nonpatients and Patients at Admission with Striving and Relationship Dimensions in Their Self-descriptions

Variable	Nonpatients (n = 40)	Patients (n = 29)	Chi-square
Agency variables			
Ambitious	67.5%	24.0%	12.65**
Successful	67.5%	37.9%	5.94*
Relatedness variables			
Articulation of relationships	92.5%	86.2%	.73
Cold/warm to others	97.5%	55.2%	18.62**
Neg./pos. other	60.0%	41.4%	2.34

*$p < .05$. **$p < .001$.

parents (e.g., Blatt et al., 1979; Bornstein & O'Neill, 1991), there was no significant difference in the overall conceptual level of the self-descriptions of patients and nonpatients. The strongest discriminator between the two groups was the extent to which different dimensions were used in the self-descriptions. The self-descriptions of nonpatients were rich and multidimensional, in contrast to those of patients, which were more flat and constricted. In addition, nonpatients had significantly longer self-descriptions than patients, suggesting a more highly developed and differentiated sense of self, as well as a capacity and willingness to share their self-view with a relatively unfamiliar person. This constriction in the descriptions of patients was also seen in the fact that significantly more patients omitted themes related to ambition, success, or the quality of relationships with others in their self-descriptions than did nonpatients.

In summary, the methodology for analyzing self-descriptions appears to be a valuable tool for assessing aspects of the sense of self across a broad spectrum, ranging from seriously disturbed patients to normal adolescents. Patients had a more negative and ineffective view of themselves; and though they also had significantly more expressions of depression in their self-descriptions, it appears that the patients do not fully include depressive feelings in their sense of self, at least at admission. Warding off such negative feelings might be part of a general tendency to avoid experiencing a more diverse and more reality-based self-view. Likewise, expressions of striving and the quality of relationships with others were often missing from patients' self-descriptions. Generally, patients' self-descriptions lacked a sense of agency and relatedness, dimensions often considered indications of psychological well-being (Blatt, 1990; Blatt & Blass, 1990). A primary difference between the two groups was the extent to which various dimensions were integrated in their self-descriptions, one of the most striking aspects being the patients' constricted, undeveloped sense of self.

These results raise the question of how the sense of self develops normally into a positive and diverse self-representation, how the sense of self becomes impaired in psychopathology, and how it changes in the therapeutic process. The data on the self-descriptions of normal adolescents and young adults provide a base-line for beginning to conceptualize the normal development of the sense of self. An informal reading of the self-descriptions of the 40 normal adolescent females in this study suggests that other people and themes of interpersonal relationships are prominent in the self-descriptions of younger adolescents, whereas among the older adolescents, there is an increased focus on agency and self-definition, with great reflectivity and expressions of internality. In even older subjects, it seems likely that these two domains would be more fully integrated (Blatt, 1990; Blatt & Blass, 1990). Although this sample is too small to test differences across age systematically, the data suggest that our methodology may provide important insight into the changes in the sense of self that occur in both males and females during adolescence and the beginning of adulthood.

Changes in the Sense of Self over Long-Term Treatment[4]

Developmental processes can be explored in longitudinal studies of normal adolescents and young adults, as well as in studies of patients over the course of long-term intensive treatment. We expected that as treatment progressed, the self-descriptions of patients would be less constricted, have a more positive tone, and contain an increasing number of modes and dimensions. Such changes should parallel independent measures of therapeutic change, that is, changes in symptoms, behavior, and styles of functioning (Diamond, Kaslow, Coonerty, & Blatt, 1990; Gruen & Blatt, 1990; Blatt, Wiseman, Prince-Gibson, & Gatt, 1991).

To illustrate the potential value of our method for understanding aspects of change during long-term intensive treatment, we evaluated changes in the self-descriptions of one seriously disturbed patient over 1½ years of inpatient treatment. The patient's admission evaluation and several treatment review protocols prepared during her hospitalization provided collateral data with which to compare changes noted in her self-descriptions over the course of treatment. Independent ratings of her treatment protocols indicate that she made substantial improvement over the 19 months of treatment. Her Global Adjustment Score (GAS) was 22 at admission and 43 at discharge. This patient was selected for study because the quality of her representations of self and others had been the focus of some of our earlier investigations (Diamond et al., 1990; Gruen

& Blatt, 1990) and because her admitting diagnosis was a severe psychotic depression.

BACKGROUND. Patient A, a single, white female, was 13 years old at the time of admission for her third psychiatric hospitalization. Prior to this admission, she had been living in a large urban center with her father and his second wife. A's mother, also a resident of that city, had been divorced from A's father since A was 3½ years old. There was a brother 2 years younger. Her father was reportedly an alcoholic, his brother suffered what was described as a "nervous breakdown," and A's maternal uncle had been hospitalized several times for unspecified psychiatric disturbances.

A's difficulties emerged from a background of chronic bitterness between her divorced parents and longstanding interpersonal and personality disturbances. When she was 4 or 5, A underwent psychiatric evaluation for difficulty separating from her mother. At about age 7 or 8 she began to believe that her body was possessed by the devil and began to have hallucinations of the devil's voice and face. By age 10 she was refusing to go to school altogether and began to abuse cannabis, alcohol, Valium, Quaalude, and IV heroin.

A was first hospitalized at age 12 after she took an overdose of Valium. She was discharged after a few days and continued to deteriorate over the next year, escalating her drug abuse and experiencing visual and auditory hallucinations. She was also chronically depressed, anxious, and suicidal, with occasional brief periods of elation and euphoria; but she refused outpatient psychotherapy. By the time of her third psychiatric admission, she was diagnosed as suffering from severe psychotic depression with marked paranoid trends, and she was given an additional diagnosis of mixed personality disorder with histrionic, compulsive, and paranoid features.

During the course of her 19-month hospitalization, it was reported in reviews of her treatment that A's self-esteem improved noticeably; she became less vulnerable to psychotic decompensation, and was more capable of using relationships with others to get through crises. She was also able to realize that her involvement with drugs was a substitute for the nurturance she felt she could not obtain in other ways. Although she was still considered to be vulnerable to psychotic regression, she was discharged from the hospital to a residential facility because of her parents' financial inability to continue intensive treatment.

SELF-DESCRIPTIONS. Patient A's self-description was obtained shortly after her admission to the hospital and every 6 months thereafter until she was discharged 19 months later. These four self-descriptions are presented in Table 6.4. Changes in Patient A's self-descriptions on our 13 scales over the course of treatment are presented in Table 6.7.

Similar to the mean for the group of patients at admission, A's self-description at admission was negative in tone, and she viewed herself as weak and ineffective. There was a mild expression of depression and a low level of differentiation. Her self-description did not include expressions of striving, and there was no mention of others or the nature of relationships. A used only two of the four modes—inner feelings and thoughts, and behavioral features—to describe herself, so her score on Substantiality was low. Though high on Conceptual level, her description at admission was relatively flat and lacking in dimensions that might portray her physical appearance or her relationships with others. The self-description at admission contained perplexing polarities: "outgoing" and "withdrawn," "conceited" and "modest." These polarities suggested her beginning recognition of contradictory aspects of herself; but the description was fragmented and unintegrated, organized around rudimentary differentiations based on binary oppositions (Lévi-Strauss, 1963). Furthermore, she described her-

TABLE 6.7. Patient A's Scores on Self-description Scales at Admission and over the Course of Treatment

Variable (range)	Admission	6 months	1 year	Discharge (19 months)
Agency variables				
Neg./pos. self (1–7)	3	4	4	4
Weak/strong (1–7)	2	3	4	3
Ambitious (1–7)	—	—	—	—
Successful (1–7)	—	5	3	3
Relatedness variables				
Articulation of relationships (1–4)	—	3	2	1
Cold/warm to others (1–7)	—	5	4	—
Neg./pos. other (1–7)	—	3	3	—
Cognitive-affective variables				
Depression (1–7)	3	4	5	6
Reflectivity (1–7)	6	5	5	6
Toleration of contradiction (1–7)	4	4	3	3
Differentiation/integration (1–7)	2	3	4	4
Use of dimensions				
Conceptual level (1–9) (developmental level)	7	7	7	8
Substantiality (1–7) (number of dimensions)	2	2	4	5

Note. A dash (—) indicates that the scale could not be scored.

self as primarily state dependent, and this description also lacked cohesion and continuity. But the syntax of her self-description and her qualification that it "depends" on context, suggested the possibility that she was capable of developing more subtle differentiations.

Some aspects of A's self-description at admission distinguished her from the other patients. Her high scores on Reflectivity, Tolerance of contradictions, and Conceptual level were distinctive and seem to point to a more inner-directed orientation and overideational style in comparison to both patient and nonpatient peers. Such self-reflective and conceptual capacities, though consistent with her depressive and paranoid character style, might also indicate that A would be relatively responsive to psychotherapy—she seemed open to thinking about herself in different ways. At admission many patients responded to the request for a self-description by saying, "I can't do it," or "I won't do it." Although A voiced a reluctance to describe herself, she went on to participate in a relatively revealing way. Her capacity to express her reservations verbally, yet still comply with the task, suggested a potential to become involved in the therapeutic process in a constructive way.

In the independent clinical evaluation at admission, A was portrayed as depressed in her appearance and behavior, notably withdrawn, with poor diet and hygiene, usually not able to sustain a conversation, not sure of what was going on around her, and hardly ever attending school. Her treatment team described a tendency for her to enact her depression rather than to communicate it verbally. It is noteworthy that her self-description at admission contained only a minimal expression of depression. She seemed unable or unwilling to allow herself access to her painful feelings; instead, she seemed to ward off awareness of her suicidality and despair. Other aspects of the independent admission evaluation corresponded to the overideational style expressed in her self-description: she was described by the clinical staff as obsessive, self-preoccupied, and ruminative, with a psychotic level of ambivalence; her major defenses against depression were intellectualization and isolation of affect.

Over the course of treatment, there were several important changes in A's self-descriptions, reflected in the various scales used to evaluate aspects of the self-description (see Table 6.5). She developed more of a balance between negative and positive aspects of herself, and viewed herself as stronger and more effective as treatment progressed. At admission and 6 months, she showed blocking and difficulties with the task of describing herself, but by 1 year she no longer discussed the task itself, and proceeded with the description. The earlier reluctance to describe herself could have been more than a resistance to participate; it could have been a rudimentary assertion or defiance against the examiner and the task as she attempted to establish some sense of self-cohesion within her fragile identity—a defense she no longer needed at 1 year.

But what was most striking was that, over the course of treatment, her expressions of depression steadily increased and seemed to parallel independent multiple indications of her improvement. At 6 months, she described herself as "vulnerable, hurt, lonely"; at 1 year as "depressed, suspicious, alone . . . hopeless . . . withdrawn, angry"; and at discharge, she expressed the opinion that "people who want to kill themselves should be allowed to kill themselves." By discharge she had begun to include her suicidal thoughts in her self-description, although in a somewhat intellectualized and distanced way. Overall, there was an inverse relationship between her talking about her depression and her behaving and appearing depressed. The increase in her verbalization of depression in her self-descriptions coincided with reports in treatment reviews that she took better care of herself, sometimes attended school, was more connected to others, and appeared less psychotic. Her growing awareness of her painful existence and her increasing capacity to verbalize her depression seemed related to improvements noted in her clinical status.

In addition to the increase in expression of depression in her self-descriptions over time, there was a dramatic change in the extent to which A's self-descriptions became more elaborated over the course of treatment. At 6 months and 1 year, her self-descriptions increased in differentiation and integration; that is, more areas of her life were included, such as relationships and activities. And at 1 year there was also a change in the number of modes she used to describe herself: inner feelings, outer personality traits, and behavioral qualities were all mentioned. Her self-descriptions became rich and varied. In sum, there was a fuller sense of interpersonal relatedness and an increased ability to include more dimensions in her sense of self, including access to dysphoric experiences. Though more in touch with her desperately unhappy existence, she appeared to be almost celebrating her discovery of herself.

At 6 months she explicitly recognized the presence of the examiner and turned to the examiner for help with the task. In addition to this dependency on another, she acknowledged that she felt "lonely," yet could be giving toward others ("considerate"). The inclusion of another person, and her comments on how she behaved toward others, indicated an emerging potential for relatedness. She was aware of an audience, of others listening to her and recording what she said, as well as of the need for some precision in her verbalizations if others were to understand her. Perhaps she had come to believe that it was worth telling others about herself, that this clarity would help others to understand her, and that what she said might have an impact on others. She was aware of being active in describing herself, and she commented on her success at gaining confidence, indicating an increased sense of agency at 6 months. Although in subsequent descriptions she saw herself as less successful, she continued to depict herself on striving dimensions.

A's self-description at discharge must be viewed in light of the interruption of her treatment because of insufficient funds. At discharge, she distanced herself from others in her self-description. By saying that one of her abnormal opinions was that people who want to should be allowed to kill themselves, she included others in her self-description, but she carefully separated herself from others by saying, "I wasn't referring to myself, either." Thus, her description of her relationships and view of others were less direct than previously. Also, she depicted herself as a little less effective, as weaker—all understandable at a time when she had to interrupt important, helpful relationships by leaving the hospital.

Although her description at termination did not continue to develop as might have been predicted from the changes seen at 6 months and 1 year, it contained many of the strengths she gained during treatment. She continued to use three modes to describe herself as she had at 1 year, and at the same time, the conceptual level increased to an even more sophisticated level: she recognized that she was "hiding behind a facade." She showed an interest in how she appeared to others versus how she felt inside; and she expressed some of her central values. She came close to mentioning the examiner and their relationship explicitly by saying "can be mature—haven't really acted it during the psych testing—I sort of fooled around." Overall, the description seemed more integrated, though perhaps less varied than before when she used largely a list of adjectives and nouns to describe herself. Although her toleration of contradictions remained unchanged, she had a greater sense of herself as a real, substantial person. Her self-description at discharge had an immediacy that differed markedly from her previous self-descriptions.

In reviewing A's protocols over the course of treatment, we notice in particular two important aspects of the process of treatment, which our self-description scales reflect. First, A's increasing capacity to articulate her depression and include it in her self-description, and second, her expanding, richer sense of self during treatment. Zetzel (1949, 1965) considered that the capacity to bear depressive affect reflects the ability to control primitive aggression without severe regression, and a mature acceptance of the inevitable. Winnicott (1963) viewed the capacity to experience and tolerate guilt, though painful, to be a mark of a developmental achievement that enables the individual to accept responsibility for aggression against love objects. Likewise, we propose that the depressive feelings that A increasingly articulated in her self-descriptions were constructive because they reflected a greater internality, an acceptance of responsibility for her reactions to others, and a greater willingness to be aware of and to share her painful experiences with others and to seek their assistance. At the same time, and perhaps as a result, she began to see herself as stronger and more effective, to turn her attention to others, to develop a sense of agency, and to identify interests and values. These changes suggest the beginning of a process in which her self-preoccupation gave way to an engagement with the external world and the future, which, if her treatment continued, could in turn strengthen her sense of self.

In summary, our methodology for assessing the self has provided a window through which to measure important dimensions of the self that are related to types of depression and that distinguish between patients and nonpatients. It has also given us the opportunity to observe substantial changes in a seriously disturbed patient's sense of self during long-term treatment. The correspondence between the self-descriptions and information reported in admission evaluation and treatment review protocols of this patient provided concurrent validity for our method of analysis of self-descriptions. We believe that this method of analysis may be useful in longitudinal studies of the development of the sense of self, as well as of changes in the sense of self during the therapeutic process. This method may also be useful for understanding more fully the sense of self in different types of psychopathology, especially depression.

CONCLUSIONS

A disrupted sense of self is a fundamental component of depression. We have identified three basic aspects of the self—self-reflectivity, the capacity to tolerate and integrate affective experiences, and a sense of personal agency—and all three are at issue in depression. Empirical investigation of the sense of self in two types of depression in normal young adults indicates that distortions in the sense of self are most apparent in self-critical depression, in which there are negative feelings about the self, a sense of guilt, and feelings of hopelessness. Self-critical depression correlated significantly in both men and women with descriptions of self as cold, negative, nonnurturing, and poorly related to others. These impairments in the sense of self occurred primarily in a self-critical depression, where we expected an introjected sense of self in which self–object differentiation and a beginning capacity for self-reflectivity have been established. Feelings of guilt in a self-critical depression, for example, require a capacity for self-reflectivity as well as some sense of trying to atone for supposed failures and/or transgressions (Blatt, 1974). But the self-reflectivity is painful and judgmental and results in intense negative feelings about the self.

We expected the sense of self in a dependent depression usually to be at a more rudimentary level in which the self is depleted, impaired, or only partially formed. Reflectivity is limited, affect is warded off, and agency is expressed primarily in distorted form as in symptomatic enactments. Dependent depressive experiences are less often expressed in verbal (symbolic) form, but more often are enacted in a frantic search for contact and gratification, such as in somatic complaints, seeking of help, or in clinging and demanding behavior. The sense of self is usually unconsolidated and insecurely established, and the person feels depleted, abandoned, or unloved if a gratifying other is unavailable. There is little constancy in the sense of self; rather, it is highly reactive to environmental events. Although dependent depression usually involves a rudimentary sense of self, it is possible that in more organized individuals with a more internalized sense of self, dependent depressive feelings may also be expressed in feelings of shame and loss concerning a specific meaningful relationship, rather than a more nonspecific and general sense of loss of gratification.

While we found significant impairments in the sense of self in self-critical depression, in our study of the relationship of aspects of self-description to two types of depressive experiences in normal young adults, we found relatively few significant relationships between aspects of the sense of self and dependent depressive experiences. This lack of substantial findings suggests that the sense of self may be less articulated in dependent depression than it is in self-critical depression. Dependent depression was significantly related only to an overall negative view of the self, and only in women. This general lack of relationships between dependent depression and many aspects of self-descriptions may also be a consequence of the limited self-reflectivity that occurs in dependent depression and of warding off and enacting affect rather than tolerating and integrating it. Another reason for the insufficient findings may be that dependently depressed individuals are less responsive to the request to describe themselves than are self-critically depressed individuals, who are generally more cognitively oriented and self-reflective.

We also compared the sense of self in normal adolescents and young adults to the sense of self in a group of seriously disturbed adolescents hospitalized in a long-term treatment facility. We expected the patients' self-descriptions, obtained early in their hospitalization, to be characterized by threats of psychological disintegration, fragmentation, and devitalization. Our data indicate that the self-descriptions of severely disturbed patients are highly constricted, with little sense of agency or relatedness to others. The self-descriptions of patients tended to be more negative than those of nonpatients, with greater expressions of ineffectiveness and depression. Although patients expressed significantly more depression in their self-descriptions than normals, the level of depression in their self-descriptions was relatively mild. They did not include significant expressions of depression in their self-descriptions, though many of these patients were clinically depressed. Affective experiences generally seemed to be omitted from their self-descriptions. Patients and nonpatients did not differ significantly in the degree of self-reflectivity in their self-descriptions, but patient self-descriptions were significantly less differentiated and integrated and had less tolerance for contradiction than those of the nonpatients. The self-descriptions of the nonpatients were rich and multidimensional, whereas those of the patients were more constricted and flat. Also, patients more often omitted any reference to striving and interpersonal relations in their self-descriptions. Though not apparent in the patients' self-descriptions, clinical evidence suggests that patients' painful negative affective experiences were warded off through a number of different forms of discharge, including somatic concerns and/or acting out (Blatt, 1991b). The failure to experience affect fully and to communicate it, and the tendency to ward off these experiences through enactments, may be a specific example of an impairment in the capacity for self-reflectivity.

In the longitudinal study of change in the self-description of one seriously disturbed, psychotically depressed patient over the course of 19 months of intensive inpatient treatment, we noted how her depression changed from enactments to a greater capacity to experience and integrate affect in her sense of self. Although her initial self-description contained only minimal depressive tones, clinically she engaged in a wide range of destructive activity. This patient's depressive concerns were more self-critical than about interpersonal loss and loneliness. Her self-descriptions early in the treatment process (at admission and 6 months later) suggested that her self-critical depression was at a more rudimentary sense of self, in which negative feelings were disavowed and projected on to others or discharged and expressed in negative and destructive actions.

Over the course of treatment, the patient's self-descriptions changed dramatically. She developed a better balance between negative and positive aspects of herself and began to feel that she was gaining greater self-confidence. Her self-descriptions became increasingly elaborate and substantial, with greater differentiation and integration of various aspects of her experiences. Through the course of treatment, she developed an increasing sense of herself as real and substantial. She became more cognizant of interpersonal relationships and expressed a fuller sense of agency. Her self-descriptions were more thoughtful, more carefully delineated, and indicated a greater capacity for self-reflectivity. Most important, she also began to express more fully aspects of her affective experiences, particularly depressive feelings.

As treatment progressed, her enactments of depression diminished, and she developed an increasing capacity to reflect on and communicate her profound feelings of depression. Her progress in treatment, in large part, can be characterized by both the emergence of a fuller sense of self as well as the capacity to tolerate depressive affect. Of particular importance were the observations that this patient's experiences of depression were central to the treatment process and were an integral part of her expanding sense of self that emerged during the treatment process. These experiences of affect, especially depression, her increased sense of agency, and her capacity for reflective self-awareness were core aspects in her development of a sense of self. Her access to depressive feelings appears to have been a crucial part of her development of a more effective sense of self. These changes in her sense of self closely parallel the clinical progress independently noted in her treatment reviews.

Although impairments and distortions of the sense of self are integral to depressive experiences, it is important to note that access to depression—the capacity to be self-reflectively aware of affective experiences and to be able to tolerate and integrate negative as well as positive affect—indicates an important developmental milestone in the process of gaining a mature sense of self in which there is increased capacity for self-reflectivity, the ability to utilize affects to enrich one's experiences, and a fuller sense of one's effectiveness and agency. It is also important to note that the capacity to experience and integrate affect, including depression, is an important part of the development of the sense of self. In some depressed patients, disruptions in the development of the self sometimes occur very early in life, before there is any significant consolidation of the sense of self. In others, disruption in the sense of self occurs somewhat later in the developmental process and results in an exaggerated, painful, and intensely critical self-reflectivity. And in some individuals, the sense of self progresses to a more mature level; experiences of agency, affect, and self-reflectivity have become an integral part of a relatively realistic and multidimensional sense of the self in which components of personal agency and interpersonal relatedness are woven together in an effective identity. Part of the goal of the treatment of depressed individuals is to enable them to acknowledge an impaired and/or distorted sense of self and to appreciate its developmental antecedents so they can proceed to develop a more realistic and effective sense of self—a sense of self in which there is reflective self-awareness of their interests in, and capacities for, interpersonal relatedness and personal agency.

NOTES

1. The sense of self as object—as the passive recipient of experience—enriches our understanding of instinctual life. The initial sense of self as the recipient or object of love and affection articulates a dimension that is often overlooked in more traditional formulations of drive satisfaction as the result of an active search for discharge and satisfaction. Recognizing the importance of receptive wishes to be the object of the other's desire, of being loved by the other, increases our awareness of the relational dimensions inherent in instinctual life.

2. This conceptualization of the self in terms of the dimensions of agency and affect are consistent with a recent reformulation (Blatt, 1990; Blatt & Blass, 1990;

Blatt & Shichman, 1983) of Erikson's psychosocial model, which notes that there are two fundamental developmental lines embedded in Erikson's linear, epigenetic, developmental model: (1) an attachment or relatedness developmental line proceeding from trust versus mistrust, to cooperation versus alienation, to intimacy versus isolation; and (2) a separation or self-definitional developmental line that proceeds from autonomy versus shame, to initiative versus guilt, to industry versus inferiority, to identity versus role diffusion. Within the attachment developmental line, the terms of the psychosocial crises of each stage are conceptualized as polar opposites (trust vs. mistrust, and intimacy vs. isolation), whereas in the self-definitional developmental line, the terms are nonpolar (e.g., autonomy vs. shame, initiative vs. guilt). Thus, Erikson's terms in the self-definitional developmental line appear to express two different dimensions: an "expressive mode of self," such as autonomy, initiative, and industry, which describes a functional-behavioral component, and a "self-feeling" mode, such as shame versus pride, guilt versus self-esteem, and inferiority versus confidence, which describes "a most basic feeling that one has regarding one's being" (Blatt & Blass, 1990, p. 117). These two dimensions embedded in Erikson's self-definitional developmental line, the expressive or functional mode of self and the self-feeling, are consistent with the two dimensions of the self: agency and affect.

3. We asked individuals to simply describe themselves, sometimes in written form in group testing of nonclinical subjects, and sometimes in verbal form recorded verbatim as part of a clinical interview.

4. This section is reprinted from Bers et al. (1993).

REFERENCES

Arieti, S., & Bemporad, J. R. (1978). *Severe and mild depression: The therapeutic approach*. New York: Basic Books.

Arieti, S., & Bemporad, J. R. (1980). The psychological organization of depression. *American Journal of Psychiatry, 137*, 1360–1365.

Balint, M. (1959). *Thrills and repression*. London: Hogarth Press.

Bannister, D., & Agnew, J. (1976). The child's constructing of self. In J. K. Cole & A. W. Landfield (Eds.), *Nebraska symposium on motivation, 24*, 99–123. Lincoln: University of Nebraska Press.

Beck, A. T. (1967). *Depression: Clinical, experimental, and theoretical aspects*. New York: Harper & Row.

Beck, A. T. (1983). Cognitive therapy of depression: New perspectives. In P. J. Clayton & J. E. Barrett (Eds.), *Treatment of depression: Old controversies and new approaches* (pp. 265–290). New York: Raven Press.

Beck, A. T., Epstein, N., Harrison, R. P., & Emery, G. (1983). *Development of the Sociotropy-Autonomy Scale: A measure of personality factors in psychopathology*. Unpublished manuscript, University of Pennsylvania, Philadelphia.

Behrends, R. S., & Blatt, S. J. (1985). Internalization and psychological development through the life cycle. *Psychoanalytic Study of the Child, 40*, 11–39.

Benvineste, E. (1971). *Problems in general linguistics* (M. E., Meek, Trans.). Coral Gables, FL: University of Miami Press. (Original work published 1966)

Bers, S. A., Blatt, S. J., Sayward, H., & Johnston, R. (1993). Normal and pathological aspects of self descriptions and their change over long-term treatment. *Psychoanalytic Psychology, 10*(1).

Blatt, S. J. (1974). Levels of object representation in anaclitic and introjective depression. *Psychoanalytic Study of the Child, 24*, 107–157.

Blatt, S. J. (1983). Narcissism and egocentrism as concepts in individual and cultural development. *Psychoanalysis and Contemporary Thought, 6*, 291–303.

Blatt, S. J. (1990). Interpersonal relatedness and self-definition: Two personality configurations and their implication for psychopathology and psychotherapy. In J. L. Singer (Ed.), *Repression and dissociation: Implications for personality theory, psychopathology and health* (pp. 299–335). Chicago: University of Chicago Press.

Blatt, S. J. (1991a). A cognitive morphology of psychopathology. *Journal of Nervous and Mental Disease, 179*, 449–458.

Blatt, S. J. (1991b). Depression and destructive risk-taking behavior in adolescence. In L. P. Lipsitt & L. L. Mitnick (Eds.), *Self-regulatory behavior and risk-taking* (pp. 285–309). Norwood, NJ: Ablex.

Blatt, S. J., & Behrends, R. S. (1987). Separation-individuation, internalization and the nature of therapeutic action. *International Journal of Psycho-Analysis, 68*, 279–297.

Blatt, S. J., & Bers, S. A. (1987). *The assessment of self-descriptions: A scoring manual.* Unpublished manuscript, Yale University, New Haven, CT.

Blatt, S. J., Bers, S. A., & Stein, J. (1985). *A manual for the assessment of qualitative and structural aspects of self-descriptions.* Unpublished manuscript, Yale University, New Haven, CT.

Blatt, S. J., & Blass, R. (1990). Attachment and separateness: A dialectic model of the products and processes of psychological development. *Psychoanalytic Study of the Child, 45*, 107–127.

Blatt, S. J., & Blass, R. (1992). Relatedness and self-definition: Two primary dimensions in personality development, psychopathology and psychotherapy. In J. Barron, M. Eagle, & D. Wolitsky (Eds.), *Interface of psychoanalysis and psychology* (pp. 399–435). Washington, DC: American Psychological Association.

Blatt, S. J., Chevron, E. S., Quinlan, D. M., Schaffer, C. E., & Wein, S., (1988). *The assessment of qualitative and structural dimensions of object representations.* Unpublished manuscript, Yale University, New Haven, CT.

Blatt, S. J., Chevron, E. S., Quinlan, D. M., & Wein, S. (1979). *The assessment of qualitative and structural dimensions of object representations* (rev. ed.). Unpublished manuscript, Yale University, New Haven, CT.

Blatt, S. J., D'Afflitti, J. P., & Quinlan, D. M. (1976). Experiences of depression in normal young adults. *Journal of Abnormal Psychology, 85*, 383–389.

Blatt, S. J., D'Afflitti, J. P., & Quinlan, D. M. (1979). *Depressive Experiences Questionnaire.* Unpublished manuscript, Yale University, New Haven, CE.

Blatt, S. J., & Maroudas, C. (1992). Convergence of psychoanalytic and cognitive behavioral theories of depression. *Psychoanalytic Psychology, 9,* 157–190.

Blatt, S. J., Quinlan, D. M., Chevron, E. S., McDonald, C., & Zuroff, D. (1982). Dependency and self-criticism: Psychological dimensions of depression. *Journal of Consulting and Clinical Psychology, 50,* 113–124.

Blatt, S. J., & Shichman, S. (1983). Two primary configurations of psychopathology. *Psychoanalysis and Contemporary Thought, 6,* 187–254.

Blatt, S. J., Wein, S. J., Chevron, E. S., & Quinlan, D. M. (1978). *The assessment of qualitative and structural dimensions of object representation.* Unpublished manuscript, Yale University, New Haven, CT.

Blatt, S. J., Wein, S. J., Chevron, E. S., & Quinlan, D. M. (1979). Parental representation and depression in normal young adults. *Journal of Abnormal Psychology, 88,* 388–397.

Blatt, S. J., Wiseman, H., Prince-Gibson, E., & Gatt., H. (1991). Object representation and change in clinical functioning. *Psychotherapy, 28,* 273–283.

Bornstein, R. F., & O'Neill, R. M. (in press). Parental perceptions and psychopathology. *Journal of Nervous and Mental Disease.*

Bowlby, J. (1969). *Attachment and loss: Vol. 1. Attachment.* New York: Basic Books.

Bowlby, J. (1973). *Attachment and loss: Vol. 2. Separation, anxiety, and anger.* New York: Basic Books.

Bowlby, J. (1980). *Attachment and loss: Vol. 3. Loss, separation and depression.* New York: Basic Books.

Bowlby, J. (1988). Developmental psychology comes of age. *American Journal of Psychiatry, 145,* 1–10.

Cane, D. B., Olinger, L. J., Gotlib, I. H., & Kuiper, N. A. (1986). Factor structure of the Dysfunctional Attitude Scale in a student population. *Journal of Clinical Psychology, 42,* 307–309.

Chodorow, N. (1978). *The reproduction of mothering: Psychoanalysis and the sociology of gender.* Berkeley, CA: University of California Press.

Chodorow, N. (1989). *Feminism and psychoanalytic theory.* New Haven: Yale University Press.

Diamond, D., Kaslow, N., Coonerty, S., & Blatt, S. J. (1990). Changes in separation-individuation and intersubjectivity in long-term treatment. *Psychoanalytic Psychology, 7,* 363–397.

Emde, R. N. (1988). Development terminable and interminable. *International Journal of Psycho-Analysis, 69,* 23–42.

Erikson, E. H. (1950). *Childhood and society.* New York: W. W. Norton.

Erlich, H. S., & Blatt, S. J. (1985). Narcissism and object love: The metapsychology of experience. *Psychoanalytic Study of the Child, 40,* 57–79.

Feffer, M. (1970). Developmental analysis of interpersonal behavior. *Psychology Review, 77,* 177–214.

Flavell, J. (1977). *Cognitive development.* Englewood, NJ: Prentice-Hall.

Freud, S. (1957). On narcissism: An introduction. In J. Strachey (Ed. and Trans.), *The standard edition of the complete psychological works of Sigmund Freud*

(Vol. 14, pp. 73–102). London: Hogarth Press. (Original work published 1914)

Freud, S. (1957). Mourning and melancholia. In J. Strachey (Ed. and Trans.), *The standard edition of the complete psychological works of Sigmund Freud* (Vol. 17, pp. 7–122). London: Hogarth Press. (Original work published 1917)

Freud, S. (1959). Inhibitions, symptoms and anxiety. In J. Strachey (Ed. and Trans.), *The standard edition of the complete psychological works of Sigmund Freud* (Vol. 20, pp. 87–174). London: Hogarth Press. (Original work published 1926)

Freud, S. (1961). Civilization and its discontents. In J. Strachey (Ed. and Trans.), *The standard edition of the complete psychological works of Sigmund Freud* (Vol. 21, pp. 64–145). London: Hogarth Press. (Original work published 1930)

Gilligan, C. (1982). *In a different voice*. Cambridge, MA: Harvard University Press.

Gilligan, C. (1988). Remapping the moral domain. In C. Gilligan, J. V. Ward, & J. M. Taylor (Eds.), *Mapping the moral domain* (pp. 3–19). Cambridge, MA: Harvard University Press.

Gruen, R. J., & Blatt, S. J. (1990). Changes in self and object representation during long-term dynamically oriented treatment. *Psychoanalytic Psychology*, *7*, 399–422.

Harter, S. (1982). A developmental perspective on some parameters of self-regulation in children. In R. Karoly & F. H. Kanfer (Eds.), *Self-management and behavior change: From theory to practice*. Elsmsford, NY: Pergamon Press.

Izard, C. (1972). *Patterns of emotion: A new analysis of anxiety and depression*. New York: Academic Press.

Katz, P., & Zigler, E. (1967). Self-image disparity: A developmental approach. *Journal of Personality and Social Psychology*, *5*, 186–195.

Kegan, R. (1982). *The evolving self*. Cambridge, MA: Harvard University Press.

Kernberg, O. F. (1976). *Object relations theory and clinical psychoanalysis*. New York: Jason Aronson.

Kernberg, O. F. (1989). An ego psychology of object relations theory of the structure and treatment of pathological narcissism: An overview. *Psychiatric Clinics of North America*, *12*, 671–694.

Klein, G. S. (1976). *Psychoanalytic theory*. New York: International Universities Press.

Kohut, H. (1971). *The analysis of the self*. New York: International Universities Press.

Kohut, H. (1977). *The restoration of the self*. New York: International Universities Press.

Lee, B., & Noam, G. G. (1983). *Developmental approaches to the self*. New York: Plenum Press.

Lévi-Strauss, C. (1963). *Structural anthropology*. New York: W. W. Norton.

Lichtenstein, H. (1977). *The dilemma of human identity*. New York: Jason Aronson.

Loewald, H. W. (1973). On internalization. *International Journal of Psycho-Analysis*, *54*, 9–17.

Miller, J. B. (1984). *Toward a new psychology of women*. Boston: Beacon Press.
Modell, A. H. (1984). Self psychology as a psychology of conflict: Comments on the psychoanalysis of the narcissistic personality. In G. H. Pollock & J. Gedo (Eds.), *Psychoanalysis: The vital issue* (Vol. 2, pp. 131–148). New York: International Universities Press.
Modell, A. H. (1985). The two contexts of the self. *Contemporary Psychoanalysis, 21*, 70–90.
Mullener, N., & Laird, J. D. (1971). Some developmental changes in the organization of self-evaluations. *Developmental Psychology, 5*, 233–236.
Piaget, J. (1962). *Play, dreams and imitation in childhood*. New York: W. W. Norton. (Original work published 1945)
Rizzuto, A. M. (1991, May). *I, me, myself: Sense of self and psychoanalysis*. Paper presented at the meeting of the Psychoanalytic Institute of New England East, Boston.
Sampson, E. E. (1985). Decentralization of identity: Toward a revised concept of personal and social order. *American Psychologist, 40*, 1203–1211.
Sampson, E. E. (1988). The debate on individualism: Indigenous psychologies of the individual and their role in personal and societal functioning. *American Psychologist, 43*, 15–22.
Schaffer, C. E., & Blatt, S. J. (1990). Interpersonal relationships and the experience of perceived efficacy. In R. J. Sternberg & J. Kolligan, Jr. (Eds.), *Competency considered* (pp. 229–245). New Haven, CT: Yale University Press.
Selman, R., & Byrne, J. (1974). A structural-developmental analysis of levels of role-taking in middle childhood. *Child Development, 45*, 803–806.
Sharpless, E. A. (1985). Identity formation as reflected in the acquisition of person pronouns. *Journal of the American Psychoanalytic Association, 33*, 861–885.
Stern, D. (1983). The early development of schemas of self, of other, and of various experiences of "self with other." In J. D. Lichtenberg & S. Kaplan (Eds.), *Reflections of self psychology* (pp. 49–84). Hillsdale, NJ: Analytic Press.
Stern, D. N. (1985). *The interpersonal world of the infant*. New York: Basic Books.
Surrey, J. L. (1984). The "self-in-relation": A theory of women's development. *Work in Progress, #2*. Wellesley, MA: Stone Center Working Papers.
Tomkins, S. (1963). *Affect, imagery, consciousness*. New York: Springer.
Weissman, A. N., & Beck, A. T. (1978, August). *Development and validation of the Dysfunctional Attitude Scale: A preliminary investigation*. Paper presented at the 1987 meeting of the American Psychological Association, Toronto, Canada.
Werner, H., & Kaplan, B. (1963). *Symbol formation: An organismic-developmental approach to language and the expression of thought*. New York: Wiley.
White, R. W. (1959). Motivation reconsidered: The concept of competence. *Psychological Review, 66*, 297–333.
Winnicott, D. W. (1960). The theory of the parent-infant relationship. *International Journal of Psycho-Analysis, 41*, 585–595.
Winnicott, D. W. (1963). The development of the capacity for concern. *Bulletin of the Menninger Clinic, 27*, 167–176.

Zetzel, E. R. (1949). Anxiety and the capacity to bear it. *International Journal of Psycho-Analysis, 20*, 1–12.

Zetzel, E. R. (1965). Depression and the incapacity to bear it. In *Drives, affects, behavior* (Vol. 2, pp. 243–274). New York: International Universities Press.

Zung, W. W. (1973). From art to science: The diagnosis and treatment of depression. *Archives of General Psychiatry, 29*, 328–337.

Commentary

ZINDEL V. SEGAL
Clarke Institute of Psychiatry,
University of Toronto

J. CHRISTOPHER MURAN
Beth Israel Medical Center,
Mount Sinai School of Medicine

PSYCHODYNAMIC FORMULATIONS OF depression have a long and scholarly history dating back to Freud's early work on distinguishing mourning from melancholia. This emphasis on the accurate capture of affective experience is echoed in the chapter by Blatt and Bers and serves as an important template in their attempts to decode the relations between self-based processes and emotional phenomena. Our commentary on this work is organized around two central issues: (1) points of convergence and divergence in our views on what constitutes a vulnerability to depression, and (2) problems with the reliance on open-ended self-descriptions as a measure of change in self constructs.

AGREEMENT ON THE VULNERABILITY BUT NOT ON THE PATH

To the uninitiated, a quick perusal of the ostensibly differing chapters in this section might be somewhat puzzling because it would reveal similar things being written about the self-views of depressed persons.

That adjectives such as "inadequate," "worthless," "failure," and "rejected" are offered by both sets of authors to characterize how depressed individuals think and judge themselves points to an important commonality that may render the specific posturing of each model less necessary. Continuing this process, an examination of descriptions of the diathesis for the development of unipolar depression could be similarly accommodated to the "no great difference between them" schema. In this case, both accounts describe the occurrence of negative events in childhood as laying the groundwork for disturbed cognitive processes later in life, which propel a reactive dysphoria into a full-blown depression. This dysphoria is seen as triggered by a type of social adversity, whose nature serves to prime or activate the reemergence of material based on these childhood experiences. Once in awareness, there is little else the person can do but ruminate unproductively on this content.

The similarities described to this point represent important areas of convergence between accounts. It would be wrong to conclude, however, that the remaining differences are less substantial as a result of this concordance, since the ways in which these models generated their insights, the implications for interventions that flow from them, and the nature of self-processes being described differ markedly.

Cognitive models of depression draw heavily from social-cognition-based accounts of normal self-development to describe how these regulatory processes go awry in depression. Although these models incorporate aspects of performance that are "unintended" or "out of awareness," they are largely shorn of the motivational underpinnings that psychodynamic accounts invoke to explain why it would be dangerous to have such information enter awareness. Rather, the description is of the cognitive skills that go into the building of a sense of self, as well as the elements or fundamental attributes that constitute it. It is not really necessary to subscribe to a particular developmental path in order to explain how these abilities develop; put another way, they can develop in a number of different ways, only one of which is the path described by Blatt and Bers.

In our view, their path seems to be overly reductionistic and constrained by events in the first years of life. Furthermore, there is a strong emphasis on the child's attachment history with the parents, and the potency ascribed to these factors is merely stated, not supported. The self of the vulnerable individual is developed to maintain a parental love that is conditional upon certain childhood behaviors (e.g., being independent and self-reliant, being obedient, and looking to others for guidance).

We find this model lacking because it seems to close the window on selfhood development too soon. Statements such as "the sense of self emerges out of the shared, reciprocal, loving relationship between parent and infant during the first 3 years of life" (p. 180) implies possession of a truly wondrous temporal specificity. Although many cognitive–behavioral theorists are impressed with the research regarding mother–infant attachment (e.g., Stern, 1985), they do not underestimate the formative impact of peer relationships on self-identity beyond the preoedipal window. Blatt and Bers acknowledge the importance of peer relations in adolescence for the development of self-identity, but they do not address the possibility that girls and boys pass through this process in fundamentally different ways. They cite the work of Gilligan and others, but the crucial gender-based distinction conveyed in this corpus is not highlighted, and we consider this an oversight, since it bears directly on questions of how vulnerability to depression develops and how one can account for the observed gender differences in this disorder.

To elaborate this point somewhat further, Gilligan's work (Gilligan, 1982; Gilligan, Lyons, & Hanmer, 1989) is particularly provocative because it highlights formative events for the creation of self-identity, which occur "outside" the cradle of parents and family (see also Harter, 1990). More specifically, it was suggested that the identity we inhabit develops, through interactions with peers, especially during adolescence, and not through exclusive interactions with an important caregiver in the early years of life. She also asserted that girls face different challenges during this transition than do boys. This is an interesting point to consider, since the starting point for the higher incidence of depression in females versus males is in adolescence (Lewinsohn, Duncan, Stanton, & Hautzinger, 1986; Sorenson, Rutter, & Aneshensel, 1991).

Gilligan discussed data that suggest that the formation of self-identity in girls is tied to the development of a strong sense of caring and response to others in their peer relationships, and that the ability to problem-solve in relationships is associated with robust self-definition in college-age women. Yet this path to selfhood for females often runs counter to prevailing social expectation. In describing the possible struggle that arises from the collision of these two trends, Gilligan and colleagues (1989) wrote:

> For girls to remain responsive to themselves, they must resist the conventions of feminine goodness; to remain responsive to others, they must resist the values placed on self-sufficiency and independence in North American culture. Thus for girls to develop a clear sense of self in relationship with others means—at least within the mainstream of North American culture—to take on the problem of resistance and also to take up the question of what relationship means to themselves, to others, and to the world. (p. 10)

We believe that the trajectory of male identity formation is probably as complex. Our aim in reviewing this work is to suggest that the formulations of self-development outlined by Blatt and Bers seems to have bypassed an important juncture, especially one that for females may have direct implications for the development of a self that is vulnerable to depression (Harter, 1990).

WEAK METHODS MAKE FOR WEAK CONCLUSIONS

Blatt and Bers devote a good deal of coverage to their research on the self in depression. This is especially laudable since the tradition they represent has often held a sceptical view of attempts to justify or document, in empirical terms, truths that have struck most adherents as self-evident. Although it is true that the psychodynamic tradition boasts a legacy of carefully crafted case reports and thoughtful descriptions of therapy process, this format remains, nonetheless, superior for purposes of documentation rather than investigation. As such, it is encouraging to read empirically based efforts in this domain, since it helps to promote and define a common ground for discussion of concepts relevant to adherents of both traditions.

The primary method chosen to study the self in both depressed patients and nondepressed samples of different ages was the collection of self-descriptions, given in response to the request, "describe yourself." These descriptions were analyzed for content differences by raters who judged them along predetermined dimensions, and differences were taken to reflect the varying patterns of self-organization in these groups. Blatt and Bers describe patients as having more negative and ineffective views of themselves, and even though their descriptions contained references to depressed mood, this was not included as a salient feature of the sense of self. Nondepressed controls' descriptions were longer, "rich and multi-dimensional," and better integrated overall.

The difficulty we have with accepting that these findings reflect differences in self-representation lies in the proliferation of equally plausible competing explanations for these results, and the relative absence of efforts to rule them out. At an intuitive level, the differences described between the patient and nonpatient samples makes good sense, but they may just as easily describe other ways in which the groups differ, without saying very much about self-representation. For example: (1) since no measure of intelligence was taken, it seems likely that the student sample had a higher verbal IQ than that of the patients; (2) the lack of a hospitalized nonclinical control group makes it difficult to know if the experience of being a patient may have influenced self-perceptions and, therefore, self-descriptions; (3) there is no control for the differing contingencies surrounding self-disclosure in a mental health versus a school setting, especially considering that such disclosure can effect variables such as length of stay for one group and not the other; (4) even if these findings were proven reliable, it would be difficult to accept them as relevant to depressive self-representation because the patient group consisted of individuals with diagnoses of schizophrenic spectrum disorders, severe personality disorders, and major affective disorders.

In the first study describing the comparisons between aspects of self-descriptions and measures of clinical depression in normal young adults, there is a good chance that item overlap between the content of the BDI, Zung, and DEQ and the 12 rating scales may have accounted for the findings reported. More specifically, some of these 12 scales may have rated items similar to those on one of the three measures of depression used to classify subjects. We wonder to what extent ratings of the punitive, judgmental, intellectual, and constructive involvement with other dimensions assess content similar to the following items on the BDI: "I feel I am being punished," "I am disgusted with myself," "I feel I am a complete failure as a person," and "I have lost all my interest in other people."

Finally, a question more fundamental to that of control and design is, What level of cognitive organization can be revealed by spontaneous, open-ended self-descriptions? We find it somewhat ironic that adherents of a theoretical orientation that questions people's ability to be accurate commentators on their own psychological processes (unless such commentary is veiled from the commentator or expressed in symbolic form) would put credence into a procedure that is sensitive to so much conscious—not to mention unintentional—editing (Uleman & Bargh, 1989). Two such important influences that deserve consideration are mood and accessibility effects.

It is a well-established finding that mood can have a direct impact on the nature of cognitive material reported, such that content that is congruent with an individual's mood will be favored over material that is mood incongruent (Teasdale & Fogarty, 1979; Williams, Watts, MacLeod, & Mathews, 1988). How can we know whether the descriptions obtained reflected subjects' true views of themselves or only the results of a production process that was biased by an existing mood state? This is especially relevant to the patient sample, since no assessments were taken under nonpathological conditions.

The same point can be made of the data for changes in self over long-term treatment. Quite apart from the explicit demands associated with asking for self-descriptions in order to track an intervention that has as one of its goals the modification of self-perceptions, could the reported changes in the patients' descriptions over the course of therapy not have been due to the alleviation of dysphoric mood states, with different reports tracking these changes? We are not suggesting that we have an answer to this question, but only that the multiplicity of self-views leaves one wondering which should be considered as primary and which as products of processes other than a cognitive structure.

A procedure that asks for spontaneous descriptions is also bound to be influenced by the relative accessibility of different constructs in mind at the time of reporting (Higgins & King, 1981). Since accessibility has been shown to be a function of the recency and frequency with which information has been brought to mind, how salient the information is, the person's affective state, and the relation of information to other accessible constructs, reporting on the self is not an entirely straightforward process. It is difficult to see how the methodology described by Blatt and Bers would allow one to determine which self-descriptions reflect the operation of "momentarily" as opposed to "chronically" activated constructs. The latter would seem most pertinent to revealing the more ingrained and enduring self-views that subjects hold, and yet we do not know which process the Blatt and Bers inquiry mirrors (or, more likely, that it reflects both processes operating simultaneously).

Another possibility is that these chronic self-views are activated in response to situations that prime or trigger them. In this case, a probe by the experimenter, or instructions that provide a context for this type of reflection, may have pointed subjects in the intended direction without constraining them too greatly.

CONCLUSION

Our aim in making these comments has been to pinpoint some of the threats to internal validity that need to be overcome in the future, so that greater confidence can be placed in this important line of investigation. As stated earlier, the recognition of distortions in depressed persons' self-views is an encouraging point of convergence between cognitive–behavioral and psychodynamic models. Other meeting grounds may be found in studying the relationship between personality, social adversity, and depression. For example, Blatt's seminal work in drawing a distinction between certain core features of depressive experience has allowed investigators from various orientations to better appreciate the phenomenology of depressed individuals. In its various guises (i.e., sociotropy/autonomy, need for approval/self-criticism, anaclitic/introjective), it has the potential to provide a more productive framework for investigating the interaction between personality functioning and symptom onset than has recently been the case. As investigators from different orientations consider this paradigm, we can expect to see a number of theoretical constructs be put to the test. Following this process of empirical triage, perhaps a clearer image of what we mean when we talk about a depressive self-schema will emerge.

REFERENCES

Gilligan, C., Lyons, N. P., & Hanmer, T. J. (1989). *Making connections: The relational world of adolescent girls at Emma Willard School*. Cambridge, MA: Harvard University Press.

Gilligan, C. (1982). *In a different voice*. Cambridge, MA: Harvard University Press.

Harter, S. (1990). Developmental differences in the nature of self-representation: Implications for understanding, assessment, and treatment of maladaptive behavior. *Cognitive Therapy and Research, 14*, 113–142.

Higgins, E. T., & King, G. A. (1981). Accessibility of social constructs: Information-processing consequences of individual and contextual variability. In N. Cantor & J. F. Kihlstrom (Eds.), *Personality, cognition and social interaction* (pp. 69–121). Hillsdale, NJ: Lawrence Erlbaum.

Lewinsohn, P. M., Duncan, E. M., Stanton, A. K., & Hautzinger, M. (1986). Age at first onset for nonbipolar depression. *Journal of Abnormal Psychology, 95*, 378–383.

Stern, D. N. (1985). *The interpersonal world of the infant*. New York: Basic Books.

Sorenson, S. B., Rutter, C., & Aneshensel, C. S. (1991). Depression in the community: An investigation into age of onset. *Journal of Consulting and Clinical Psychology, 59*, 541–546.

Teasdale, J. D., & Fogarty, S. J. (1979). Differential effects of induced mood on the retrieval of pleasant and unpleasant events from episodic memory. *Journal of Abnormal Psychology, 88*, 248–257.

Uleman, J. S., & Bargh, J. A. (Eds.). (1989). *Unintended thought*. New York: Guilford Press.

Williams, J. M. G., Watts, F. N., MacLeod, C., & Mathews, A. (1988). *Cognitive psychology and emotional disorders*. New York: Wiley.

IV

Eating Disorders

7

Self-representation in Eating Disorders: A Cognitive Perspective

KELLY BEMIS VITOUSEK
LINDA S. EWALD
University of Hawaii

ANOREXIA NERVOSA IS fundamentally both a cognitive disorder and a disorder of the self. After the psychopathological process has been initiated, the lives of anorexics are progressively dominated by a central, overdetermined idea about one aspect of the self: that the self's worth is represented in—or at least delimited by—the weight and shape of the body. This belief arises from a complex interaction among more basic views of the self and a sociocultural context that supports the linkage between weight and personal values. Once formed, the dominant anorexic idea gives rise to subsidiary beliefs and behaviors, characteristic information-processing errors, and starvation-induced physiological changes, which all serve to maintain and reinforce the underlying premise.

Cognitive models of the eating disorders differ from cognitive models of other disorders in several important respects (Garner & Bemis, 1982, 1985). Perhaps the most obvious and significant of these is the prominence of material on the *motivation* for, and *function* of, symptomatic behavior. Cognitive theories of psychopathology usually disavow dynamic notions of motivated symptomatology, emphasizing instead the *automaticity* of the information-processing errors that derive from lawfully and unintentionally acquired schemas. However, cognitive theories of the eating disorders (Bemis, 1983; Fairburn & Garner, 1988; Garner & Bemis, 1982, 1985; Vitousek & Hollon, 1990) have tended to stress the motivated, functional aspects of anorexic beliefs and behaviors—to at least as great an extent as the psychodynamic theories of the eating disorders (Bruch, 1973, 1978;

Goodsitt, 1985), which they most closely resemble. When confronted with the fiercely egosyntonic nature of symptoms in anorexia nervosa, all observers—whatever their general theoretical predilections—are forced to contend with questions of purpose and meaning. Individuals with other forms of psychopathology generally see their disorders as interfering with the attainment of important objectives; most anorexics view their illness as a fulfillment of cherished values and goals. In many senses, anorexia is not only an expression of core elements of the self, but an active attempt to *create* a self. It is, moreover, in spite of all of its aversive consequences, a partially *successful* attempt that carries some adaptive advantages for affected individuals—and helps to account for their resistance to treatment.

It is misleading to discuss "the eating disorders" collectively, or even to characterize "anorexia nervosa" as a unitary phenomenon. We endorse a multidimensional perspective (Garfinkel & Garner, 1982), recognizing considerable diversity in initiating and maintaining variables between and within individuals with these conditions. In this chapter, we largely restrict our discussion to the "classic" or "primary" form of anorexia nervosa: a modal subtype that has been recognized with substantial reliability over time and by many observers (Bemis, 1978; Bruch, 1973; Dally, 1969; King, 1963; Strober, 1991). We assume that many elements of the cognitive model we present also apply to less typical forms of anorexia nervosa and to the kindred disorder, bulimia nervosa, but we adopt the conservative course of limiting our generalizations to the most cohesive and best understood subgroup of eating-disordered individuals.

THE DEVELOPMENT AND MAINTENANCE OF ANOREXIA NERVOSA

Figure 7.1 outlines a simplified model of the onset and maintenance of anorexia nervosa drawn from the cognitive theories of Garner and Bemis (1982, 1985) and Vitousek and Hollon (1990), and closely related models formulated by Slade (1982) and Casper (1983). Both to avoid reiterating previously published material and to conform to the specialized interests of the book, we will selectively emphasize those elements of the model that are most relevant to self-representation. It should not be assumed that our allocation of space is proportionate to the hypothesized importance of various theoretical components.

Distal Conditions

As illustrated graphically in Figure 7.1, the cognitive model declines to take a strong position on the contribution of specific genetic and familial variables to the etiology of anorexia nervosa. This is neither an ahistorical nor

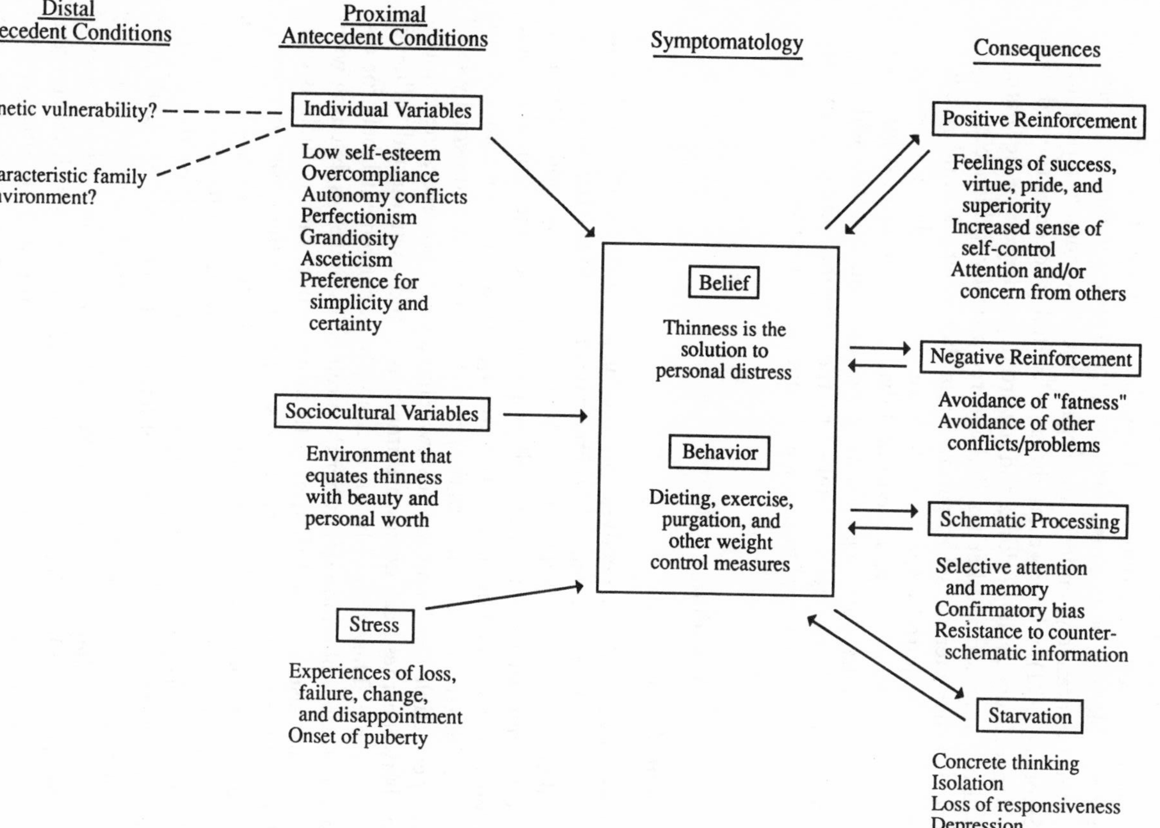

FIGURE 7.1. A cognitive model of anorexia nervosa.

an antidevelopmental stance; indeed, it is assumed that the stable individual characteristics necessary for symptom onset have their origin in the interplay between these two sets of variables. If forced to hazard a guess about the role of remote causal factors in the genesis of anorexia nervosa, we would (tentatively) endorse the organismic-developmental perspective of Strober (1991), who postulated that inherited tendencies toward harm avoidance, low novelty seeking, and reward dependence may be shared by the future anorexic and her family,[1] and reciprocally influence the emergence of a characteristic self-organization in the vulnerable child. We have, however, an acquired respect for the diversity of family backgrounds in cases of anorexia nervosa, a theoretical disinclination for post hoc reconstructions of unstudied events, and a personal distaste for adding the specter of the "anorexigenic family" to the "schizophrenigenic mother" and "refrigerator parent" ghosts who haunt our collective past.

Proximal Conditions

Individual Variables

Across theoretical perspectives, the modal pre-anorexic personality has been characterized in remarkably similar terms: young girls who are at risk are likely to have been insecure, avoidant, conforming, and excessively "good" children who are not well-prepared to become competent and independent adults. For clarity, we have organized our list of characteristic features into three clusters, with the general themes of the "unworthy self," the "perfectible self," and the "overwhelmed self"; however, the boundaries between these categories are imprecise, and their mutual influence considerable. They should be viewed simply as convenient labels for discussing related phenomena, rather than reified as subselves dwelling within. It must also be noted that, as with more remote factors such as early childhood experience, aspects of the self *preceding* the onset of symptomatology can only be identified retrospectively. Investigators who obtain low scores on self-concept questionnaires administered to anorexic samples can merely guess that such negative views of the self predated—and perhaps contributed to—symptom onset; researchers who record the persistence of such characteristics after symptom resolution can still only speculate that they represent durable traits rather than residual traces of illness. We can at least derive some reassurance from the much shorter time interval between the hypothesized proximal factors and the emergence of symptoms, and from the unusually high interobserver and cross-theoretical reliability of these dimensions. None of them is uniquely associated with the cognitive model.

The first cluster of variables implicated in the development of anorexia nervosa—the "unworthy self"—subsumes profound feelings of ineffectiveness, inadequacy, inferiority, and impotence (Bruch, 1973, 1978; Casper, 1983; Crisp, 1980; Garner & Bemis, 1985; Goodsitt, 1985; Guidano & Liotti, 1983; Lerner, 1986; Strober, 1991). Bruch wrote that these individuals "suffer from a deep fear of being incompetent—a 'nothing'—and of not getting or even deserving respect" (Bruch, 1985, pp. 10–11). Lacking a clear, cohesive sense of self, they are preoccupied by the agonizing, absorbing question of their own value. Anxiously scanning the environment for cues about how they should calculate their intrinsic worth, they become utterly dependent on external frames of reference and hyperattuned to the negative judgments of others (Garner & Bemis, 1985; Guidano, 1987; Riebel, 1985). One client evocatively described the sense of despair she experienced whenever her inner doubts were confirmed by another's criticism: "It's a sense of general darkening and dismay, like being under water and sinking deeper and deeper, and your only hope to ever emerge again is to obtain the other person's approval; and that seems more and more unlikely and beyond hope" (Guidano, 1987, p. 166).

The exaggerated need for approval is often manifested in extreme overcompliance. As Lerner (1986) noted, "like chameleons, [anorexics] quickly and accurately attune to the expectations of others and mold themselves, their behavior, and feelings accordingly" (p. 41). For these individuals, normal adolescent conflicts surrounding issues of dependence versus independence are magnified. Profound longings for closeness and excessive reliance upon external affirmation conflict with values that exaggerate the need for autonomy and self-sufficiency, resulting in an intense ambivalence in relation to others.

The characteristics that constitute the "unworthy self" should be measurable as (1) *low self-esteem*, (2) *feelings of helplessness and ineffectiveness*, (3) a *poorly developed sense of identity*, (4) a *tendency to seek external verification*, (5) *extreme sensitivity to criticism*, and (6) *conflicts over autonomy/dependency*.

The second cluster—the "*perfectible self*"—includes a superficially opposite set of attitudes about the supreme significance and moral probity of the self. If the anorexic individual chronically doubts her own worth, she has few uncertainties about her importance. "Grandiose fantasies of omnipotence and invulnerability" awkwardly coexist with the terrible sense of ineffectiveness (Goodsitt, 1985, p. 76), vying with it on a moment-to-moment basis for ascendance in the individual's self-concept, and causing dizzying alternations in her mood state.

Slade is probably correct that "of all the premorbid, predisposing factors reported in the literature, the one which is most commonly endorsed and most evident is that of obsessive–compulsive traits or perfectionistic tendencies" (Slade, 1982, p. 171). According to most commentators, the perfectionistic style of anorexics is a compensatory mechanism that develops in an attempt to cope with the more fundamental underlying sense of inadequacy. As Guidano (1987) noted, "if the problem consists of drawing a sense of self out of others' judgments, perfectionism logically becomes the way to provide a positive solution to the problem" (p. 164). If one can avoid committing any errors, consistently anticipating, fulfilling, and even surpassing the expectations of the audience, one may both avoid censure and secure reassurance about one's basic worth. As a brilliant adolescent client once remarked to the first author:

> "I remember when I first heard someone quote Abraham Lincoln about 'you can please all of the people some of the time, and some of the people all of the time, but you can't please all of the people all of the time.' I thought: Why *not*? Why *not*? If you *can* please everyone some of the time, why shouldn't it be possible to satisfy them all of the time, if you just get very good at it? At any rate, I felt determined to try."

In the finest psychodynamic tradition, the client failed to recognize her own substitution of the verb "to please" for the original verb "to fool"—an insertion that reveals a great deal about the futility of the perfectionistic strategy. Even if one is successful in pleasing others, the possibility remains that one may simply have fooled them. Feeling like an imposter (Barnett, 1986) or an impersonator (Story, 1976), the anorexic derives little sense of accomplishment from her attainments, and obtains no real reassurance about her personal worth. Moreover, she becomes trapped in the inflationary cycle of perfectionism (Mahoney, 1974), resetting the minimum standard for acceptable performance to a higher level as soon as a previously set goal has been reached, and failing to adjust her expectations to the increasingly competitive reference groups to which success may expose her. The client quoted above insisted that in order to feel satisfied with her achievements, she would need to outperform all contenders with whom she might be compared; even if she were invited to join a special study group composed of the 10 brightest high school students collected from throughout the English-speaking world, she would need to prove herself the best among the best or "risk jeopardizing everything I am."

The sublime grandiosity expressed in such statements suggests that the perfectionism of the anorexic individuals is not altogether a secondary defensive development that helps to compensate for feelings of inadequacy. Their perfectionism also expresses their commitment to their own perfectibility. Secretly, many seem to treasure the notion that they are extraordinary beings, charged with a unique mission whose precise nature has yet to be revealed. Disdaining the average and ordinary, they do not so much crave reassurance about their basic worth as recognition of their innate superiority.

The set of anorexic beliefs about the importance of the self is distinguishable from more classically narcissistic beliefs. Anorexic individuals cast their aspirations in *moral* terms, and expect to have to demonstrate their accomplishments. Like modern-day Calvinists, they seem to believe that their status as one of the elect or one of the damned has already been determined by predestination; if they cannot enhance their preordained worth through good works, their conduct may nonetheless betray the underlying truth. Thus, another reason for the anxious avoidance of error is a desperate wish to prevent the discovery, by themselves as well as others, that they may not be all that they aspire to be.

Many anorexics endorse stringent and austere codes of conduct; they establish "high moral standards and have a keen sense for what is right and wrong" (Casper, Offer, & Ostrov, 1981, p. 660). They often profess the virtues of asceticism (Bemporad, Ratey, O'Driscoll, & Daehler, 1988; Bruch, 1973; Garner & Bemis, 1982, 1985; Goodsitt, 1985; Lawrence, 1979; Mogul, 1980; Selvini-Palazzoli, 1978; Story, 1976; Strober, 1991; Thoma, 1967), and long to attain transcendent strength and goodness. Many have a "sense of being concerned with the higher things in life" and despise the worldliness of others (Mogul, 1980, p. 162). Self-discipline and self-denial are prized, while the pursuit of the merely pleasurable is dismissed as frivolous and self-indulgent (Garner & Bemis, 1985; Goodsitt, 1985; Strober, 1991). If there is a distinctive cognitive style in anorexia nervosa, equivalent to the negative biasing of memory and expectations in the affective disorders and the vigilant monitoring of threat cues in the anxiety disorders, it seems to take the form of the New Year's resolution: "I must just do X, so that Y will come to pass—and I shall be the better person for my efforts" (Vitousek & Hollon, 1990).

It is hypothesized, then, that the "*perfectible self*" includes the elements of (1) *perfectionism* (including both *high standard-setting* and the *avoidance of error*), (2) *grandiosity*, (3) *asceticism*, and (4) a "*New Year's resolution*" cognitive style of self-exhortation.

The third cluster of characteristics can be labeled the "*overwhelmed self*." Anorexic individuals describe a sense of being intolerably burdened by the multiplicity of expectations, responsibilities, and choices that impinge upon them, as on all other participants in contemporary society. Some confess that they feel "dazed," "muddled," or "in a fog" much of the time, often insisting that this distressing state had become familiar long before the initiation of dieting, which could produce starvation pathology. As they make their way through the routines of daily life, they feel bombarded by an excess of stimuli and bewildered by complex or ambiguous situations; when confronted with major life choices, they are paralyzed with indecision.

In an attempt to control this highly aversive confusional state, individuals vulnerable to anorexia nervosa appear to develop a longing for simplicity, clarity, certainty, and predictability, which is manifested in many different forms (Vitousek & Hollon, 1990). One recovered client related the following anecdote about her experience prior to the onset of her eating disorder:

> "Before every birthday and Christmas, I used to give my mother a list of items specifying the things I did *not* want her to give me. Over time, it got so long that it took a lot of ingenuity for her to come up with any possibilities I hadn't already excluded. Why did I do it? Because I was trying so hard to make my life less complicated and tiring. If I were given clothes, I would have to remember to wear them regularly, so that I wouldn't hurt my parents' feelings, and because it's wasteful for clothes to hang unused in the closet. If I were given a new stuffed animal, I would have to add it into my bedtime ritual of kissing each of them goodnight in just the right way, and it was already so burdensome to complete. Love carried so many obligations—you end up owing things both to the gift you are given and the person who gives it to you. It isn't that I felt somehow 'unworthy' of gifts—they were just so much work, and I wanted the relief of having less to worry about."

The cause of this preference for simplicity is unclear. It is conceivable that it may be a consequence of the (possibly heritable) tendencies toward low novelty seeking and harm avoidance that Strober (1991) implicates in the etiology of anorexia nervosa; it is possible that these tendencies are "hard-wired" in the form of difficulties in processing rich or contradictory sets of information. It also seems plausible that this reductionism is, at least to some extent, secondary to the perfectionism of the anorexic individual and the labor-intensive lifestyle it forces her to adopt. As illustrated in the preceding excerpt, if an individual assumes responsibility for everything in the immediate environment and expects excellence in all pursuits, it becomes adaptive to restrict the range of variables that must be taken into account.

Several other prominent features associated with anorexia nervosa may also be linked, in part, to the intolerance for uncertainty. Most of these young women are extremely uncomfortable with both the experience and the expression of strong affect, which seems to be destabilizing, in part because of its unpredictability. Social relationships, and particularly heterosexual relationships, are inherently complicated and fraught with ambiguities. Finding them difficult to predict or control, and unsure of what is expected of her within them, the vulnerable individual may find it less taxing to withdraw into a self-contained isolation. As discussed in a subsequent section, the transitions from childhood into adolescence and adolescence into young adulthood (which represent the bimodal peak ages of onset for anorexia nervosa) also tend to be experienced as confusing and overwhelming for these individuals; their wish to retreat into the simpler and more orderly world of childhood may again be partially attributable to a basic deficit in managing complex stimulus sets.

The following characteristics could be expected to cluster together as aspects of the "*overwhelmed self*": (1) a *preference for simplicity* (manifested in a focused cognitive style and a tendency to reduce complex information), (2) a *preference for certainty* (manifested in a desire for predictability, clear task demands, and a high degree of personal control), and (3) a *tendency to retreat from complex or intense social environments* (manifested in discomfort with strong affect, interpersonal avoidance and anxiety, and fears of psychosexual maturity).

These aspects of the self seem to represent the general self-schemas of individuals who develop anorexia nervosa; however, it is not clear that these variables are in any sense unique to the psychopathology of this specific disorder. Certainly, the pervasive sense of ineffectiveness, perfectionistic striving, narcissistic self-preoccupation, hypersensitivity to criticism, ambivalence about attachment and autonomy, and social avoidance implicated here and elsewhere in the etiology of anorexia nervosa are strongly associated with other forms of psychiatric disturbance, particularly subtypes of the affective, anxiety, and personality disorders. Indeed, in the rare instances when appropriate control groups have been included, it has sometimes been discovered that these "general" beliefs about the self are precisely that—concomitants of diverse forms of psychopathology rather than features that selectively predispose to, or correlate with, the eating disorders (Cooper, Cooper, & Fairburn, 1985). Some of the postulated variables, including asceticism and the New Year's resolution cognitive style, have yet to be investigated in comparative research, and it remains possible that more specific associations will eventually be identified. For the moment, it should be emphasized that the apparent lack of exclusivity between postulated aspects of the self and eating disorder symptomatology does not imply that these variables are unimportant; it merely underscores that etiological models of anorexia nervosa must explain why individuals with similar views of the self might seek different specific solutions and develop varying forms of psychopathology (Vitousek & Hollon, 1990).

Sociocultural Variables

A great deal has been written about the role of cultural factors in the development of eating disorders (see Polivy, Garner, & Garfinkel, 1986, and Rodin, Silberstein, & Striegel-Moore, 1985, for extended reviews). The emphasis on thinness in our society has significantly shaped the attitudes, beliefs, and behavior of many young women. The message that slenderness is the standard for which to strive is delivered not only by the fashion industry, but by the general media, and has been accompanied by a proliferation of weight-loss centers, diet products, and self-help guides to weight control. In a culture preoccupied with appearance, one of the most conspicuous manifestations of this absorption is the pronounced dissatisfaction with even mild obesity, and the pursuit of an extremely slim figure. The majority of American women are dissatisfied with their weight, and it has been estimated that 56% diet on a regular basis (Schlundt & Johnson, 1990). Additionally, in the last few years there has been heightened pressure on women to attain bodies that are not only thin, but firm and toned, which has led to increases in the use of compulsive exercise as an adjunct to dieting.

The equation of slenderness and happiness is a delusion that anorexics share with many other members of Western society. In our culture, thinness has come to symbolize competence, success, control, sexuality, and a kind of androgynous independence (Bennett & Gurin, 1982), while obesity is equated with laziness, gluttony, lack of intelligence, and low social status (Frankenburg, Garfinkel, & Garner, 1982). Thus, in many ways anorexia nervosa is not only an egosyntonic disorder, but a culturally syntonic disorder. In a society that links one's worth as a person to one's weight and shape, anorexic attitudes are "a clear product (albeit magnified) of our society's attitude toward obesity. . . . [Anorexics] learn from the adulation of skeletal women that to be thin is essential for acceptability, and from the omnipresent 'how-to-diet' articles that thinness is well within their grasp" (Frankenberg et al., 1982, p. 471).

Stress

Shortly before the onset of their anorexic symptoms, the self-schemas of vulnerable individuals seem to undergo a challenge that threatens their fragile equilibrium. The stressors precipitating this crisis are rarely catastrophic events; more typically, they represent ordinary points-of-passage such as reaching menarche, entering a new school, moving away from home, or getting married (Levine & Smolak, 1989). The shift from childhood into adolescence is often the pivotal event; in most cases, its disruptive effects have less to do with the specifically sexual implications of puberty than with the cognitive and social changes that it entails.

Normal cognitive development in adolescence involves increasing complexity and differentiation in views of the self, and a heightened preoccupation with others' opinions (Harter, 1990). Since different observers have contrasting perspectives, all adolescents must struggle to reconcile diverse views of themselves into a consistent and coherent whole. Girls in particular tend to experience conflict and uncertainty about the true nature of the self during this period, and the "self as chameleon" may be the normative pattern of middle adolescence (Harter, 1990).

It is not surprising that this transitional period is especially stressful for young girls whose developmental course has left them intolerant of ambiguity and dependent on external frames of reference. These perfectionistic individuals have learned the rules of childhood by rote; suddenly, in adolescence, it seems that there are no rules, or that the rules are relative, shifting, and contradictory. Adept at conforming conscientiously to the standards of correct deportment established by parents and teachers, they feel disoriented in a world where social skills and autonomy are valued more than compliance. As one client expressed it:

> "During elementary school, I was always pretty much on top of things. I generally knew more than my classmates—and I felt years and years older than the rest of them. All at once, in seventh grade, they seemed to know so many answers—how to act, what to wear, what music to listen to, how to get other people to like them—when I hadn't even figured out the important questions. I kept wondering, how did they *learn* all these things—and where was I when they were learning them? It was scary—in everything I did, I ran the risk of being wrong and not even knowing it."

What appears consistent in most cases is the occurrence of some event or period of transition that places the provisional self-concept of these young women in jeopardy (Casper & Davis, 1977). The "unworthy self" is confirmed by repeated experiences of self-defined failure, the "overwhelmed self" is swamped by the multiplicity of possible roles and identities, and the "perfectible self" scrambles frantically to restore a sense of order and purpose. On the verge of adulthood, these individuals come to an impasse in their lives; to go on as before seems impossible (Bruch, 1978), and they long for direction and a renewed sense of competence (Casper, 1983).

Beliefs and Behavior

In the midst of their confusion and self-doubt, those who will become anorexic arrive at the idea that losing weight will somehow alleviate their distress. The origin of this belief seems to vary from case to case and may receive supplementary support from several sources in each individual client.

In its interpretation of the proximal causes of anorexia nervosa, the cognitive model is entirely consistent with Bruch's characterization of the disorder as a "desperate struggle for a self-respecting identity" (Bruch, 1973, p. 250), a late stage in a long-standing effort "to be 'perfect' in the eyes of others" (p. 251). Consistent with their predilection for oversimplifying, these individuals interpret fashion's demand for minimal proportions in an exaggerated, concrete manner, truly believing that they will merit respect if they aspire to extreme thinness (Bruch, 1978). Selvini-Palazzoli's (1978) book contains the following passage written by an anorexic patient about the onset of her symptoms:

> I started to think hard about what it was everyone disliked about me. I didn't have to look too far: it could only be my body. My face was all right, and so were my large eyes and my thick black hair, but my hips were really much too broad and my ankles too thick. . . . I suddenly felt a sense of great relief. At last I had hit upon the reason for my loneliness and my despair. And I could do something positive to remedy it. I would go on a strict diet. It was like a sudden illumination, and I felt perfectly content. (p. 147)

The body seems to be selected as the focus of the self-reformist campaign for a number of reasons. The experience of puberty is always associated with an intensified focus on the body—and the most salient aspect of puberty for the human female is a substantial increase in the deposition of body fat. This "fatness spurt" moves the maturing young girl away from current cultural ideals for feminine attractiveness, and may draw teasing or critical commentary, all at a time when she is increasingly concerned with popularity and attractiveness (Levine & Smolak, 1989).

More abstractly, the preanorexic may see the shaping of her body as the "first possible move in defining the dimensions (literally) of what one will be" (Rakoff, 1983, p. 38). It is the most accessible territory that can be conquered by the self—and may be one of the few aspects of life over which it is really possible to obtain the "absolute control" or contemplate the "total success" that Slade (1982) believed anorexics crave. The choice of dieting as a vehicle for self-improvement is further strengthened by the association between self-deprivation and self-control, which possess their own intrinsic value for these ascetic individuals.

Thus, through a variety of means, the "great anorexic lie" (Selvini-Palazzoli, 1978) becomes established: the belief that "being too fat" is the cause of all personal misfortunes, and therefore must be corrected (Bruch, 1973; Garner & Bemis, 1982). The cognitive model does not insist on temporal precedence for this central belief over the dieting behavior. In some novice anorexics, the idea that thinness is a solution to personal distress does seem to be formulated in advance of dieting behavior, which is then undertaken with a specific objective in mind. Others, however, formulate the central premise only after they have experienced the reinforcing consequences of weight loss that was initially achieved casually, or even accidentally. Whatever the sequence, the anorexic conviction soon begins to exert powerful effects on the thoughts, feelings, and behavior of the individual who holds it. More desultory attempts at weight control are replaced by a strict dietary regimen, a program of rigorous exercise, and often a variety of elimination tactics such as vomiting and the abuse of laxatives and diuretics. The business of serious weight loss begins. Over time, a host of secondary irrational beliefs about the magical properties of food and the consequences of weight gain or loss starts to devolve from the central premise, and ruminations about intake and output come to dominate most of the anorexic's cognitive experience.

Consequences

Figure 7.1 charts four classes of consequences that are hypothesized to result from—and, reciprocally, to maintain—anorexic beliefs and behaviors. Because each of these has been extensively discussed elsewhere (Bemis, 1983, 1986; Garner & Bemis, 1982, 1985; Garner, Rockert, Olmsted, Johnson, & Coscina, 1985; Vitousek & Hollon, 1990), we shall review them only briefly before turning to a consideration of the belief systems postulated to account for their functional effects.

Positive Reinforcement

In the early stages of dieting, many anorexic individuals receive direct social reinforcement in the form of praise for their slender appearance and remarkable self-control. As the disorder progresses and the applause dies down, some anorexics may begin to be rewarded by a different form of environmental feedback: the concern and attention that their condition elicits from friends and family members. However, such external reinforcement seems to play a relatively minor role in most cases of anorexia nervosa (Crisp, 1977; Garner & Bemis, 1982; Slade, 1982). Thinness may retain a "signaling" value that is intended to convey a variety of messages to the world (Rakoff, 1983), but it is not necessary that these be received or that specific reinforcement be returned for the pattern to persist. Once the basic postulate about the importance of thinness has been firmly established, the complex of anorexic beliefs and behaviors becomes functionally autonomous (Garner & Bemis, 1982), operating almost independently of environmental input.

The cognitive model postulates that positive *self*-reinforcement makes a much more significant and persistent contribution to the maintenance of symptomatology (Bemis, 1983, 1986; Garner & Bemis, 1982, 1985; Slade, 1982). Individuals with anorexia nervosa do not experience their disorder as an affliction but as an accomplishment, in which they feel a complete emotional and moral investment (Casper et al., 1981). They "do not complain about their condition—on the contrary they glory in it," believing that in their thinness they have secured "the perfect solution to all their problems" (Bruch, 1978, p. 137). Every morsel of food refused, every inch in diameter eliminated, every pound of weight shed become occasions for self-congratulation. When asked to characterize their reactions to weight loss, anorexics report that they feel delighted, inspired, triumphant, proud, and powerful; at such moments, they see themselves as special, superior, and deserving of the respect and admiration of others (Bemis, 1986). The potency of the intrinsic positive reinforcement attached to dieting and weight loss can only be understood against the barren background in which it occurs; for the anorexic individual, her symptoms represent "successful behavior in the context of perceived failure in all other areas of functioning" (Slade, 1982, p. 173).

Negative Reinforcement

Diagnostic criteria for anorexia nervosa specify the presence of an "intense fear of gaining weight" (American Psychiatric Association, 1987), an element so prominent in the anorexic experience that the disorder is sometimes referred to as a "weight phobia" (Crisp, 1980). The negative reinforcement of avoiding feared stimuli contributes significantly to the maintenance of the anorexic syndrome (Bemis, 1983, 1986; Garner & Bemis, 1982, 1985; Slade, 1982). Anorexic, bulimic, agoraphobic, and simple phobic subjects all furnish similar descriptions of their subjective experience during imaginal exposure to personally relevant, feared situations, indicating that they feel frightened, guilty, and isolated (although physical symptoms of anxiety and expectations of danger figure less prominently in the accounts of eating-disordered subjects). When describing their responses to the successful avoidance of feared stimuli, all groups also report a strong sense of relief and enhanced security—the affective concomitants of negative reinforcement (Bemis, 1986).

The cognitive model suggests that the characteristics of avoidance behaviors as a general class may go a long way in accounting for the progressive deterioration observed in anorexia nervosa, and its remarkable imperviousness to modification (Garner & Bemis, 1982, 1985). By continuing to avoid anxiety-provoking stimuli, individuals insulate themselves from potentially disconfirmatory data, and are eventually controlled principally by cognitive sets that generate idiosyncratic internal contingencies (Bandura, 1978; Beck, 1970). Over time, a "margin of safety" principle seems to develop: anorexics come to believe that they must put ever greater distance between themselves and the frightening numbers on the scale that signify obesity (Crisp, 1980; Russell, Campbell, & Slade, 1975). The game of staying just a few pounds below this critical or "magic" weight rapidly turns sinister, as the new lower numbers chosen for extra security are converted into the absolute upper limit, and a still lower margin of safety is required.

Some specific features of the feared stimuli in anorexia nervosa further expedite the process of isolation that occurs in other disorders of avoidance. In anorexia nervosa, the most frightening stimulus is the *self* at unacceptable weight levels, and the only means of evading this object is to exert rigorous control over the impulse to eat, which is constantly stimulated by internal drives and widespread environmental cues (Garner & Bemis, 1982). The single-minded devotion to achieving their goal pulls anorexics away from the tempering influence of others into a tense and task-oriented world. At the same time, this all-encompassing preoccupation may itself serve as a form of avoidance behavior (Slade, 1982), since it enables the anorexic individual to concentrate her anxieties on a single issue, avoiding direct confrontation with the problems that may have contributed to the development of anorexic behavior in the first place. Moreover, many aspects of the avoidance pattern—even including the anxiety and distressing cognitions that accompany concerns about food and weight—may be experienced as positive, valued, and functional for affected individuals, since they subserve the unchallenged premise about the importance of thinness (Garner & Bemis, 1982).

Schematic Processing

The cognitive model hypothesizes that individuals with anorexia nervosa (and bulimia nervosa) develop organized cognitive structures around the issues of weight and its implications for the self that profoundly influence their perceptions, thoughts, affect, and behavior (Vitousek & Hollon, 1990). Once weight-related self-schemas have developed, they may act to prolong symptoms in a relatively automatic way, affecting the manner in which eating-disordered individuals perceive and interpret their experience. The existence of a schema in a given domain tends to produce systematic errors in the processing of material relevant to that domain, through mechanisms such as overuse of the schema, selective attention and memory, perseverance, illusory correlation, confirmatory bias, egocentric bias, false consensus, and availability and representativeness heuristics (Nisbett & Ross, 1980; Tversky & Kahneman, 1974). Just as these mechanisms have been implicated in the maintenance of depressive and anxiety disorders, it is postulated that they serve to support the maladaptive behavior manifested in the eating disorders.

Anorexic individuals live in a world dense with weight-related meanings, and their response to external stimuli is largely determined by their own salient concerns. Other people are judged not on the basis of personal qualities but their status as thinner or fatter than the self; activities are evaluated not for their potential to produce pleasure or growth but their tendency to facilitate or interfere with weight control. Anorexics' views of themselves are also tied to their weight-related schemas. Experiences that lead to self-evaluation or self-criticism produce an intensified focus on body size and shape (Striegel-Moore, McAvay, & Rodin, 1986), while shifts in weight dramatically influence affect and cognition.

In addition to the automatic effects that schema-driven processing seems to exert on the maintenance of symptomatology, Vitousek and Hollon (1990) have suggested that schematic principles may help to explain why anorexic symptomatology serves a valued *function* for affected individuals. Schematic processing, in general, acts to simplify, organize, and stabilize the perceiver's experience of the self and the external environment. Because anorexics seem to have a particularly urgent need for these simplifying, organizing, and stabilizing functions, it may be that their focus on weight is "chosen," valued, and defended in part because it has unusually powerful schematic properties. Individuals with eating disorders—like individuals with paranoid delusions and those who embrace extreme religious or political creeds—may actually welcome the dominance of monolithic cognitive structures that reduce the complexity and ambiguity of daily life.

Starvation

Another variable that is both a consequence of, and a contributor to, eating disorder symptomatology is the impairment of psychological functioning associated with starvation. The starvation process is known to have a variety of adverse cognitive and emotional effects on normal individuals, including poor concentration, concrete thinking, rigidity, withdrawal, obsessive-compulsive behavior, and depression (Keys, Brozek, Henschel, Mickelsen, & Taylor, 1950). In anorexia nervosa, the prolonged restriction in food intake and profound weight loss may affect cognitive "hardware," thinking style, and level of cognitive activity, as well as thought content (Vitousek, Garner, & Hollon, 1991). Some recent suggestive findings have linked starvation sequelae to cognitive perseveration (Demitrack et al., 1990) and to impairments in information-processing capacity and control functions (Laessle, Bossert, Hank, Hahlweg, & Pirke, 1989), all of which may serve to perpetuate the restrictive patterns from which they result. Unable to reason clearly, progressively more detached from others, and engaged in an escalating battle to subdue their own tyrannical hunger, anorexics become increasingly susceptible to the influence of their own distorted perceptions. Psychologically as well as physically, "the starving organism is like a closed system that goes on functioning indefinitely at a reduced level" (Bruch, 1978, p. 90).

The Functions of Anorexia Nervosa

The effects of the aforementioned four classes of maintaining variables are interpretable only through consideration of the belief systems of anorexic individuals. Restrictive eating and weight loss are not intrinsically reinforcing, either positively or negatively; behaviors that impair cognitive processing capacity and promote social and sexual disinterest are not universally self-perpetuating. To make sense of anorexics' extraordinary responsiveness to these events, we must understand what they *mean* to these young women and what functions they come to serve for those affected. It is not enough to recognize the positive valence and significance attached to thinness by the wider culture, since the disorder does not afflict the vast majority of individuals who endorse the same views. Nor is it sufficient to sketch out a purportedly toxic family profile and to list the personal inadequacies that are hypothesized to ensue, since—at best—such accounts can do no more than suggest a general vulnerability to distress and dysfunction. Any comprehensive theoretical model of anorexia nervosa must attempt to explain both "Why this particular individual?" *and* "Why this specific disorder?" The cognitive model suggests that the core symptoms of anorexia nervosa acquire their reinforcing properties because they express or fulfill central components of the belief systems of vulnerable individuals. It is the linkage between varied aspects of the self and the consequences of dieting and weight loss that cause the disorder to serve an adaptive function for the anorexic individual.

Some possible associations between key elements of the self and the functions of anorexic behavior are charted in Table 7.1; several of these are discussed in more detail below. A few caveats are in order. First, although the aspects of the self that are listed in the table have substantial cross-theoretical reliability in clinical accounts of anorexia nervosa, only a few have been investigated empirically; moreover, as noted earlier, it has not been established whether these elements precede or follow the onset of symptomatic behavior.

Second, in few cases is it considered likely that an individual would be vulnerable in all the areas listed in the left-hand column, or probable that her eating disorder would fulfill each of the functions listed on the right. It is in fact the assumption of the cognitive model (in concordance with many other etiological theories of anorexia nervosa) that the disorder is multiply determined within individuals, that symptoms can serve several functions simultaneously, that no single contributing factor is present in every case, and that the significance and relative importance of different reinforcement systems can change over the course of the illness (Bemis, 1986; Casper & Davis, 1977; Garfinkel & Garner, 1982; Solyom, Thomas, Freeman, & Miles, 1983; Yager, 1982). There are a variety of reasons why a young female in our culture might turn to weight control in search of a solution to her personal distress and sense of inadequacy; once weight loss is commenced, there are a variety of variables capable of sustaining the maladaptive behavior pattern. This heterogeneity in the motives for, and functions, of weight reduction is noted clinically by many therapists who work with large samples of anorexics. Selvini-Palazzoli (1978) observed that some of her patients seemed to be primarily concerned with emaciation as an *escape from* nonacceptance, criticism, and sexual advances, whereas others seemed to have more of a *pull toward* emaciation in the belief that it helped them attain freedom, beauty, intelligence, and morality. It is hoped that researchers will also be sensitive to the presence of individual differences in the intent and function of anorexic behavior; indeed, these differences should be sought and studied in their own right,

TABLE 7.1. The Adaptive Function of Anorexic Symptoms for Aspects of the Self

Aspects of the self	Functions of anorexic symptomatology
"Unworthy self"	
Low self-esteem	Weight loss leads to feelings of pride and accomplishment Scale permits daily assessment of personal worth
Feelings of helplessness and ineffectiveness	Personal control established over one area of functioning Self-denial enhances sense of self-efficacy Control over others increases
Poorly developed sense of identity	Identity of an anorexic is acquired Thinness and fasting help to define boundaries of self Complex issues surrounding adult identity are bypassed
Tendency to seek external verification	Weight becomes template for determining correct conduct Social endorsement of thinness and self-control
Extreme sensitivity to criticism	Teasing about weight avoided Importance of weight decreases sense of vulnerability in other domains
Conflicts over autonomy and dependence	Disorder allows defiant assertion of independence while simultaneously eliciting concern, nurturance, and attention from others
"Perfectible self"	
Perfectionism	Weight, calories, and exercise offer quantifiable standards for achievement Strivings focus on a domain amenable to exercise of will
Grandiosity	Visibly surpass others in a domain highly valued by others Sense of uniqueness and superiority derived from disorder
Asceticism	Bodily urges suppressed through self-control and starvation Sins of overeating can be atoned for through fasting, purgation, and exercise
New Year's resolution cognitive style	Preference for dichotomous good/bad rule systems satisfied Disorder sets attainable series of challenges
"Overwhelmed self"	
Preference for simplicity	Cognitive focus narrowed by starvation and schematic processing Weight control provides simple, predictable rule system
Preference for certainty	Belief in thinness exempt from mistrust of experience Weight and calories provide quantifiable feedback
Tendency to retreat from complex social environments	Dieting and starvation aid retreat into self Social demands and expectations become less relevant Conflict created by sexual maturation is alleviated
Avoidance of strong affect	Emotions blunted by starvation Eating, purging, and exercise used to regulate emotion

rather than being seen as unwelcome variance that obscures the identification of universal variables.

Finally, it should not be assumed that dieting and weight loss are undertaken *deliberately* with the goal of achieving specific objectives, or that eating-disordered individuals are always *aware* of the postulated connections between underlying aspects of the self and symptomatology. There appear to be individual differences in the purposefulness of anorexic behavior—and certainly in the insight and honesty these individuals can bring to bear upon their self-examination. But the egosyntonic nature of anorexic symptomatology should assuage the discomfort of any theorist who hesitates to impute motivation to pathological behavior. The proposition that this disorder serves a valued function is one that most anorexics would vigorously defend.

One of the functions that the disorder seems to fulfill is the gratification of the *ascetic* and *moralistic* elements of the "perfectible self." On principle, anorexics often esteem abstinence, discipline, and self-denial, while their aesthetic sense values minimalism and parsimony (Vitousek & Hollon, 1990). The anorexic pattern affords an economical opportunity to express these tendencies. Daily, the disorder offers many occasions for the satisfying experience of successfully "doing without." It defines a specific set of sins (the consumption of the wrong sorts or quantities of food) that can be atoned for through the practice of specific acts of contrition (fasting, purging, and exercise). Eventually, it embodies the penitent in an ethereal form that proclaims her virtues abroad.

Lawrence (1979) is correct that the disorder is better understood as a moral quest than as a silly cosmetic obsession; however, the moral code it subserves does not bear close scrutiny. Anorexics clearly derive an altogether worldly sort of pleasure from their self-restraint. For these individuals, "asceticism provides the way to an exhilarating sense of power" (Mogul, 1980, p. 161). They are immensely proud of their unusual facility in repudiating their physical needs, and offer up their thinness to the glory of themselves. A few draw vague connections between their self-deprivation and their sensitivity to the plight of humankind; when asked to identify the advantages of being anorexic, one client sanctimoniously replied, "It makes me feel like I'm in touch with the sufferings of the world." The moral bankruptcy of claiming kinship with the involuntarily starved through the self-centered pursuit of thinness altogether escaped her. There is in fact a blithe sort of hypocrisy to the asceticism of anorexia nervosa. Anorexics seek at once to excel in the culturally sanctioned business of weight control, and to transcend the petty preoccupations of a superficial society. Their weight loss is to be both enviable and sublime; if it can serve simultaneously to enhance physical attractiveness and spiritual purity, so much the better (Garner & Bemis, 1982).

Indeed, the anorexic's experience of moral and ascetic gratification through thinness seems closely allied to another aspect of the self: *grandiosity*. As Bruch (1978) noted,

> The longer the illness lasts and the more weight they lose, the more anorexics become convinced that they are special and different, that being so thin makes them worthwhile, significant, extraordinary, eccentric, or outstanding; each one has a private word to describe the superiority she strives for. Then they feel they are no longer able to communicate with ordinary people, who won't understand. (p. 74)

In addition to the secret pleasures Bruch described, there is often an exhibitionistic quality to the expression of symptoms. More than 50 years ago, it was observed that "once [anorexics] became thin, they made a virtue of it, and paraded their emaciation and took pride in their uniqueness" (Rahman, Richardson, & Ripley, 1939). One client of the first author's expounded on the practical advantages of anorexia nervosa as a highly visible form of accomplishment:

> "When you are out shopping in a store, or attending a meeting, or going to a party, no one can tell if you get straight A's in school. You don't get to have your transcript emblazoned on your forehead. But everyone can see, immediately, that you are the thinnest person in the room. They all know what you have achieved, and you don't even have to bring it to their attention."

This distinction is so prized by some anorexics that it may be pursued to the point of death. For the Danish author Karen Blixen (Isak Dinesen), who may have qualified for a diagnosis of anorexia nervosa intermittently throughout her life, fasting was, "even when she was an old woman dying of emaciation, an ironic, powerful, and essentially feminine act of heroism" (Thurman, 1982, p. 66). Shortly before her death, she spoke of her gratification at finally having become the "thinnest person in the world." If it were necessary for a woman to age, she wrote, the most dignified way to do it was "to become a skeleton, a skull, a memento mori. . . . Then I should still be an inspiring figure. . . . I should still inspire them with horror" (Thurman, 1982, p. 387).

One aspect of the "overwhelmed self" that is linked to the benefits of symptomatology is the *preference for simplicity*. This characteristic may represent the basic theme, or "cognitive essence," of anorexia nervosa (Vitousek & Hollon, 1990); certainly, the disorder caters to it extremely well. One of the principal effects is a "narrowing down of the world"—an effect that operates across all of the four categories of consequent events. Both positive and negative reinforcement are experienced when the complexities of life can be bypassed with rules and rituals, and the reward system shrinks to a few weight-relevant variables: schema-driven processing channels information in more manageable and predictable ways, semistarvation encloses the individual in self-sufficient isolation.

Although the "narrowing" function of the disorder has been implicated in its perpetuation by both cognitive and dynamic theorists (Goodsitt, 1985; Strober, 1991; Vitousek & Hollon, 1990), there is little empirical evidence for the construct. There has been one intriguing suggestion that anorexics' difficulty in coping with complex stimuli and preference for narrow-band input may be associated with information-processing deficits. One study determined that although anorexics equalled or surpassed their normal peers on effortful learning and memory tasks, they performed significantly worse on measures of automatic processing that reflect awareness of information peripheral to the focus of attention (Strupp, Weingartner, Kaye, & Gwirtsman, 1986). The investigators speculated that anorexics may value the pursuit of thinness as one domain in which an intense and focused cognitive style can find expression and further the attainment of a desired goal. Another study found evidence of a need for immediate closure and a concrete, dichotomous thinking style in the conceptual organization of eating-disordered subjects (Johnson & Holloway, 1988). The authors hypothesized that since these individuals possess only a few categories for the classification of incoming data, they must reject or simplify information that fails to fit existing structures.

The wide array of adaptive functions outlined in Table 7.1 may make it appear that anorexics are amply compensated for their symptomatology, and should be left alone to enjoy its benefits without therapeutic interference. The cognitive model most emphatically does *not* contend that anorexia nervosa is a satisfactory resolution to the problems that confront the vulnerable individual. In fact, it is recognized that the disorder causes "appalling unhappiness" (Lawrence, 1979) that immeasurably exceeds the advantages it can deliver. Even though the disorder may be experienced initially as voluntary, it is in reality no more freely chosen than other forms of psychopathology; when it reaches the chronic phase, many individuals become aware of their inability to control its progression. Although weight loss does supply anorexics with intermittent positive and negative reinforcement and does allow the expression of some underlying aspects of the self, it can never confer the sense of identity, competence, and emotional equilibrium anorexics expected it to provide (Casper, 1983). Whatever weight they reach "in this struggle for self-respect and respect from others, it [is] 'not right' for giving them inner reassurance" (Bruch, 1973, p. 101). Rather than concluding that they have embarked on the wrong route to personal validation, they decide that they simply have not gone far enough—perhaps the elusive goal they seek is just around the corner (Bemis, 1986; Lawrence, 1979). They are caught up in the self-perpetuating cycle of anorexic behavior, trapped by its laws, dependent on its rewards, unable to challenge its central premise. The key difference between individuals with anorexia nervosa and individuals with other forms of disordered behavior is that the latter generally recognize their problem as such, whereas the former are deluded into viewing it as part of the solution. This small difference has profound ramifications for the understanding and treatment of anorexia nervosa—and accounts for the cognitive model's uncharacteristic emphasis on the *functions* of this particular disorder.

THE ASSESSMENT OF THE COGNITIVE MODEL

As the eating disorder field embarks on a long-overdue transition from model building to model testing, from descriptive to experimental psychopathology, it will become increasingly important to devise means of confirming or refuting our hypotheses about the functional relationships supporting anorexia nervosa (Vitousek, Daly, & Heiser, 1991). The cognitive model of anorexia nervosa—like most other theoretical accounts of the disorder—assigns a crucial role to variables to which only the subject has direct access. If theorists tend to concur that the key elements are private ones, they unfortunately also generally agree that eating-disordered individuals make extremely unsatisfactory informants.

Because of their investment in preserving their symptomatology, anorexics are prone to deliberate, instrumental distortion in self-report; paradoxically, their tendency toward overcompliance may also lead to misrepresentations, as they strive to conform to the subtly communicated biases of their therapists (Bruch, 1978). Finally, anorexics' capacity to report on their inner experience may also be limited by inadvertent distortion caused by poor introspective skills. Because of these difficulties and other technical problems unique to the study of the eating disorders (see Vitousek et al., 1991, and Vitousek, Garner, & Hollon, 1991, for discussions), the field faces a formidable challenge in attempting to assess the experience of the anorexic individual. However daunting, it is a challenge that must be met; at the present developmental stage of eating disorder research it is no longer acceptable to support etiological models with nothing more than claims of superior insight or extensive clinical experience.

As noted earlier, the empirical status of most elements of the cognitive model remains unestablished. A recent burst of activity has been restricted, for the most part, to the assessment of self-statements about eating and weight, while higher-order cognitive elements are rarely examined. Moreover, the quality of this research has not kept pace with the rapid increments in quantity. Only a handful of studies incorporate psychiatric control groups, which are necessary for establishing the specificity of hypothesized components; even fewer include comparison subjects such as chronic dieters or restrained eaters, necessary to control for the effects of restricted food intake and hunger. The "eating disorder" subjects are sometimes drawn from large samples of normal high school or college students on the basis of deviant scores on screening instruments; in some reports, the resulting groups are designated, without qualification, as "anorexic" or "bulimic."

A few of the postulated aspects of the self have been measured and do appear to characterize the anorexic population—at least after the onset of disorder and in comparison to normal control subjects. Anorexic and bulimic samples possess lower levels of self-esteem across most domains of functioning (Casper et al., 1981; Dykens & Gerrard, 1986; Weinreich, Doherty, & Harris, 1985) and obtain higher scores on indices of perfectionism (Garner, Olmsted, & Polivy, 1983; Slade & Dewey, 1986). They are more likely than normal individuals to endorse irrational beliefs (Ruderman, 1986; Steiger, Fraenkel, & Leichner, 1989; Steiger, Goldstein, Mongrain, & Van der Feen, 1990) and to commit processing errors such as overgeneralization and dichotomous thinking (Fremouw & Heyneman, 1983; Strauss & Ryan, 1988), even when the content of the items is unrelated to eating and weight. However, other hypothesized aspects of the self have yet to be assessed; while some would undoubtedly prove difficult to operationalize, most seem to merit a formal attempt, if only on the basis of their prominence in clinical accounts of the eating disorders.

The food- and weight-related beliefs of eating-disordered individuals have received considerably more attention from researchers. At least seven inventories have been assembled for the purpose of identifying disorder-specific self-statements; because most of these can be used with both anorexic and bulimic subjects, they will be discussed collectively. These include the Anorectic Attitude Scale (Goldberg et al., 1980), the Bulimic Cognitive Distortions Scale (Schulman, Kinder, Powers, Prange, & Gleghorn, 1986), the Attitude and Belief Survey (Scanlon, Ollendick, & Bayer, 1986), the Food and Weight Cognitive Distortions Scale (Thompson, Berg, & Shatford, 1987), the Anorectic Cognitions Scale (Mizes & Klesges, 1989), and two separate instruments entitled the Bulimic Thoughts Questionnaire (Franko, Zuroff, & Bendiksen, 1988; Phelan, 1987).

Although each subsumes slightly different content areas, most of these instruments were intended to serve similar purposes, and many bear a striking resemblance to one another. Four of them incorporate items from a table on anorexic beliefs compiled by Garner and Bemis (1982). Particularly popular entries include "Gaining five pounds would push me over the brink," "If I eat a sweet, it will be converted instantly into stomach fat," and "When I see someone who is overweight, I worry that I will be like her." The authors of virtually all of these questionnaires have established that their inventories differentiate bulimics and/or anorexics from normal individuals; some have additionally shown that scores decrease over the course of treatment, predict response to treatment, and correlate with other indices of eating disorder symptomatology.

The problem is that while such variables can be operationalized much more neatly than underlying aspects of the self and are certainly more accessible than schematic processing, they are also considerably less crucial to an examination of the cognitive model (Vitousek & Hollon, 1990). Presumably, psychodynamic and behavioral theorists would be completely comfortable with the proposition that the thought content of those who worry a great deal about eating and weight differs from the thought content of those who do not. The confirmation that this is so does little to support the validity of the comprehensive cognitive theory of anorexia nervosa.

A more promising direction for future research may be the use of methods and analyses derived from cognitive science, which are currently being applied to the study of many forms of psychopathology (see discussions in Markus, 1990; Safran, Segal, Hill, & Whiffen, 1990; Segal, 1988). Techniques designed for the study of information processing may be used to confirm self-report data through less transparent means, to draw nonobvious conclusions from the superficial content of the eating disorders, and to connect such material with elements of "deep" cognitive structure. Vitousek and Hollon (1990) have recently outlined 10 general strategies for the investigation of information processing in the eating disorders. They suggest that individuals with weight-related self-schemas may differ from others in the following ways: (1) the ease and speed with which food- and weight-related stimuli are processed, (2) the elaboration of meaning around the construct of weight, (3) the intrusion of weight-related content into unrelated or ambiguous situations, (4) the possession of differentiated knowledge structures in connected domains, (5) an enhanced memory for schema-consistent information, (6) the ability to retrieve schema-relevant behavioral evidence, (7) the degree of confidence in judgments and predictions about food and weight, (8) the specific relevance of weight concerns for the self, (9) the level of cognitive and affective involvement in weight-related events, and (10) the resistance to counterschematic information.

Each of these predictions can be investigated through the use of experimental or correlational designs, many of which are less dependent than traditional questionnaire studies on the veracity of direct self-report. A variety of information-processing studies are currently underway, and data bearing on a few theoretical points—generally with bulimic subjects—are already available. In a dichotic listening paradigm, for example, bulimics were found to exhibit increased perceptual sensitivity and physiological responsiveness to information relevant to body weight concerns (Schotte, McNally, & Turner, 1990). In another study, bulimics in whom negative mood had been induced showed more heart-rate deceleration when viewing slides of forbidden foods, an effect that was not obtained with restrained eating controls (Laberg, Wilson, Eldredge, & Nordby, 1991).

Three groups of investigators have adapted the Stroop color-naming test to examine concerns about food, weight, and shape. Using slightly different stimulus materials, all have determined that anorexics and/or bulimics are significantly slower in naming the colors of the ink in which food-related words are printed; more equivocal results have been obtained when weight-related words are presented (Ben-Tovim, Walker, Fok, & Yap, 1989; Channon, Hemsley, & de Silva, 1988; Fairburn, Cooper, Cooper, McKenna, & Anastasiades, 1991). Each of these studies, however, failed to consider the possibility that *hunger* might be the most parsimonious explanation for the disruption in processing associated with food cues (Vitousek & Hollon, 1990). In fact, when the Stroop test was administered to normal subjects who had fasted for 24 hours, it was found that short-term deprivation also interfered with response time to food words (Channon & Hayward, 1990). It appears that in the eating disorders, the Stroop task may measure statelike salient concerns as well as more stable attentional biases, just as temporary concerns about health (Cook, Jones, & Johnston, 1989) can produce Stroop response patterns similar to those obtained with anxiety disorder samples (Hope, Rapee, Heimberg, & Dombeck, 1990; Mathews & MacLeod, 1985; Mogg, Mathews, & Weinman, 1989).

Another cautionary tale about the delicacy of information-processing paradigms is contained in the results of a more recent study by Vitousek, Ewald, Mew, and Manke (1991). In previous research, clinically anxious subjects have revealed an apparent bias toward threatening versus neutral interpretations of ambiguous stimuli by producing more threat-relevant spellings of homophones such as "pain/pane" in comparison to normal controls (Mathews, Richards, & Eysenck, 1989). It was hypothesized that eating-disordered individuals would manifest an equivalent differential attentiveness toward those meanings of homophones and homographs that were related to their specific psychopathology, reflecting a more general predisposition to abstract weight-related material from situations containing equivocal cues. As predicted, anorexic and bulimic subjects did choose food- or weight-related interpretations more frequently than did normal or subclinical subjects. On post-test questionnaires, however, clinical subjects reported more awareness of the study's concealed purpose than did controls, and some acknowledged intentional avoidance of eating or weight responses. The nature of the experiment had been disguised from all subjects with a false rationale and some distractor tasks, but it appeared possible that anorexics and bulimics were "tipped off" by the logical assumption that they had been included in the study because of their symptomatic status. To examine this possibility, an additional control group was "primed" before the experimental session with the knowledge that the study concerned the eating disorders. These normal subjects produced responses similar to those of clinical subjects and, like the clinical subjects, more often discerned the purpose of the investigation. It appears that this paradigm measures the influence of contextual cues instead of (or in addition to) more stable and meaningful differences in information processing.

The assessment of some of the most central hypotheses of the cognitive model—that the eating disorders serve specific functions related to underlying aspects of the self—is likely to prove particularly challenging. Unfortunately, while it may be possible to identify cognitive variables commonly associated with anorexic patterns after symptom onset, it is likely to be exceedingly difficult to verify that they are *causally* related to the maintenance of the disorder. By definition, stimuli cannot be designated as positive or negative reinforcers unless their presentation or removal alters the frequency or intensity of the target behavior; within the functional analysis approach, it is insufficient to state that certain variables are present without demonstrating their causal effect (Cullen, 1983). Many of the factors that the cognitive model proposes as maintaining variables cannot be manipulated in a manner that would clearly establish their *control* over the relevant maladaptive behaviors. For example, it is certainly feasible—and would be highly desirable—to assess patients' beliefs about the importance of weight as a measure of self-worth; it may not be possible to vary these attitudes or the intrinsic positive reinforcement hypothesized to result from them without an extended and highly confounding course of psychotherapy. Since definitive experimental tests of the "functional" hypotheses of the cognitive model may never be forthcoming, it may be necessary to build a case for its theoretical propositions by assembling a variety of supportive-but-not-conclusive pieces of evidence.

In spite of all the perils of self-report, one of these lines of inquiry may involve asking anorexics themselves to characterize their own subjective experience of the functions of their eating disorder. In one direct attempt to examine subjects' consciously recognized investment in their symptomatology, eating-disordered individuals were asked to respond to the Concerns About Change Scale, a measure designed to assess a variety of fears and concerns that psychiatric patients may have about giving up or recovering from their presenting problem (Bemis, 1986). It was determined that the anorexic group accumulated the highest total score, significantly exceeding the scores obtained by three clinical comparison groups composed of bulimic, agoraphobic, and simple phobic subjects. Discrepancies between anorexic and comparison group scores were particularly pronounced for those subscales intended to measure concerns about the potential loss of perceived *benefits* (such as a feeling of accomplishment and a sense of identity) that subjects associated with the disorder.

One possible interpretation of these data is that anorexics should be credited with considerable insight into a variety of factors that clinicians have implicated in their resistance to change, including abstract fears of adulthood and intimacy, which are supposed to be smoldering far below the surface of their conscious awareness. Other possibilities are that these subjects were lying or were parroting theoretical biases acquired from either their therapists or the widely available (and avidly consumed) popular accounts of the eating disorders. Some threats to the validity of self-report may be reduced by separating research from the therapeutic context and by using disinhibiting instructional sets (Vitousek et al., 1991); we are also experimenting with several novel assessment strategies that partially conceal the nature of the inquiry into the functions of symptomatology. No matter how successful such attempts prove, however, they cannot guarantee that the "functional" variables nominated by anorexics actually contribute to the regulation of anorexic behavior. It remains useful to know what our clients think, since they are undoubtedly influenced by their own causal models; moreover, the material obtained by self-report may suggest promising directions for additional research.

TRANSLATING THE COGNITIVE MODEL INTO TREATMENT

Protocols for the implementation of cognitive–behavioral therapy in anorexia nervosa have been presented elsewhere (Garner & Bemis, 1982, 1985). Since one of the distinguishing features of this orientation is an allegiance to methodological behaviorism, attempts have been made to specify treatment methods in sufficient detail so that they can be replicated by other therapists and researchers. Space limitations prohibit an extended description of recommended procedures in this chapter; therefore, our brief overview will again highlight those features most closely related to the topic of this book.

All the elements specified in the etiological model shown in Figure 7.1, from proximal antecedent conditions through starvation effects, become explicit targets of therapeutic intervention. In general, the treatment sequence addresses these in reverse order (although some issues related to each category are dealt with at every stage of therapy). Thus, the restoration of normal food intake and weight is the first order of therapeutic business, followed by attention to the distortions caused by schematic processing, to internal contingencies maintaining anorexic beliefs and behaviors, to sociocultural influences, and, finally, to underlying aspects of the self. Across all phases, the *functional* or *adaptive* quality of eating disorder pathology is strongly emphasized.

In most therapeutic encounters, client and therapist begin with the shared assumption that the former is seeking the help of the latter toward the mutual goal of symptom remission, even though they often disagree about the definition, scope, or preferred mode of treatment of the problem. Because of the egosyntonic nature of symptomatology, this assumption is rarely mutual from the outset of therapy in anorexia nervosa. As the mother of one client wryly expressed it: "Anorexics being offered treatment act like fish being thrown a life preserver—they just don't think they need to be rescued." Clearly, the most critical therapeutic task in the initial stage of intervention is that of enlisting an often wary and resistant client as a collaborator who has at least a tentative interest in exploring the validity of her beliefs.

The establishment of a sound, supportive therapeutic relationship is viewed as a prerequisite for success in this endeavour, since its quality profoundly influences the client's willingness to confront the terrifying prospect of weight gain. Later in treatment, the relationship also serves as a prototype for examining beliefs about other interpersonal issues in the client's life (Garner & Bemis, 1985; Guidano & Liotti, 1983). However, the therapeutic relationship is not hypothesized to be curative in its own right, and must be managed delicately to prevent it from becoming the focus of treatment. Clients are gently dissuaded from transferring their tendency to seek external verification to the person of the therapist—the goal of treatment is not for them to adopt the standards of another, but to develop the capacity to evaluate, select, and fulfill their own.

During the early phases of therapy, the anorexic's current personal goals are not called into question; rather, she is asked to take a closer look at the *means* she has been using to secure her objectives, and the full range of consequences that have resulted. It is explicitly acknowledged that weight loss must confer some significant benefits that would be missed if normal weight status were restored, and it should be emphasized that since the aim of therapy is to make the *client* feel better, it would be unsuccessful if she were not fully compensated for these losses. Much of the first few sessions of therapy is devoted to helping the client construct an exhaustive list of both the pros and the cons of her eating disorder, *in her own terms*, and begin the process of exploring their implications. Without disparaging cherished beliefs, the therapist questions the client about how well her attempted coping mechanisms are really working out in practice: Is weight loss fulfilling the purposes she intended it to serve when dieting was first initiated? Is the price that she must pay higher than she anticipated? Is she compromising any other values in following this course, or closing out any other options?

This deliberate emphasis on the *functional* aspects of the anorexic's attitudes and behaviors seems to penetrate barriers that arguments about their *correctness* cannot breach (Garner & Bemis, 1982, 1985). When they come to appreciate that the therapist is interested in *all* of the consequences they have experienced in living with their disorder, rather than selectively confronting them with its risks and disadvantages (as family members and physicians tend to do), they will usually provide surprisingly candid material about the costs of anorexia. They are often weary of their hunger, distressed by their continual preoccupation with the trivia of weight control, troubled by some of the physical and psychological symptoms of starvation, and torn between competing and incompatible goals.

Once this line of inquiry has begun to nurture some incipient doubts about the value of the anorexic pattern, the therapist can begin to engage the client in the effort to develop some more satisfying alternatives that may better serve her own interests. Throughout treatment, the anorexic is taught to test the validity of the assumptions and perceived reinforcement contingencies that influence her, rather than accepting her own or her therapist's view of reality. She is encouraged to experiment with new strategies for achieving her goals, new sources of positive reinforcement for experiencing pleasure and pride, and new standards for gauging her self-worth. Over the course of therapy, attention gradually shifts away from the focal symptomatology of anorexia nervosa to the more general aspects of the self that may have predisposed the individual to the development of her disorder. At no point, however, is her obsession with eating and weight seen as a superficial phenomenon that obscures a view of the "real" issues; in fact, because of the close correspondence between aspects of the self and the functions of an eating disorder, specific anorexic ideas provide a window to understanding the client's broader system of self-evaluation (Garner & Bemis, 1985).

Cognitive therapy for anorexia nervosa—like classic cognitive therapy for depression (Beck, Rush, Shaw, & Emery, 1979)—is highly structured and labor-intensive, with the therapist taking a very active role in the conduct of sessions. A wide variety of therapeutic techniques is employed in the typical 1- to 2-year course of treatment; however, the approach is not theoretically or strategically eclectic, but is always guided by a cognitive model that emphasizes the systematic examination of the accuracy and utility of beliefs. Thus, behavioral techniques are used to help clients gather data about how events influence their cognitions and affect, and to offer opportunities for practicing different ways of interpreting the environment. Psychoeducational techniques are employed to provide counterschematic information about the effects of dieting and weight loss, and to disabuse clients of the notion that their disorder makes them unique and special. Interpersonal techniques are included to help clients examine their expectations about others and to experiment with other means of securing social approbation.

Although the cognitive–behavioral method appears to be fairly widely used in the treatment of anorexia nervosa, particularly in university-affiliated specialty clinics, there is little compelling evidence for its efficacy. In contrast, the case for cognitive–behavioral treatment in bulimia nervosa is already considerably better established, in spite of the disorder's more recent professional debut (see Garner, Fairburn, & Davis, 1987, for a review). Bulimia researchers have earned the right to begin investigating second-generation questions about the comparative value, active ingredients, and therapeutic mechanisms of cognitive therapy (Bemis, 1988). The approach has in fact proven so popular that its originator has begun to caution against a premature crystallization of theoretical models and treatment techniques for bulimia nervosa (Fairburn, 1987).

The persistent lack of data in the case of anorexia nervosa is certainly embarrassing for an approach with a commitment to empiricism, but it is, at least, nothing singular for the field. Astonishingly, there are virtually no controlled studies on psychotherapy of any kind for anorexia nervosa. A number of explanations can be advanced to account for this phenomenon. The disorder is rare, and its "crisis" phase of short-term weight restoration seems to distract research attention away from the long course of therapy that must follow. The extended period of treatment that virtually all commentators, regardless of theoretical orientation, believe necessary for the remediation of anorexia nervosa is daunting for two reasons: It increases the likelihood of subject attrition that will further reduce sample size and undo randomization, and it places investigators reinforced for publication frequency on a schedule of dysfunctionally deferred gratification. While these considerations make the absence of data more understandable, none provides an acceptable excuse. Formal trials of the utility of the cognitive approach to anorexia nervosa are long overdue.

The only controlled study published to date that includes a cognitive–behavioral condition yielded equivocal evidence for its relative efficacy (Channon, de Silva, Hemsley, & Perkins, 1989). At end-of-treatment and 6- and 12-month follow-up, most patients showed clinical improvement, but, few differences were obtained between cognitive–behavioral and behavioral interventions. It did appear, however, that the cognitive modality was more acceptable to clients and was associated with higher rates of compliance—a finding that the authors noted was of some interest because of the notorious difficulty of engaging anorexics in treatment. However, while the investigators stated that the cognitive condition was patterned after Garner and Bemis (1982, 1985), it is not clear how closely it did conform to recommended procedures. It appears that the primary focus of cognitive treatment was the identification and challenge of food- and weight-related irrational beliefs. In discussing the failure of cognitive–

behavioral therapy to demonstrate incremental benefit over behavioral treatment, Channon et al. (1989) suggested that in future it might be "more appropriate to focus on the relative importance of thinness as a life goal relative to other goals . . . rather than attempting to modify individual cognitions" (p. 534). Since the former is precisely what Garner and Bemis strongly advocate on both practical and theoretical grounds, it is puzzling that this crucial component of cognitive therapy was apparently omitted from a test of the method's utility.

CONCLUSION

Most experts in the field of the eating disorders agree that the central and distinguishing psychopathology of these conditions is a pathological overconcern with weight and shape. The merging of personal identity with body dimensions seems to represent a conversion of more general vulnerabilities and views of the self into a highly specific form that is in some ways adaptive for the affected individual. In the study and treatment of these critical elements, a cognitive analysis holds promise for furthering our understanding of these conditions. Cognitive assessment strategies may help the researcher not only to catalog the content of eating disorder beliefs, but to examine the processes through which these dominant beliefs develop, proliferate, and become increasingly impervious to corrective feedback. Cognitive treatment strategies may assist the therapist in learning how to get inside these structures and facilitate a more adaptive reconstruction of beliefs. Although cognitive interventions are clearly not the only available means for changing the dysfunctional attitudes of eating disorder clients (Fairburn, 1987; Garner & Bemis, 1982), an examination of the mechanisms through which they do work may also advance our knowledge of the variables that maintain eating disorder symptomatology. Many elements of the cognitive etiological model and associated therapeutic approach can be operationalized and tested; in the next decade, it is anticipated that the field will continue to do so with increasing rigor and sophistication.

NOTE

1. Because 90–95% of individuals with anorexia nervosa are female (Bemis, 1978), feminine pronouns are used to refer to anorexics in this chapter.

REFERENCES

American Psychiatric Association. (1987). *Diagnostic and statistical manual of mental disorders* (3rd ed., rev.). Washington, DC: Author.

Bandura, A. (1978). The self-system in reciprocal determinism. *American Psychologist, 33*, 344–358.

Barnett, L. R. (1986). Bulimarexia as a symptom of sex-role strain in professional women. *Psychotherapy, 23*, 311–315.

Beck, A. T. (1970). Role of fantasies in psychotherapy and psychopathology. *Journal of Nervous and Mental Disease, 150*, 3–17.

Beck, A. T., Rush, A. J., Shaw, B. F., & Emery, G. (1979). *Cognitive therapy of depression*. New York: Guilford Press.

Bemis, K. M. (1978). Current approaches to the etiology and treatment of anorexia nervosa. *Psychological Bulletin, 85*, 593–617.

Bemis, K. M. (1983). A comparison of functional relationships in anorexia nervosa and phobia. In P. L. Darby, P. E. Garfinkel, D. M. Garner, & D. V. Coscina (Eds.), *Anorexia nervosa: Recent developments in research* (pp. 403–415). New York: Alan R. Liss.

Bemis, K. M. (1986). *A comparison of the subjective experience of individuals with eating disorders and phobic disorders*. Unpublished doctoral dissertation, University of Minnesota, Minneapolis.

Bemis, K. M. (1988). The evolution of cognitive–behavioral therapy for anorexia nervosa and bulimia nervosa. *International Cognitive Therapy Newsletter, 4*(3), 11–14.

Bemporad, J. R., Ratey, J. J., O'Driscoll, G., & Daehler, M. L. (1988). Hysteria, anorexia and the culture of self-denial. *Psychiatry, 51*, 96–103.

Bennett, W., & Gurin, J. (1982). *The dieter's dilemma*. New York: Basic Books.

Ben-Tovim, D. I., Walker, M. K., Fok, D., & Yap, E. (1989). An adaptation of the Stroop test for measuring shape and food concerns in eating disorders: A quantitative measure of psychopathology? *International Journal of Eating Disorders, 6*, 681–687.

Bruch, H. (1973). *Eating disorders: Obesity, anorexia nervosa, and the person within*. New York: Basic Books.

Bruch, H. (1978). *The golden cage: The enigma of anorexia nervosa*. Cambridge, MA: Harvard University Press.

Bruch, H. (1985). Four decades of eating disorders. In D. M. Garner & P. E. Garfinkel (Eds.), *Handbook of psychotherapy for anorexia nervosa and bulimia* (pp. 7–18). New York: Guilford Press.

Casper, R. C. (1983). Some provisional ideas concerning the psychologic structure in anorexia nervosa and bulimia. In P. L. Darby, P. E. Garfinkel, D. M. Garner, & D. V. Coscina (Eds.), *Anorexia nervosa: Recent developments in research* (pp. 387–392). New York: Alan R. Liss.

Casper, R. C., & Davis, J. M. (1977). On the course of anorexia nervosa. *American Journal of Psychiatry, 134*, 974–977.

Casper, R. C., Offer, D., & Ostrov, E. (1981). The self-image of adolescents with acute anorexia nervosa. *Journal of Pediatrics, 98*, 656–661.

Channon, S., de Silva, P., Hemsley, D., & Perkins, R. (1989). A controlled trial of cognitive-behavioural and behavioural treatment of anorexia nervosa. *Behaviour Research and Therapy, 27*, 529–535.

Channon, S., & Hayward, A. (1990). The effect of short-term fasting on processing of food cues in normal subjects. *International Journal of Eating Disorders, 9*, 447–452.

Channon, S., Hemsley, D., & de Silva, P. (1988). Selective processing of food words in anorexia nervosa. *British Journal of Clinical Psychology, 27*, 259–260.

Cook, J. A. M., Jones, N., & Johnston, D. W. (1989). The effects of imminent minor surgery on the cognitive processing of health and interpersonal threat words. *British Journal of Clinical Psychology, 28*, 281–282.

Cooper, Z., Cooper, P. J., & Fairburn, C. G. (1985). The specificity of the Eating Disorders Inventory. *British Journal of Clinical Psychology, 24*, 129–130.

Crisp, A. H. (1977). The differential diagnosis of anorexia nervosa. *Proceedings of the Royal Society of Medicine, 70*, 686–690.

Crisp, A. H. (1980). *Anorexia nervosa: Let me be*. London: Academic Press.

Cullen, C. (1983). Implications of functional analysis. *British Journal of Clinical Psychology, 22*, 137–138.

Dally, P. J. (1969). *Anorexia nervosa*. New York: Grune & Stratton.

Demitrack, M. A., Lesem, M. D., Listwak, S. J., Brandt, H. A., Jimerson, D. C., & Gold, P. W. (1990). CSF oxytocin in anorexia nervosa and bulimia nervosa: Clinical and pathophysiologic considerations. *American Journal of Psychiatry, 147*, 882–886.

Dykens, E. M., & Gerrard, M. (1986). Psychological profiles of purging bulimics, repeat dieters, and controls. *Journal of Consulting and Clinical Psychology, 54*, 283–288.

Eldredge, K., Wilson, G. T., & Whaley, A. (1990). Failure, self-evaluation, and feeling fat in women. *International Journal of Eating Disorders, 9*, 37–50.

Fairburn, C. G. (1987, April). *The uncertain status of the cognitive approach to bulimia nervosa*. Paper presented at the Symposium on the Psychobiology of Bulimia Nervosa, Ringberg Castle, Germany.

Fairburn, C. G., Cooper, P. J., Cooper, M. J., McKenna, F. P., & Anastasiades, P. (1991). Selective information processing in bulimia nervosa. *International Journal of Eating Disorders, 10*, 415–422.

Fairburn, C. G., & Garner, D. M. (1988). Diagnostic criteria for anorexia nervosa and bulimia nervosa: The importance of attitudes to shape and weight. In D. M. Garner & P. E. Garfinkel (Eds.), *Diagnostic issues in anorexia nervosa and bulimia nervosa* (pp. 36–55). New York: Brunner/Mazel.

Frankenberg, F., Garfinkel, P. E., & Garner, D. M. (1982). Anorexia nervosa: Issues in prevention. *Journal of Preventive Psychiatry, 1*, 469–483.

Franko, D. L., Zuroff, D. C., & Bendiksen, I. (1988, April). *Further validation of the Bulimic Thoughts Questionnaire*. Paper presented at the Third International Conference on Eating Disorders, New York.

Fremouw, W. J., & Heyneman, N. E. (1983). Cognitive styles and bulimia. *The Behavior Therapist, 6*, 143–144.

Garfinkel, P. E., & Garner, D. M. (1982). *Anorexia nervosa: A multidimensional perspective*. New York: Brunner/Mazel.

Garner, D. M., & Bemis, K. M. (1982). A cognitive–behavioral approach to anorexia nervosa. *Cognitive Therapy and Research, 6*, 123–150.

Garner, D. M., & Bemis, K. M. (1985). Cognitive therapy for anorexia nervosa. In D. M. Garner & P. E. Garfinkel (Eds.), *Handbook of psychotherapy for anorexia nervosa and bulimia* (pp. 107–146). New York: Guilford Press.

Garner, D. M., Fairburn, C. G., & Davis, R. (1987). Cognitive-behavioral treatment of bulimia nervosa. *Behavior Modification*, *11*, 398–431.

Garner, D. M., Olmsted, M. P., & Polivy, J. (1983). Development and validation of a multidimensional eating disorder inventory for anorexia nervosa and bulimia. *International Journal of Eating Disorders*, *2*, 15–34.

Garner, D. M., Rockert, W., Olmsted, M. P., Johnson, C., & Coscina D. V. (1985). Psychoeducational principles in the treatment of bulimia and anorexia nervosa. In D. M. Garner & P. E. Garfinkel (Eds.), *Handbook of psychotherapy for anorexia nervosa and bulimia* (pp. 513–572). New York: Guilford Press.

Goldberg, S. C., Halmi, K. A., Eckert, E. D., Casper, R. C., Davis, D. M., & Roper, M. (1980). Attitudinal dimensions in anorexia nervosa. *Journal of Psychiatric Research*, *15*, 239–151.

Goodsitt, A. (1985). Self psychology and the treatment of anorexia nervosa. In D. M. Garner & P. E. Garfinkel (Eds.), *Handbook of psychotherapy for anorexia nervosa and bulimia* (pp. 55–82). New York: Guilford Press.

Guidano, V. F. (1987). *Complexity of the self: A developmental approach to psychopathology and therapy*. New York: Guilford Press.

Guidano, V. F., & Liotti, G. (1983). *Cognitive processes and emotional disorders*. New York: Guilford Press.

Harter, S. (1990). Developmental differences in the nature of self-representations: Implications for the understanding, assessment, and treatment of maladaptive behavior. *Cognitive Therapy and Research*, *14*, 113–142.

Hope, D. A., Rapee, R. M., Heimberg, R. G., & Dombeck, M. J. (1990). Representations of the self in social phobia: Vulnerability to social threat. *Cognitive Therapy and Research*, *14*, 177–189.

Johnson, N. S., & Holloway, E. L. (1988). Conceptual complexity and obsessionality in bulimic college women. *Journal of Counseling Psychology*, *35*, 251–257.

Keys, A., Brozek, J., Henschel, A., Mickelsen, O., & Taylor, H. I. (1950). *The biology of human starvation* (Vol. 2). Minneapolis: University of Minnesota Press.

King, A. (1963). Primary and secondary anorexia nervosa syndromes. *British Journal of Psychiatry*, *109*, 470–479.

Laberg, J. C., Wilson, G. T., Eldredge, K., & Nordby H. (1991). Effects of mood on heart rate reactivity in bulimia nervosa. *International Journal of Eating Disorders, 10*, 169–178.

Laessle, R. G., Bossert, S., Hank, G., Hahlweg, H., & Pirke K. M. (1989). Cognitive processing in bulimia nervosa: Preliminary observations. *Annals of New York Academy of Sciences*, *575*, 543–544.

Lawrence, M. (1979). Anorexia nervosa: The control paradox. *Women's Studies International Quarterly*, 2, 93–101.

Lerner, H. D. (1986). Current developments in the psychoanalytic psychotherapy of anorexia nervosa and bulimia nervosa. *The Clinical Psychologist*, *39*, 39–43.

Levine, M. P., & Smolak, L. (1989, November). *Toward a developmental psychopathology of eating disorders: The example of the middle school transition.*

Paper presented at the eighth National Conference of the National Anorexic Aid Society, Columbus, OH.

Mahoney, M. J. (1974). *Cognition and behavior modification*. Cambridge, MA: Ballinger.

Markus, H. (1990). Unresolved issues of self-representation. *Cognitive Therapy and Research*, *14*, 241–253.

Mathews, A., & MacLeod, C. (1985). Selective processing of threat cues in anxiety states. *Behaviour Research and Therapy*, *23*, 563–569.

Mathews, A., Richards, A., & Eysenck, M. (1989). Interpretation of homophones related to threat in anxiety states. *Journal of Abnormal Psychology*, *98*, 31–34.

Mizes, J. S., & Klesges, R. C. (1989). Validity, reliability, and factor structure of the Anorectic Cognitions Questionnaire. *Addictive Behaviors*, *14*, 589–594.

Mogg, K., Mathews, A., & Weinman, J. (1989). Selective processing of threat cues in anxiety states: A replication. *Behaviour Research and Therapy*, *27*, 317–323.

Mogul, S. L. (1980). Asceticism in adolescence and anorexia nervosa. *Psychoanalytic Study of the Child*, *35*, 155–175.

Nisbett, R. E., & Ross, L. (1980). *Human inference: Strategies and shortcomings of social judgment*. Englewood Cliffs, NJ: Prentice-Hall.

Phelan, P. W. (1987). Cognitive correlates of bulimia: The Bulimic Thoughts Questionnaire. *International Journal of Eating Disorders*, *6*, 593–607.

Polivy, J., Garner, D. M., & Garfinkel, P. E. (1986). Causes and consequences of the current preference for thin female physiques. In C. P. Herman, M. P. Zanna, & E. T. Higgins (Eds.), *Physical appearance, stigma, and social behavior: The Ontario Symposium* (Vol. 3, pp. 89–112). Hillsdale, NJ: Lawrence Erlbaum.

Rahman, L., Richardson, H. B., & Ripley, H. S. (1939). Anorexia nervosa with psychiatric observations. *Psychosomatic Medicine*, *1*, 335–365.

Rakoff, V. (1983). Multiple determinants of family dynamics in anorexia nervosa. In P. L. Darby, P. E. Garfinkel, D. M. Garner, & D. V. Coscina (Eds.), *Anorexia nervosa: Recent developments in research* (pp. 29–40). New York: Alan R. Liss.

Riebel, L. (1985). Eating disorders and personal constructs. *Transactional Analysis Journal*, *15*, 42–47.

Rodin, J., Silberstein, L., & Striegel-Moore, R. (1985). Women and weight: A normative discontent. *Nebraska Symposium on Motivation*, *32*, 267–307.

Ruderman, S. (1986). Bulimia and irrational beliefs. *Behaviour Research and Therapy*, *24*, 193–197.

Russell, G. F. M., Campbell, P. G., & Slade, P. D. (1975). Experimental studies on the nature of the psychological disorder in anorexia nervosa. *Psychoneuroendocrinology*, *1*, 45–56.

Safran, J. D., Segal, Z. V., Hill, C., & Whiffen, V. (1990). Refining strategies for research on self-representations in emotional disorders. *Cognitive Therapy and Research*, *14*, 143–160.

Scanlon, E., Ollendick, T. H., & Bayer, K. (1986, November). *The role of cognitions in bulimia: An empirical test of basic assumptions*. Paper presented at the annual meeting of the Association for Advancement of Behavior Therapy, Chicago.

Schlundt, D. G., & Johnson, W. G. (1990). *Eating disorders: Assessment and treatment*. Boston: Allyn and Bacon.

Schotte, D. E., McNally, R. J., & Turner, M. L. (1990). A dichotic listening analysis of body weight concern in bulimia nervosa. *International Journal of Eating Disorders*, *9*, 109–113.

Schulman, R. G., Kinder, B. N., Powers, P. S., Prange, M., & Gleghorn, A. (1986). The development of a scale to measure cognitive distortions in bulimia. *Journal of Personality Assessment*, *50*, 630–639.

Segal, Z. V. (1988). Appraisal of the self-schema construct in cognitive models of depression. *Psychological Bulletin*, *103*, 147–162.

Selvini-Palazzoli, M. (1978). *Self-starvation: From individual to family therapy in the treatment of anorexia nervosa* (rev. ed.). New York: Jason Aronson.

Slade, P. (1982). Towards a functional analysis of anorexia nervosa and bulimia nervosa. *British Journal of Clinical Psychology*, *21*, 167–179.

Slade, P. D., & Dewey, M. E. (1986). Development and preliminary validation of SCANS: A screening instrument for identifying individuals at risk of developing anorexia and bulimia nervosa. *International Journal of Eating Disorders*, *5*, 517–138.

Solyom, L., Thomas, C. D., Freeman, R. J., & Miles, J. E. (1983). Anorexia nervosa: Obsessive-compulsive disorder or phobia? A comparative study. In P. L. Darby, P. E. Garfinkel, D. M. Garner, & D. V. Coscina (Eds.), *Anorexia nervosa: Recent developments in research* (pp. 137–147). New York: Alan R. Liss.

Steiger, H., Fraenkel, L., & Leichner, P. P. (1989). Relationship of body image distortion to sex-role identifications, irrational cognitions, and body weight in eating-disordered females. *Journal of Clinical Psychology*, *45*, 61–65.

Steiger, H., Goldstein, C., Mongrain, M., & Van der Feen, J. (1990). Description of eating-disordered, psychiatric, and normal women along cognitive and psychodynamic dimensions. *International Journal of Eating Disorders*, *9*, 129–140.

Story, I. (1976). Caricature and impersonating the other: Observations from the psychotherapy of anorexia nervosa. *Psychiatry*, *39*, 176–188.

Strauss, J., & Ryan, R. M. (1988). Cognitive dysfunction in eating disorders. *International Journal of Eating Disorders*, *7*, 19–27.

Striegel-Moore, R., McAvay, G., & Rodin, J. (1986). Psychological and behavioral correlates of feeling fat in women. *International Journal of Eating Disorders*, *5*, 935–947.

Strober, M. (1991). Disorders of the self in anorexia nervosa: An organismic-developmental paradigm. In C. Johnson (Ed.), *Psychodynamic treatment of anorexia nervosa and bulimia* (pp. 354–373). New York: Guilford Press.

Strupp, B. J., Weingartner, H., Kaye, W., & Gwirtsman, H. (1986). Cognitive processing in anorexia nervosa: A disturbance in automatic information-processing. *Neuropsychobiology*, *15*, 89–94.

Thoma, H. (1967). *Anorexia nervosa*. New York: International Universities Press.

Thompson, D. A., Berg, K. M., & Shatford, L. A. (1987). The heterogeneity of bulimic symptomatology: Cognitive and behavioral dimensions. *International Journal of Eating Disorders, 6,* 215–234.

Thurman, J. (1982). *Isak Dinesen: The life of a storyteller.* New York: St. Martin's Press.

Tversky, A., & Kahneman, D. (1974). Judgment under uncertainty: Heuristics and biases. *Science, 185,* 1124–1131.

Vitousek, K., Daly, J., & Heiser, C. (1991). Reconstructing the internal world of the eating-disordered individual: Denial and distortion of self–report. *International Journal of Eating Disorders, 10,* 647–666 .

Vitousek, K., Ewald, L. S., Mew, L., & Manke, F. (1991). *The interpretation of ambiguous stimuli in eating disorders: The importance of contextual cues.* Unpublished manuscript, University of Hawaii, Honolulu.

Vitousek, K., Garner, D. M., & Hollon, S. D. (1991). *The assessment of cognitive processes in the eating disorders.* Unpublished manuscript, University of Hawaii, Honolulu.

Vitousek, K., & Hollon, S. D. (1990). The investigation of schematic content and processing in eating disorders. *Cognitive Therapy and Research, 14,* 191–214.

Weinreich, P., Doherty, J., & Harris, P. (1985). Empirical assessment of identity in anorexia and bulimia nervosa. *Journal of Psychiatric Research, 19,* 297–302.

Yager, J. (1982). Family issues in the pathogenesis of anorexia nervosa. *Psychosomatic Medicine, 44,* 43–60.

Commentary

HOWARD D. LERNER
University of Michigan

THE CONCEPT OF "self" in psychoanalytic theory stands at the cross-currents of several traditional philosophical and psychological issues, which Grossman (1982) formulates as lying along two axes. The first axis considers the everyday, "personal experience" of self—self-awareness, self-consciousness, and self-esteem—and with this, the philosophical issues of mind–body, free will, and the relationship between the self and the world of things. The other axis embodies the psychoanalytic dimension, with the concrete events of the clinical situation and the subjective experience of the patient at one end of the continuum, and its systematic, "theoretical concepts" at the other end. The concept of self joins these coordinates and the different perspectives they offer. The essential tension in understanding any psychoanalytic theory of the self is between the subjective and objective points of view regarding experience.

The origins of the concept of self can be traced to Freud's ambiguous use of the word *"ich,"* which he used indiscriminately to refer to both a psychic agency of the mind (the ego) and to a personal, subjectively experienced sense of self. Strachey translated *"ich"* as "ego," thus shifting usage to the more impersonal, intrapsychic, systemic meaning of the term. Hartmann (1950/1964) distinguished the ego from the self and redefined narcissism as the libidinal investment not of the ego but of the self, thereby separating the subjective/personal from the objective/impersonal. Hartmann's formulations, however, were ambiguous. On the one hand, he used the term *self* to refer to the whole person, including both bodily and psychological dimensions. On the other hand, he formulated the self in terms of the aggregation of self-representations, implying that such an aggregate is a subcategory of the ego's representational function.

Presently, there are three lines of psychoanalytic theorizing about the self. One line, represented by Grossman (1982), regards the self as a fantasy formation. From this perspective, the self is seen as a compromise formation involving the dynamic interplay of drive, defense, morality, and reality. Whereas *ego* is seen as a technical term for classifying behavior, fantasies, and defenses, *self,* by contrast, is a term of immense significance for the individual in that it provides an organization, or frame of reference, for internal experience.

A second line of theorizing regards the self as an integrated structure of self-representations, with particular reference to the internalization process, in general, and introjection, in particular. Following from Hartmann (1950/1964), Kernberg (1975) defined the self as "an intrapsychic structure consisting of multiple self-representations and the related affect dispositions. Self-representations are affective cognitive structures reflecting the person's perception of her/himself in real and fantasized interactions with others" (pp. 315–316). From this frame of reference, the self is regarded as part of the ego.

The third line of theorizing about the self is that of Kohut (1971, 1977), who conceived of the self as a superordinate, unified, coherent constellation, with drives and defenses that evolve out of a developmental line of narcissism. Essentially, the self develops from the empathic mirroring and idealizing activities of parental figures. According to this perspective, which has come to be known as self psychology, the self is conceptualized as a superordinate structure subsuming within it the id, ego, and superego. Repeatedly, Kohut distinguished between the self as experience-near, and the structural entities if id, ego, and superego as experience-distant, implying that the self occupied a different level of conceptual and experiential organization.

Blatt (1974) and Behrends and Blatt (1987) noted that a concept of self provides a place in psychoanalytic theory for considering a personal self as an active and originating source of personal activity, and as such, allows for a more complete account of complex experiential states. A concept of self also offers a conceptual frame of reference for formulating a theory of object relations, as well as a vehicle for conceptualizing personal qualities and capacities that involve an integration of various substructures of the personality.

In my chapter I emphasized the representational aspect of the self, seen as a complex compromise formation. Based on developmental research, theory, and clinical experience, I traced the development course of individuals with subclinical eating disorders and focused on the miscarriage of empathy and the repair of communicative mismatches resulting in an "omnipotent self" composed of a system of magical thinking and power, which interferes with the normative evolution of reality testing and the development of reality-based self-esteem and competence. As a result, all events and happenings are experienced magically as caused or controlled by the omnipotent self: limits and commitments, as well as separations implying loss, are experienced as intolerable through all phases of development; the experience of growing up and the achievement of autonomy, in which the experience of pleasure is achieved in reality through effort and mature relationships become unsatisfying. From this perspective, disturbances in eating behavior, such as fluctuations in weight, bingeing, and excessive exercising, emanate from an omnipotent self, a compromise formation representing strivings to achieve perfection, reunion with mother, defense against feelings of helpless rage and humiliation, and a pathological source of self-esteem. I then discussed the patients' need to protect the omnipotent self in relationship to the staunch resistance that these individuals present at each phase of psychotherapy.

I found the chapter by Vitousek and Ewald to be crisply clear, rich, and decisive in the stance taken. I at once resonated with the clinical descriptions of the patients described and wanted to learn more about them. These descriptions were in accord with my clinical experience. For example, the description of the Danish author Karen Blixen as she spoke of the gratification of becoming the "thinnest person in the world . . . to become a skeleton, a skull, a memento mori. . . . Then I should still be an inspiring figure. . . . I should inspire them with horror" (p. 240) encapsulates the hostile omnipotent strivings and intense masochism of many eating-disordered patients. In what follows, I will focus on differences between the cognitive and psychodynamic perspectives as it bears on values, the role of theory, the role accorded to dynamics, developmental variables and the unconscious, research, the role accorded to sexuality and aggression, and finally, treatment.

The difference between the cognitive and psychoanalytic perspectives begins most basically with values. The cognitive approach embodies a value structure of empiricism and "methodological behaviorism," with an emphasis on quantitative research and staying close to more surface, observational data. Psychoanalysis is both a method of psychological inquiry and a theory of personality. The method is a simple one in which the patient is asked to state whatever comes to mind as freely as possible without attempting to edit, while the analyst directs his/her attention as exclusively as possible to the task of understanding the nature and origins of the patient's psychological conflicts and experience, and of communicating that understanding to the patient. This method provides access to the truly important domains of an individual's mental life—to uniquely personal motives, memories, and current experiences—and makes possible an independent, objective appraisal of those aspects of psychic life. Like other empiricists, psychoanalysts infer functional and causal relations among the data obtained from this method, avoiding, if possible, generalizations that are inconsistent with one another as well as those that are incompatible with well-supported conclusions from other branches of science. These generalizations or hypotheses constitute psychoanalytic theory. Some of those psychoanalytic hypotheses that have been substantiated both within and outside of psychoanalysis include the ubiquity of psychic conflict and unconscious mental processes, the universality of transference in all interpersonal relationships, the role of infantile sexuality and aggression in the shaping of development, and the power of the past in determining the present and the future. Although psychoanalytic hypotheses are certainly scientifically testable outside of the clinical situation, research from other disciplines can serve to support, inform, or revise psychoanalytic theory. The ultimate test for the usefulness of data, however, is its usefulness clinically.

The cognitive approach to eating disorders appears to accord less significance to the role of theory than does psychoanalysis. Vitousek and Ewald, for example, postulate three selves—the "unworthy self," the "perfectable self," and the "overwhelmed self"—but do not attempt to integrate these selves into an overall theory of personality or to demonstrate either dynamically or empirically how these selves are interrelated. Rather, they infer a self-structure from clusters of character traits that appear to be descriptive and discontinuous. There is little attempt to spell out the dynamic relationship between these selves or their developmental origin. For example, in reference to the three selves, the authors state: "These aspects of the self seem to represent the general self-schemas of individuals who develop anorexia nervosa" (p. 229). The psychoanalytically informed reader may attempt to relate these selves dynamically; that is, the unworthy and perfectable selves may involve the superego activities of the conscience and ego ideal, respectively, whereas the "overwhelmed" self represents the ego activity of integration. There is also an absence of a developmental tracing of the self-representation or its precursors. Although distal and proximal conditions for the development of eating disorders are considered, developmental factors are only hinted at and never seriously considered. Blatt and his colleagues as well as several contemporary psychoanalytic authors have concluded independently that developmentally salient aspects of psychological structure and functioning stem from the early mother–child relationship. In terms of its application to an understanding of the origin, vicissitudes, multiple dimensions, and treatment of eating disorders, a developmental perspective provides an assimilative and unified focus, within which multiple approaches can be organized. The developmental perspective is rooted deeply in psychoanalysis and embraces all aspects of psychological functioning—the relationship between past experience and present functioning (temporal progression), between early trauma and present symptoms, and between historical events and psychic reality. In addition, a developmental focus provides a framework for discerning the relative etiological weights of constitutional and experiential factors. The developmental approach, especially as it has been built upon the systematic naturalistic and longitudinal study of infants, infant–mother interactions, and children, provides a potential methodological link between psychoanalysis and cognitive approaches, as well as a possible resolution of extant tensions between clinical and research approaches to psychopathology. It appears that the wealth of empirical, quantitative research available in the areas of developmental psychopathology, infant development, and attachment can serve to inform cognitive–behavioral approaches in the same way that it has psychoanalysis.

A major difference between the psychoanalytic and cognitive approaches involves the acknowledgment of the *unconscious*. While Vitousek and Ewald assume that dieting and weight loss are not undertaken "deliberately," that eating-disordered individuals are not necessarily "aware" of the linkage between underlying aspects of the self and symptomatology, and that there appear to be individual differences in the "purposefulness" of anorexic behavior, the role of awareness, purposefulness, and nonawareness are neither accounted for nor elaborated. The assumption appears to be that the individual is aware of a multitude of selves and that the self as it is conceptualized within cognitive theory is treated as a conscious construct. The unconscious is a construct that is central to psychoanalytic theory and refers to mental contents and processes, including self and object representations that are outside conscious awareness at any given moment. The psychoanalytic approach to cognition referring to any process through which an individual becomes aware of or obtains knowledge (e.g., perceiving, imagining, symbolizing, judging, thinking, reasoning, and learning) takes into account the unconscious. All these processes can take place outside of conscious awareness and are profoundly influenced by affective states. Psychoanalysis has historically identified two interrelated but distinctly different modes of thought processes: primary and secondary. The primary process mode of thought is characterized by concreteness, condensation, displacement, visual imagery, and symbolism; it is thought to be largely unconscious and the instrument for the expression of inner subjectivity. Primary process modes of thinking are manifest through conscious and unconscious fantasy, dreams, magical thinking, slips of the tongue, jokes, and artistic/creative activities. In contrast, secondary process modes of thinking can be conscious or unconscious and are characterized by rationality, order, and logic, relying heavily on verbal symbolism, lexical modes of communication, and functioning chiefly at the service of adaptation to reality. It appears that cognitive–behavioral treatment theory focuses exclusively on secondary process mentation.

Closely related to the role accorded the unconscious in psychoanalytic theory is the appreciation of *fantasy*. Fantasy is defined psychoanalytically by Laplanche and Pontalis (1973) as an imaginary scene in which the subject is a protagonist, representing the fulfillment of an unconscious wish in a manner that is distorted to a greater or lesser extent by defensive processes. Conscious and unconscious fantasizing combine the interaction of self and object representations, primary and secondary modes of thought processes, both sexual and aggressive drive derivatives, elements of affective expression, defensive activity, the inner world of subjective reality, adaptation to external reality, and moral judgment and punishment. The analysis of fantasy can be considered the sine qua non of psychoanalytic treatment. What Vitousek and Ewald refer to as "the unworthy self . . . confirmed by repeated experiences of self-defined failure" and "the overwhelmed self . . . swamped by the multiplicity of possible roles and identities" (p. 224) are considered psychoanalytically as fantasies and are analyzed in terms of their wish-fulfilling, defensive, representational, moral, and adaptational functions and meanings. Likewise, these authors focus on the immense significance of physiological changes in the body at puberty, as well as on research on the physiological consequences of starvation, but isolate these monumental events from the psychological level of abstraction. For example, pubertal changes contribute to important transformations of masturbation fantasies, which clinical research indicates to be expressions of significant self and object representations, particularly reflective of relationship paradigms between the subject and the parents (Laufer & Laufer, 1984).

It appears that the cognitive–behavioral approach, as compared to the psychoanalytic approach, is based on a relatively narrow view of research. Only quantitative, empirical data is deemed admissible, and clinical observation—or, for that matter, the intensive study of the individual—is not considered a valid source of data. Recognizing that the cognitive models of eating disorder assign a crucial role to variables that are "private," and that eating-disordered individuals make unsatisfactory informants, Vitousek and Ewald should be applauded for addressing the problem of reliance on self-report data and inventories, and for suggesting strategies for investigating information processing as an alternative. A suggested assessment instrument and research tool would be projective tests such as the Rorschach, which are ideally suited for the study of both the objective and subjective dimensions of schemas in general, and self and object representations in particular (Blatt & Lerner, 1983).

While the theoretical status of sexuality and aggression has changed considerably since Freud's early libido theory, their roles—whether conceptualized as instincts, energy sources, motives, affects, or drive derivatives—are considered by most analysts to be central dimensions of personality development, self and object representations, and psychic conflict. The cognitive model has little to say about the ubiquitous role of sex and aggression in psychopathology in general, and eating disorders in particular.

The conceptual differences between the psychoanalytic and cognitive–behavioral approaches to eating disorders are magnified when considering treatment. Areas of common ground include the emphasis on therapeutic alliance, the therapeutic focus on function and adaptation, and, in terms of technique (although this is not spelled out conceptually in their chapter but more through clinical vignettes), the movement from surface to depth in addressing problems. The major differences revolve around the conceptualization of treatment as essentially "problem solving" and the avoidance of transference–countertransference; the use of a "fixed agenda" regarding restoration of normal food intake as the goal of treatment; and the use of therapeutic techniques such as "dissuasion," "nurturing incipient doubts," and "teaching," which most psychoanalysts would regard as manipulative.

Although the therapeutic relationship in cognitive approaches to treatment serves as a prototype for examining treatment issues, it is not hypothesized to be curative in its own right, and according to Vitousek and Ewald, "must be managed delicately to prevent it from becoming the focus of treatment" (p. 248). The authors go on to say the clients are "gently dissuaded from transferring their tendency to seek external verification to the person of the therapist," which is seen by these authors as a resistance in terms of attempting to "adopt the standards of another" (p. 248). In essence, there is little acknowledgment of—and certainly no clinical work with—the *transference,* and psychopathology is assumed to be independent of relationships in general, and the therapeutic relationship in particular. In this way, treatment can be conceptualized as "problem solving." There is little continuity between the cognitive model of psychopathology and the therapeutic relationship.

Within psychoanalysis, the transference is broadly defined as an inherent human tendency to impose the organizing of prior perception of experience upon the present (Freud, 1925/1961; Stern, 1977; McLaughlin, 1991); is regarded as fundamental to shaping psychic reality, interpersonal perception, and experience; and is viewed within psychoanalysis as the major vehicle for mutative change, not through manipulation but through analysis. In essence, transference is an unconscious tendency to shift emotional interest and investment toward significant others in the present, with the hope of reexperiencing earlier objects or of succeeding where one formerly failed. It is maladaptive to the extent that new experiences and individuals are perceived according to earlier formative experiences and relationships, which are repeated. The transference is potentially adaptive to the extent that it reflects an urge to master the past and provides repeated opportunities to do so.

The role of transference in psychoanalytic psychotherapy can also be conceptualized in terms of self and object representations. Formulations about therapeutic action in psychoanalytic psychotherapy increasingly emphasize the therapeutic matrix as a significant interpersonal relationship in which the therapeutic relationship is mediator for the patient's development of increasing levels of organization (Blatt & Erlich, 1981; Loewald, 1960). If the internalization of object relations results in the formation of psychic structures (including self and object representations) during normal development, then the internalization of significant interactions between the patient and the therapist must play an important role in the therapeutic process. The therapist becomes available as a new object in terms of eliminating, step by step, the transference distortions that interfere with the establishment of new relationships (Loewald, 1960). It is the internalization of new and relatively undistorted relations with the therapist that leads to therapeutic change.

Based on their etiological model of eating disorders, Vitousek and Ewald outline a specific sequence of issues that are addressed in what they describe as a "highly structured" treatment regimen. The restoration of normal food intake and weight is thought to be the first order of therapeutic business, followed by attention to distortions caused by schematic processing, internal reinforcement contingencies that maintain anorexic beliefs and behaviors, sociocultural factors, and, finally underlying aspects of the self. Across all phases, according to the authors, the *functional* and/or *adaptive* quality of eating disorder psychopathology is emphasized. From a psychoanalytic vantage point, the emphasis on the functional and adaptive qualities of eating disorder pathology favor a view of the disorder as a complex compromise formation involving the components that I have previously described. However, the emphasis on what may be considered a fixed therapeutic agenda, including the restoration of normal food intake as an early goal, may, in my clinical experience, gratify the patient's defensive wishes and amplify the patient's resistance to change. The highly structured quality of the treatment, the relatively fixed agenda, and the use of techniques involving dissuasion, the nurturance of incipient doubts, and teaching would be seen by many analysts as too rigid, infantilizing of the patient, and running the danger of fostering a dependency.

In comparing cognitive and psychoanalytic approaches to eating disorders, there appears to be an agreement on the descriptive level concerning eating-disordered patients, as well as in treatment, on an emphasis on the therapeutic alliance, a focus on the function and adaptational qualities of the symptoms, and in terms of technique in moving from surface to depth. As for the conceptual formulation of the disorder and other treatment considerations, there are significant differences between the approaches. Differences in value structure, the role of theory, development, and dynamics, as well as the acknowledgment of the unconscious and an appreciation of fantasy and transference, distinguish the two approaches.

REFERENCES

Behrends, R. S., & Blatt, S. J. (1987). Internalization and psychological development throughout the life cycle. *Psychoanalytic Study of the Child, 40,* 11–39.

Blatt, S. J. (1974). Levels of object representations in anaclitic and introjective depression. *Psychoanalytic Study of the Child, 29,* 107–158.

Blatt, S. J., & Erlich, S. (1981). Levels of resistance in the psychotherapeutic process. In P. Wachtel (Ed.), *Resistance in psychodynamic and behavioral therapies* (pp 69–91). New York: Plenum Press.

Blatt, S. J., & Lerner, H. (1983). Investigations in the psychoanalytic theory of object relations and object representations. In J. Masling (Ed.), *Empirical studies of psychoanalytic theories* (Vol. 1, pp. 189–249). Hillsdale, NJ: Analytic Press.

Freud, S. (1961). Negation. In J. Strachey (Ed. and Trans.) *The standard edition of the complete psychological works of Sigmund Freud* (Vol. 19, pp. 235–243). London: Hogarth Press. (Original work published 1925)

Grossman, W. I. (1982). The self as fantasy: Fantasy as theory. *Journal of the American Psychoanalytic Association, 30,* 919–938.

Hartmann, H. (1964). Comments on the psychoanalytic theory of the ego. In *Essays on ego psychology: selected problems in psychoanalytic theory* (113–141). New York: International Universities Press. (Original work published 1950)

Kernberg, O. (1975). *Borderline conditions and pathological narcissism.* New York: International Universities Press.

Kohut, H. (1971). *The analysis of the self.* New York: International Universities Press.

Kohut, H. (1977). *The restoration of the self.* New York: International Universities Press.

Laplanche, J., & Pontalis, J. B. (1973). *The language of psycho-analysis.* New York: W.W. Norton.

Laufer, M., & Laufer, M. (1984). *Adolescence and developmental breakdown.* New Haven, CT: Yale University Press.

Loewald, H. (1960). On the therapeutic action of psychoanalysis. *International Journal of Psycho-Analysis, 41,* 483–504.

McLaughlin, J. T. (1991). Clinical and theoretical aspects of enactment. *Journal of the American Psychoanalytic Association, 39,* 595–614.

Stern, D. (1977). *The first relationship: Infant and mother.* Cambridge, MA: Harvard University Press.

8

Self-representation in Eating Disorders: A Psychodynamic Perspective

HOWARD D. LERNER
University of Michigan

OVER THE PAST 25 years, there has been an increasing coverage, both in scientific and popular publications, of eating disorders, particularly anorexia and bulimia, but more recently, what I have termed, *subclinical eating disorders* (Lerner, 1991). The individuals affected represent an intriguing and poorly understood subgroup of eating-disordered patients who present the paradoxical picture of high academic achievement and enviable talents, alongside very primitive features in other areas of their functioning. These individuals, mostly female undergraduate and graduate students, present clinically with disturbances in eating, self-regulation, and control among other symptoms. Although these patients seldom meet rigorous diagnostic criteria for either anorexia or bulimia, they often suffer from episodes of bingeing, vomiting, a history since puberty of fluctuations in weight, excessive exercising, perfectionistic strivings, and reliance on the body as a vehicle for expressing affects and exerting control over the environment. The core clinical feature that this group of patients share is a marked unevenness in psychological functioning; that is, a discontinuity in maturational levels of functioning.

In the course of my clinical work with this subgroup I found that, beyond the symptoms, there was something profoundly similar occurring in the transference and countertransference. This similarity derived from their having in common a specific traumatic disturbance in an essential aspect of their relationship with their mother; that is, the needs of the mother were the dominant focus of the relationship, with little significance placed on the feelings, needs, and competencies of the child. In what follows, I offer an early developmental formulation of this aspect of these patients by drawing upon recent formulations derived from various lines of conceptual development within psychoanalytic theory that bear on this particular syndrome. I focus on object relations theory and related disciplines (developmental and cognitive psychology), with a view toward formulating a more comprehensive psychodynamic understanding of patients presenting with subclinical eating disorders. A brief review of major trends in psychoanalytic theory is followed by a clinical description of these individuals, including the observation that they all have in common a "false self" ego style characterized by hypersensitivity, vigilance, passivity, and compliance; a masochistic orientation linked to the disturbed mother–child relationship; a core unconscious fantasy that is played out in psychotherapy; and a vexing resistance involving a specific ego defect—a delusion of omnipotence (Novick & Novick, 1991). Aspects of the mother–child relationship, the role of magical, omnipotent thinking as a resistance, and a core unconscious masochistic fantasy is then explored using clinical data. I conclude with an overview of treatment issues.

CONTEMPORARY TRENDS IN PSYCHOANALYTIC THEORY

Psychoanalytic theory is not a static body of knowledge; rather, it is in a state of constant evolution. Historically, psychoanalytic theory has evolved from an early concentration on the identification of the instincts and their development, to a focus on the functions of the ego, to a current interest in the early mother–child dyad and its decisive influence on ego development and object relations. The comparatively recent integration of a systematic psychology of the self, a broadened psychodynamic developmental theory, and a modern object relations theory into the mainstream of psychoanalytic structural theory is now providing the conceptual basis for more comprehensive and phenomenological clinical theory. This evolution is in concert with the movement away from an "experience-distant" metapsychology couched in a mechanistic, natural science framework of impersonal structures, forces, and energies, to a more "experience-near" clinical theory primarily concerned with the representational world as a core focus (Klein, 1976). Contemporary psychoanalytic theorists, researchers, and clinicians are progressively focusing on the complex interactions in early, formative interpersonal relationships and in how these transactions result in the formation of intrapsychic structures throughout development, which can best be understood in terms of the quality of the representational world. These concepts or representations of self and others, in turn, shape and direct subsequent interpersonal relationships.

Kohut (1971, 1977) has laid the theoretical foundation for a systematic psychoanalytic psychology of the self. In a formulation with significant diagnostic implications, Kohut distinguished between more classical neurotic psychopathology and what he called "pathology of the self." Unlike neurosis, which is presumed to originate in later childhood at a time when there is self–other differentiation and when the various agencies of the mind (id, ego, superego) have been firmly established, self pathology begins in earlier childhood and at a point when psychic structures are still in formation. Stemming from the absence of a cohesive sense of self, symptoms are assumed to occur when an insecurely established self is threatened by the dangers of psychological disintegration, fragmentation, and devitalization. In psychoanalytic treatment, neurotic patients are thought to develop a "transference neurosis" in which the analyst is experienced as a new edition of the parents, to whom libidinal and aggressive urges are directed. By contrast, patients with so-called self pathology develop a transference relationship in which the analyst is used to correct or carry out a function that should be managed internally, termed by Kohut a "selfobject." The differences in transference phenomena between neurotic psychopathology and self pathology reflect developmental differences in self–other differentiation and self-cohesiveness.

A second major development in psychoanalysis has been the elaboration of an empirically based, dynamic, developmental theory. Mahler (1971) and her colleagues (Mahler, Pine, & Bergman, 1975) have observed and described the steps in the separation–individuation process. The first subphase of the process begins with the infant's earliest sign of differentiation, or "hatching," from a symbiotic fusion with the mother. This is followed by the "practicing" subphase, a period in which the infant becomes absorbed in his/her own autonomous functioning to the near exclusion of the mother. The all-important period or crisis of "rapprochement" ensues, in which the child, precisely because of a more sharply perceived state of separateness, is prompted to redirect attention back to the mother. The successful negotiation of rapprochement leads to an early sense of self, individual identity, and object constancy.

A third major advance within psychoanalytic theory is modern object relations theory, which represents an integrative thrust, including a convergence of attachment theory (Bowlby, 1969), cognitive psychology (Werner, 1948; Piaget, 1954), and traditional ego psychology (e.g., Hartmann, 1958; Rapaport, 1967), all within a developmental framework (Pine, 1985). The recent focus within object relations theory is on the development of a differentiated, cohesive, and integrated representational world that develops within the context of a maternal or primary matrix, termed by Winnicott (1960/1965) "a holding environment." The primary caretaking agent is seen as the mediator of psychological organization. Defined broadly, object representation refers to the conscious and unconscious mental schemas, including cognitive, affective, and experiential dimensions of objects encountered in reality (Blatt, 1974). Beginning within an interpersonal matrix as vague, diffuse, variable sensorimotor experiences of pleasure and unpleasure, these schemas gradually expand and develop into differentiated, consistent, and relatively realistic representations of the self and the object world. Earlier forms of representation are based more on action sequences associated with need gratification; intermediate forms are based on specific perceptual features; and higher forms are more symbolic and conceptual. Whereas these schemas evolve from, and are intertwined with, the developmental internalization of object relations and ego functions, the developing representations provide a new organization for experiencing object relations (Blatt, 1974).

The profusion of recent psychoanalytic thought embodied in self psychology, developmental psychoanalysis, and object relations theory has been countered by a fourth advance in psychoanalytic thinking; that is, by both developments within as well as a rebuttal from what may be termed *modern structural theory,* or what many critics regard as classical psychoanalytic theory. Taking as its starting point Freud's (1923/1961) tripartite model of id, ego, and superego, and dispensing with concepts of psychic energy, modern structural theory remains as the mainstream hypothesis of modern psychoanalysis (Boesky, 1989). Modern structural theory takes as its premise the ubiquitous nature of internal psychic conflict and a view that this conflict can be conceptualized best through the interaction of the id, ego, and superego. According to Brenner (1983), psychic conflict is at the heart of psychoanalytic theory and treatment, the components and interaction of which result in "compromise formations." All thought, actions, plans, fantasies, and symptoms are compromise formations and are thought to be multidetermined by the components of conflict. Specifically, all compromise formations represent a combination of a drive derivative (a specific personal and unique wish of the individual, originating in childhood, for gratification); of unpleasure in the form of anxiety or depressive affect, and their ideational contents of object loss, loss of love, or castration associated with the drive derivative; of defense, which functions to minimize unpleasure; and various manifestations of superego functioning such as guilt, self-punishment, remorse, and atonement. From the vantage point of structural theory, self and object representations are seen as the result of compromise formation as well as an important influence on compromise formation. From a developmental perspective, modern structural theory emphasizes interrelatedness and process rather than chronological age, and moves away from the notion of psychosexual or libidinal phase-specificity.

Psychoanalytic formulations of eating disorders parallel the development of psychoanalytic thought. The early psychoanalytic literature conceptualized eating disorders psychosexually in terms of conflicting drives and as a defense against fantasies of oral impregnation. Later formulations emphasized the role of ego functions such as ego weakness, perceptual distortions, and interpersonal disturbances. More recent psychoanalytic conceptualizations focus on the symbioticlike attachments eating-disordered patients have with their parents, the incompleteness of the separation–individuation process, and the core depression that underlies the syndrome. Despite their differences in emphasis and conceptual points of departure, most contemporary psychoanalytic clinicians, theorists, and researchers consider eating disorders to represent a developmental arrest. Attendant upon the arrest and the failure to traverse successfully the normative phases of separation from mother, theorists detail the patient's ego defects, impaired sense of self, failure to achieve autonomy, and impaired perspective on the body. Most authors emphasize the pathogenic role of the mother and her experience of the developing child. Highly enmeshed mother–child relationships are depicted, in which the mother either does not permit separation or perceives the child as an extension of her own self. As Schwartz (1986) noted, "the child is seen literally as her 'right arm' without a psychic life of his own" (p. 443). Finally, most authors view eating disorders as residing on a broad spectrum of character development and character pathology.

CLINICAL ASPECTS OF PATIENTS WITH SUBCLINICAL EATING DISORDERS

In the group of subclinical eating-disordered patients I will describe, I have found a distinct clinical presentation, a particular type of resistance in psychotherapy, and a specific dynamic configuration involving the roles of masochism and omnipotence. Striking in each of these patients is a passive attitude toward the environment, a constant and unremitting state of hypervigilance, heightened sensitivity, and excessive vulnerability. Their vigilance and sensitivity are used as a radar screen to scan the immediate outer environment in search of potential dangers, especially threats to their fragile self-esteem. Accompanying this vigilance and sensitivity is a tendency toward compliance and accommodation in interpersonal relationships. Like chameleons, they quickly, and at times accurately, attune to the expectations of others and mold themselves, their behavior, and their affects accordingly; this sensitivity and accommodation, however, are defensive and in the service of warding off potential dangers to their self-esteem. Because such accommodation is without emotional investment, the other is often left with a sense that something crucially important but ineffable is missing. Intimately related to the compliance is a presentation of fragility. The fragility is disarming, and one quickly senses that the wrong word, the forgotten act, the slightest hint of disapproval will strain an already tenuous relationship to a point beyond repair. Underlying this profound vulnerability to external influences and the perception of the outside world as cold, hostile, and ungiving, is a core defect in the cohesion, continuity, strength, and harmony of their self-representation. These patients have an uncanny ability to emphasize with drive derivatives from others; that is, their hypersensitivity, vigilance, and peculiar empathy for others can be strikingly disarming, as in the following example:

Recently, my office building "went condo" and it became necessary for me to purchase my unit. As I was briskly walking down the street to the bank for the closing, I became aware of feeling surprisingly good, quite confident, and particularly grown-up. I was aware of standing up straight and swinging my briefcase as if I had places to go, things to do, and people to meet. Thoughts came to my mind of how years earlier I had nervously and clumsily negotiated a mortgage for a home I bought. I recalled how anxious and insecure I felt in terms of dealing with bankers, and how at times I felt like a little kid in an adult world. As I was walking along, I was very aware of how much had changed for me in recent years and how I actually felt very good and quite self-assured about this closing. I felt proud of how I had negotiated the loan with the bank. I could experience the purchase as an investment as opposed to a loss. I savored the moment, thinking that it was one of those times that I could remember in terms of feeling mature, masculine, and satisfied. A few weeks later, during a session with Ms. A., a 22-year-old patient who was initially referred to me two years previously for depression, fluctuations in her weight with episodic bingeing, and an inability to experience sexual intercourse or pleasure in dating despite being stunningly attractive. Within the throes of becoming disillusioned with me, and holding an image of me as a frustrating, uncaring parent, Ms. A. observed the following: Recently she was driving through town and saw me walking down the street. She observed how masculine I looked and how confident I appeared, walking in such a brisk manner, looking so well dressed, as if I had "places to go, things to do, and people to meet." I was, in her eyes, the ideal man, successful and attractive. She said, in a depressive tone, that I know who I am and that any woman would be attracted to me. She then became visibly saddened and complaintive, saying that she did not like that because it made her feel that she was not "special" to me. She felt she was "just another patient." Ms. A. could not tolerate feeling nonspecial in a relationship, and as such, she could think of no reason to stay in treatment. When she felt special she felt "up," and when she felt "just like another patient" she experienced profound feelings of hopelessness, helplessness, and despair. Her vigilance and hypersensitivity had many dimensions, including an uncanny ability to make me laugh. Ms. A., like other patients in this group, had a knack for accurately seizing the smallest cue as to whether she was being attended to, as well as subtle changes and fluctuations in my own moods and feeling states.

Developmentally, the chronic frustration of normative childhood needs (e.g., to be noticed, responded to, and understood by the mother, to have an effect) interfered with the formation of essential psychological structures, especially those bearing on the capacity of these patients to derive pleasure from their often impressive skills and abilities. Paradoxically, they were intelligent and verbally advanced as children, who held a rather "special" and important position in relationship to their mothers. Underlying this, however, their part of the relationship was characterized by a joyless compliance and pseudoindependence. Academic success and athletic talent often served as an organizing feature, one that gave little sense of pleasure. Paradoxically, it was often the experience of success in these areas that precipitated panic and, consequently, the outbreak of subclinical symptoms that lead them to seek treatment.

The interpersonal relationships of these individuals tend to reflect a stream of disappointing "crushes," massive inhibitions, or a painful love that can be neither consummated nor relinquished. Their self-perception is often one of being fragmented, unreal, and out of control. In this regard, these patients present what Winnicott (1960) has conceptualized as a "false self" and what Krohn (1978) terms, "ego passivity"; that is, an attempt to disown, both internally and interpersonally, responsibility in the broadest sense for thoughts, acts, and impulses. The false self can be understood most generally as an attempt to compensate for feelings of ineffectiveness by pretending to be mature, competent, and self-assured.

Treatment with these patients often begins under a cloak of great vigilance, with a readiness on their part to be distrustful of all aspects of the therapist, including a careful scrutiny of his/her attire, tone of voice, or shifting of body. For example, if the therapist recalls an incident or memory mentioned sessions before, or responds in a particularly empathic manner, the patient feels unusually integrated and whole and considers the therapist as an ally; but if the therapist cancels a session or responds with the slightest trace of irritation, the patient reacts with intense hurt and pain and regards the therapist as hostile, distant, and uncaring. With these patients, the therapist often feels as if he/she is being viewed under a microscope. Not only is every movement closely monitored, often with incredible accuracy, but comments are carefully scrutinized, reconnoitered, and regarded as evidence to evaluate carefully before allowing the relationship to continue and possibly deepen. This stance evokes a marked countervigilance and hypercaution in the therapist. Realizing that interpretations will be met with an overreaction and will frequently be taken as a personal attack, therapists are often less spontaneous, less relaxed, and painfully careful with interventions.

MASOCHISM

An important aspect of the clinical presentation of these patients is intense masochism. These patients are accustomed to putting their worst foot forward, and initially one tends to regard them as being more disturbed than they really are.

Mr. W., on his initial contact, sounded like a panicked and desperate individual. When I asked him if he felt that it was an emergency, he said yes, and I quickly arranged my schedule to meet with him. He initially appeared in my office looking like a nervous wreck. Through pressured speech and stuttering, he was able to tell me that he was preoccupied with his girlfriend in another city, with whom he was unable to have intercourse because of premature ejaculation; that he was in danger of flunking out of graduate school, where he was pursuing an advanced degree in literature; and that over the past few years he had amassed more than five incompletes in his courses. He exercised compulsively, played basketball at breakneck speeds, jogged five miles a day, and would frequently binge on junk food, occasionally vomiting. His speech, anxiety level, disheveled appearance, and barely coherent thought process was alarming and made me think that he was in the midst of a psychotic episode. My worst fears were intensified when he began to tell me about his childhood and adolescence and how, between the ages of 12 and 17, he played an imaginary baseball game with a marble and pencil in which he kept elaborate statistics and simultaneously did a play-by-play broadcast. Further, he used to—and still does—spend hours shooting baskets, keeping statistics involving himself playing against NBA superstars. My own reaction/counterreaction involved high levels of anxiety and intrusive thoughts about the need for possible hospitalization. Following this initial presentation, Mr. W. gradually let me know that he had graduated from an Ivy League school, was co-captain of the track team, and could speak six languages. What was perhaps most telling, and yet was only on the periphery of my awareness, was—from the first session—the impression that this patient bore a remarkable and uncanny resemblance to John McEnroe. It was only later that many features commonly associated with John McEnroe became manifest in his treatment.

After long, tedious, and often confusing and painstaking clinical work with these patients, I came to realize that their case histories, traumas that led to treatment, and major transference–countertransference enactments and actualizations in the clinical context involved the playing out of what Novick and Novick (1987, 1991) refer to as "the essence of masochism"; that is, an underlying structure or configuration of self and object representations in which masochistic impulses are organized as conscious and unconscious fantasies that are fixed, resistant to modification by experience, serve multiple ego functions, and take the form (although not necessarily the content) of a beating fantasy.

> In the fantasies, the subject is an innocent victim who achieves through suffering, reunion with the object, defense against aggressive destruction and loss of the object, avoidance of narcissistic pain, and instinctual gratification by fantasy participation in the oedipal situation. (Novick & Novick, 1987, p. 382)

Rather than being seen as a developmental arrest or fixation at a particular subphase of psychosexual development or of separation–individuation, the complex structure of the underlying beating fantasy, a compromise formation involving a particular configuration of self and object representations, is seen as having determinants from all levels of development. Novick and Novick (1991) define masochism as the active pursuit of psychic or physical pain, suffering, or humiliation in the service of adaptation, defense, and gratification at all levels of development. Masochism is a clinical concept whose observational and experiential grounding can be found in transference–countertransference reactions in the treatment situation. The patient's quest for pain or humiliation weaves its way into the transference, often in subtle reactions to interpretations. Counterreactions of the therapist often provide the first clue of the existence of an underlying masochistic fantasy. The therapist's impulse to be sarcastic, impatient, inappropriately joking, or heavy handed in response to the patient's subtle and often not so subtle provocations (frequently around treatment frame issues such as separations or threats to leave treatment) often provide the first glimpse of the existence of the underlying masochistic fantasy.

After repeatedly experiencing Ms. C. taking trips, or in one way or another missing sessions, either directly before or immediately after I did, I came to realize that this meek, willowy, and exquisitely fragile young woman was inviting me to engage in a sadomasochistic struggle around who was in charge, who was on top, and who was going to win. Only much later in her treatment did we realize that she was wanting me to force her to come to sessions as a way to feel wanted and cared about.

Intimately linked to the transference of patients with subclinical eating disorders and to the underlying masochistic fantasy structure is the nature of resistance one encounters in doing psychoanalytic/clinical work with this population. Based on extensive clinical studies of masochistic patients, and consistent with my own clinical experience, there is, "like a thread linking knots of fixation points at oral, anal, and phallic-oedipal phases . . . *a delusion of omnipotence* which infuses the patient's past and current functioning" (Novick & Novick, 1991, p. 309, emphasis added). This nonpsychotic delusion can include the wish to be both sexes; a profound sense of personal responsibility for death, divorce, and marital conflict; a wish for sexual parity with the oedipal parents; and magical beliefs about success, causality, and the frightening meanings attributed to sexuality and anger. One function of this delusion is to serve as a defense against profound feelings of helplessness. Beginning in infancy and through subsequent periods of development, these patients turned away from their preprogrammed capacities to interact effectively with the real world and began to use the experience of helpless rage and pain magically to predict, control, and organize their chaotic experiences. Within this magical, delusional world, safety, attachment, and control were magically associated with pain.

Mr. W., as a child, imagined himself as a fleet halfback who could not be tackled. He could defy gravity. Although he had mastered six languages, he recently became depressed when, at a party, someone said, "Learning Japanese is like learning five languages." Mr. W. decided to learn Japanese rather than complete his course work and take his qualifying exam. Class discussions for him became fights to the death. He had to be perfect, the best, number one. When he was a child, his mother called him "Apollo." His incompletes were in part because of his need to turn in "perfect papers," but he never had enough time.

Through a developmental formulation and clinical data, my investigation into the relationship of the delusion of omnipotence to subclinical eating disorders leads me to contend that it is the omnipotent self (i.e., omnipotence of thought and actions) that constitutes a major resistance, which is so vexing in doing clinical work with these patients. It is often responsible for treatment impasse and leads well-intentioned therapists to make heroic efforts toward working with these patients, which all too often fall short and end up in negative therapeutic reaction.

Beginning with Freud and Ferenczi and through the work of Klein and later Kohut and Mahler, there has been a consensus within psychoanalysis that the child comes to acknowledge the reality of the external world through repeated experiences of phase-appropriate, nontraumatic disappointments, frustrations, and delays; thus, the child gradually and reluctantly gives up a magical omnipotent system and accepts reality.

Based upon the work of the Novicks (1987, 1991), I have found in patients with subclinical eating disorders a pervasive delusion of omnipotence—an omnipotent self—which takes the form of an ego deficit that significantly interferes with reality testing. These patients do not meet rigorous diagnostic criteria for anorexia, bulimia, or obesity, nor do they present with disturbed dietary behavior as the sole presenting problem. Rather, they enter treatment with intense aggressive and sexual impulses they cannot regulate, which contributes to producing the nonpsychotic delusion that only they are powerful enough to inhibit their own omnipotent impulses. However, this can only be accomplished by resorting to masochistic means such as deadening their feelings, starving themselves, recklessly bingeing, provoking attack, repeatedly putting themselves in danger situations, or even attempting to kill themselves.

As Novick and Novick (1991) pointed out, there is an inconsistency between the state of omnipotence posited in theory to the infant, and adult clinical manifestations of fantasies of omnipotence. Most major psychoanalytic theorists (e.g., Freud, Mahler, Kohut) portray an image of the contented infant, cradled in its mother's arms and surrounded by admiring adults. They regard the infant to be in a state of infantile omnipotence, a solipsistic delusion of being the center of the universe, with unlimited power. This view is derived less directly from observational studies and more from reconstructions of adult cases in psychoanalysis. As for fantasies of omnipotence in patients with subclinical eating disorders, omnipotence is seen less in normatively derived musings and much more in hostile fantasies of control and domination and a staunch refusal to accept reality constraints. Omnipotent fantasies are validated by hostility in action and fantasy. Far from what Freud referred to as "His Majesty The Baby" (1914/1966b, p. 91), the experience from working clinically with these patients is of omnipotent fantasies enmeshed with rage and envy to compensate for profound feelings of helplessness, hopelessness, and shame.

DEVELOPMENTAL CONSIDERATIONS

The combined research of infant observation provides a description of the affective dialogue within the "good enough mother–infant unit" (Winnicott, 1971). While the "good enough" mother provides sufficient supplies of devotion to her infant, the "good enough" infant is able to respond differentially from birth to the real, salient features of the caretaking environment. It is thought that the neonate has an inborn capacity to elicit preprogrammed empathic responses from caretaking agents (Stern, 1985). A complex infant–mother transactional system is initiated in which attachment is fostered by "contingent responding by the caregiver" (Demos, 1985, p. 556). Several factors can interfere with the establishment of the infant–mother preprogrammed empathic relationship. Physical illness in the infant or depression, anxiety, psychosis, substance abuse, or intrafamilial conflict can all disrupt the pleasurable interaction and transactional system between mother and infant. A sense of *competence,* an essential ingredient of reality-based self-esteem is shattered because of a failure in reality. In essence, these individuals have suffered severe deprivation in the areas of self-competence and object relations. Although the mothers of these patients have all declared their sensitivity to their children's needs, they have been experienced as nonresponsive, distracted, or aloof. A confusion ensues within these patients: Does one believe what one is told, what is perceived, or what one wishes to perceive? The reality testing of emotional resonance breaks down.

According to Novick and Novick (1987), there is a marked and significant disturbance in the pleasure economy from birth. In these cases, an external perception takes the place of a growing awareness of the self in relationship to the mother, and as a result, the development of an internal sense of competence and effectiveness is seriously impeded. Normatively, the infant's real capacity to evoke appropriate responses from the caregiver is the root of feelings of competence, effectance, and reality-based positive self-esteem. The capacity of the mother–infant couple to repair inevitable miscommunications in the empathic tie is a significant source of feelings of competence and self-esteem, from which a range of positive feelings becomes associated with competent interactions, which in turn come to initiate and signify empathic attunement. Pleasure in this regard is dependent on and regulated by the capacity of each partner for realistic perception and interaction with the other, which leads to the experience of having an *effect* on the other (Novick & Novick, 1991).

Failures in empathic attunement and in the capacity to repair communicative mismatches is experienced as an "impingement" (Winnicott, 1971)—an unspeakable sense of premature separation from the mother, accompanied by feeling intensely helpless and dangerously exposed and unprotected—seriously disrupting the continuity and harmony of the self in relationship to the mother, and promoting the development of premature defenses, which crystallize in a "false self" within the context of a passive ego. The false self can be seen as a stable and complex compromise formation, including a defensive constellation characterized by compliance with the expectations of others and coexisting with an ego defect involving the delusion of omnipotence. These individuals exhibit a pervasive passivity of the ego, are highly receptive and compliant, and are more than ready to assimilate any stimuli from the external world, including subtle shifts in their mothers' moods.

The specific qualities of these disruptions in holding and empathic attunement communicate the unique psychological makeup, present state, and active conflicts of the mother and are globally "taken-in" by the infant. These unique qualities of the maternal impingement are experienced and taken-in as a self-protective response to premature separateness; they are internalized as the basic mark of the self—a "false self"—and are used as a model and foundation for the later development of object relations and other internal psychological structures. The potential of a reality-based "competent self" is subverted because essential communicative mismatches cannot be repaired. I have often heard patients say, "I just don't know any other way," after once again experiencing frustration, undermining themselves, or provoking crises. The child's involvement with pain at this earliest level is a learned association. According to Stern (1985), it is the actual shape of interpersonal reality that determines the developmental course. Coping occurs as reality-based adaptations. While Tronick and Gianino (1986) have demonstrated the stability of the child's earliest coping styles, Escalona (1968) has shown that it is maladaptive infant behavior that tends to persist through development. Therefore, the association of mother with unpleasure and pain leads to the early adoption of an autoplastic, rather than an alloplastic, mode of coping with internal and external stimuli, which affect all later developmental phases.

By carefully reconstructing repeated, painful, frustrating, provocative patient–therapist interactions in the clinical setting, in which I continually found myself in a position of feeling hopeless, incompetent, and ineffective, I gradually came to understand that these experiences were a clinical indication of a history and relationship pattern relevant to this form of identification. Under the cumulative impact of empathic failures, these patients, beginning in infancy, turned away from their natural, preprogrammed capacities to interact efficaciously with the real world and, as Novick and Novick (1991) wrote,

> instead began to use the experience of helpless rage and pain magically to predict and control their chaotic experience. The failure of reality-oriented competence to effect empathic attunement force the child into an imaginary world where safety, attachment, and omnipotent control were magically associated with pain. (p. 313)

Infancy is a phase of quantum leaps in the development of skills and control as the child becomes increasingly competent in regulating tension states, feeding, and bowel and bladder control. In normative development, the parents' capacity to help empathically to modulate and regulate their infant's assertive impulses is crucial for the infant's growing confidence and pleasure in these new skills. Later, however, patients with subclinical eating disorders egocentrically struggle to maintain the illusion that it was they, through their own sense of power, magic, and control, who created the discordant moods and conflicting feelings they were perceiving, even though the states were originating outside of them. As one patient said, "World hunger—my fault." In contrast to normative infancy, these patients were made to feel omnipotently responsible for their mother's and their own pain, rage, and helplessness. Disruptions in normal, reality-based, competent interactions secondary to maternal impingement coalesce with cognitive egocentricity so that the intensity of painful feelings generated in the mother–child dyad become associated with, and represent a constant affirmation of, omnipotence. Because there is an absence of self–other differentiation, attacks on the self become a powerful weapon for attacking the mother.

Some patients with subclinical eating disorders deny their hostile feelings toward their mothers. Repeated failure to elicit an empathic response and an unwillingness to sacrifice the "special" position of importance often assigned by the mother leads to a split. The affective perception is disavowed and an illusory idealization of the relationship with the mother results. The child rejects the possibility of an empathic relationship, but to avoid entirely losing the relationship, defensively converts it into one that is wished and longed for. Mother's failings and shortcomings are invariably attributed to the patient's own aggression. This is one way the child maintains a sense of omnipotent control over pain. Masochism, in this context, can be seen as an attempt to protect the self against destructive impulses directed against the mother by turning the aggression against the body.

The persistence of the child's involvement with pain and omnipotent thinking is a central thread going through the fabric of development, undergoing various transformations. According to the classical psychoanalytic view, it is the failure of normative infantile omnipotence that forces the child to turn to reality (Freud, Ferenczi, and Mahler). According to the Novicks (1991), it is the failure of reality that forces the child to turn to omnipotent solutions. The omnipotent self is neither a development arrest nor a fixation point at any one particular stage of development. Research with infants has consistently demonstrated that competence is rooted in the attunement between the child's signals and the caretaker's response. As Papousek and Papousek (1975) demonstrated, repeated failures in the mother–infant interactional dyad are frustrating and quickly lead to expressions of helplessness and confusion. Such communicative failures have been observed to produce signs of psychic pain, which are soon followed by signs of anger, such as gaze aversion. The source of pain is initially denied, and this denial is maintained by the transformation of pain into, first, a sign of attachment, and subsequently into a sign of specialness, unlimited destructive power, equality in every way with the oedipal parents, and the omnipotent capacity to coerce parents to gratify all infantile wishes.

Entry into the phallic-oedipal phase brings with it the sexualization of masochism. In normal development, oedipal disappointments are cushioned by a solid base of self-esteem and competent interactions with good enough parents. Normative aggressive infantile sexual theories of parental intercourse and the narcissistic knocks of oedipal exclusion from the parental dyad are all modified by loving respect and empathic sexual information. Patients in this sample of subclinical eating disorders experience the oedipal phase masochistically, that is, tied exclusively with their mothers and experiencing the recognition of real physical and generational differences between children and adults as yet another failure of their own, leaving them in states of helplessness and rage. Experiences such as overstimulation, inappropriate physical contact (e.g., frequent administration of enemas, sleeping with the child), and parental neglect are all transformed into fantasies of triumph, oedipal victory, and an affirmation of the child's omnipotent self and power to coerce the parents into gratifying all needs. According to Novick and Novick (1991), parental collusion with the child's need to deny oedipal exclusion adds a particular quality to omnipotence that becomes a standard by which all achievements are measured. According to these authors, the omnipotent oedipal triumph feels "quick and effortless." Any achievement requiring time and effort becomes devalued.

Ms. E., a 21-year-old student, was referred to treatment because of binge-eating and painful obsessing over breaking up with her boyfriend, a star hockey player.

The daughter of a corporate-lawyer father and a business-executive mother who subsequently divorced, Ms. E. recalled always having difficulties sleeping and being alone. As a child, she often slept with the au pair. She recalled once waking up in the middle of the night and terrified at finding herself alone, because she usually slept with the au pair, Ms. E. searched the house only to find the au pair in the parents' bedroom having intercourse with an older man.

Research in brain development, behavior, and maturation indicates that there is rapid integrative growth of auditory-visual functioning that coincides with maturing temporospatial orientation around the age of 7 years, or the transition into latency (Shapiro & Perry, 1976). Ego development, including cognitive developments, have been found to be involved in the development of moral thinking and socialization during this period. The greater stability and invariance of mental process and the new cognitive structures facilitate the inhibition and control of drives as well as the postponement of action. Latency is a time when the child becomes more firmly established and is enjoying the possibilities of competent interactions in the real world through the exercise of ego functions. The normal pleasures during the latency period frequently associated with achievement did not take place in the patients in this sample. In fact, achievements in reality were a source of little pleasure for them. Rather, fantasies of omnipotent control and triumph, often occasioned by the experience of pain, characterize this period. In contrast to a system of competence based on work and achievement experienced by most children, these patients established a magical omnipotent system in which any achievement, skill, or positive accomplishment was interpreted as a result of their own omnipotence rather than to work (Novick & Novick, 1991). Holding the ideal that achievements should be "quick and effortless," adult patients with subclinical eating disorders often exhibit either a reluctance to work or what appears to be an enormous expenditure of effort with little result. For many of these patients, success and achievement came to be associated with destructiveness and hostile triumph over others and often led to provoking punishment and inhibition.

Ms. F., an overweight, binge-eating, 45-year-old widow, lost her mother in childbirth at age 4, and after being shuffled between different homes, sexually molested, and separated from her younger sister, was shipped overseas to a convent boarding school, where she achieved impressive academic success. Years later, on the verge of being offered a prestigious college scholarship, she boasted to friends about her sexual exploits with an older military officer. Word quickly spread to the nuns, and Ms. F. was promptly expelled. Several years later when she was deemed the "star" of her graduate program and was academically courted by senior faculty, she panicked while taking her qualifying exam and purposely and unnecessarily answered a question outside of her area of expertise, failed the exam, and with a sense of relief dropped out of the program. An insistent dynamic in treatment was Ms.

F.'s compulsion to make herself a victim whenever she got close to feelings of activity, responsibility, and competence. Whenever she recognized herself as an active, powerful person in reality, who made things happen, she needed to destroy and spoil it because of enormous guilt over her own omnipotently destructive wishes. In treatment, spoiling became a vehicle for making me, in the transference, responsible for her hardships, a way of gaining control, and a quest for safety. Ms. F., for example, harbored a stoic rage, where she lived life vicariously through fantasies of my blissful life with my wife and children, while resentfully nursing her anger alone, drinking and bingeing.

Reality achievements threaten the magical system, and there is a need for misery and helplessness in order to feel magical. Pain and magic are mutually dependent upon each other in these patients.

All of these individuals experienced difficulty during adolescence. The greatest threat to the fantasies of omnipotence was the experience of pleasure, especially pleasure derived from adult activity such as sexuality. According to Novick and Novick (1991), the omnipotent system leaves no place for pleasure in reality, in that pleasure leaves these individuals feeling ordinary and not special. All the patients in my sample had a disturbed late adolescence based on a failure to take ownership of their own bodies and minds and to integrate adult sexuality into their self-image (Laufer & Laufer, 1984). The quest for perfection leaves no room for reality-based self-esteem and pleasure.

These patients need the experience of misery and helplessness to feel magical; that is, they use their masochism assertively as a way of experiencing their own omnipotent power. They fear success in reality because success carries with it the meaning of annihilation and destruction of objects that are loved (oedipal triumph); they attribute omnipotent power to their own feelings, fantasies, and accomplishments. Inhibition and spoiling successful experiences and accomplishments become a major vehicle for maintaining infantile relationships, protecting themselves against their own fantasies of aggressive destruction and the loss of others, the avoidance of narcissistic pain such as shame and humiliation, and gratification by fantasy participation in forbidden relationships. The development of fantasies of destructive omnipotence, as well as the delusion of omnipotence, represents simultaneously a defense against feelings of helpless rage and humiliation and a pathological source of self-esteem.

TREATMENT IMPLICATIONS

In patients with subclinical eating disorders, derivatives from all stages of development contribute to the formation of the omnipotent self. It is neither a developmental arrest nor a regression to a particular phase-specific fixation point. The delusion of omnipotence, which is a major component of an underlying masochistic beating fantasy, becomes manifest in treatment as a major source of resistance. Treating the delusion of omnipotence as a resistance and an ego defect of reality testing as a major focus helps organize interventions that are mutative. During the early phases of treatment, the omnipotent self becomes manifested as a resistance around the need to control all impulses for fear that they will lead to the destruction of both objects and the self. One way of accomplishing this is by assuming an infantile position in relation to the therapist. Many patients project their omnipotent self onto the therapist as a means of insisting that the parent/therapist take responsibility for managing issues of weight and eating behavior. This is often a preview of a deeper, more intense wish for the therapist to take control of their lives in a definitive and forceful way, communicated by pressuring the therapist for information, suggestions, and ideas. Parental collusion sometimes keeps the patient in this position. A subtle sign of this phenomenon frequently involves arrangements for payment of the fee, in which the patient will insist that the bill be sent directly to the parents. Removing the issue of money and the business aspect of treatment from the patient–therapist relationship infantilizes the patient, distorts the reality that the therapist is paid for professional as opposed to personal services, and contributes to the delusion of omnipotence, which interferes with the therapeutic task of assisting the patient in growing up.

Following the early phase of treatment, resistance revolves around the dangers of pleasure and the threats that pleasure and reality pose to the omnipotent self. Fear of success, intense guilt, and a desperate clinging to pain are common. With the growing recognition and expression of sexual and aggressive impulses comes the fear of not being able to stop. Spoiling becomes a powerful defense to convert pleasure to pain. One patient remarked, "Before the session I had such a delicious sandwich." Moments later she complained of a stomach ache. She experienced a "delicious" session of hard work and insight in the same manner. What is ultimately therapeutic is pitting the omnipotent self against the reality principle. In this regard, many interventions based on the so-called holding environment, such as offering extra sessions, sending postcards during vacations, or actually phoning the patient, is not only unhelpful but is actually harmful. These well-intentioned provisions support the omnipotent self of infantile relationships, limitless supplies, and magical control and treatment based on personal care rather than professional competence. They make patients feel out of control because they sense that there are no limits. These individuals require firm and empathic control, with unwavering attention to the transference and resistance. As treatment deepens, according to Novick and Novick (1988), working with the delusion of omnipotence as a resistance brings into clinical focus fixed masochistic beating fantasies, which can be analyzed in terms of their attempt to (1) maintain a preoedipal tie to the mother, (2) protect the object against destructive impulses, and (3) participate in a sadomasochistic relationship.

Working with the preoedipal object tie is quite difficult because it involves examining the parents' pathology, especially their opposition to permitting the patient to grow up. Dealing with the preoedipal tie between mother and patient is crucial for subsequent change in the patient's underlying pathology and eating disorder to take place.

In his classic paper "A Child Is Being Beaten" (1919/1966a), Freud outlined three stages of the beating fantasy that occur transiently during normal development and that become fixed in patients with masochistic pathology (Novick & Novick, 1987). In the first phase (sadism) of the beating fantasy, a disliked sibling is beaten by the father. This is thought to gratify the child's jealousy and is driven by sexual and narcissistic interests. The fantasy during the second phase is of being beaten by the father. This is a direct expression of guilt, which transforms the sadism to masochism. The fantasy is not only a punishment for forbidden sexual impulses but also a regressive substitute for it. This is where masochism and the beating fantasy become sexualized. Clinically, it can often be uncovered through analyzing masturbation fantasies. The third phase represents a turn toward sadism in terms of an oversensitivity and antagonism toward father figures. This fantasy structure is woven into the treatment process in complex ways.

Ms. W. had often lamented that her family motto was "food equals love and love equals food." After once again planning a trip in response to my previously announced plans to be away, she reluctantly offered the view that I hated her for discussing vacation plans. This was within the context of feeling miserable during the weekend, feeling excluded from her roommate's relationship with another woman, and feeling unappreciated at work. She did not know why this was coming up now or what it was about, and when I said I think I do, Ms. W. said, "You can tell me why I hate you." I replied, "Because you want me to stop you from going away." She enthusiastically responded, "I should change the family motto—'force plus food equals love.'" Her associations led to how she was in a sense "force-fed" by her mother and how she had a dream last night that she planned her trip and I was glad to see her go.

After interpreting Ms. F.'s beating fantasy—the wish that I would force her to grow up, to lose weight, and have sex—she reported during a Friday session that she was feeling more sexual, in part because her housemate had given her a Hungarian porno novel about an older woman and a younger man and, in part, because she was feeling more genuinely, as opposed to mockingly, attracted to me. Referring to me as the captain of the football team, she said she was worried that if she had me should would want the whole team. Later she modified this to mean that if she had a little of me she would want all of me, it would never be enough, and this was depressing to her. She then reported the fantasy of her car crashing and me being an adulterer. On Monday she reported that she drank heavily over the weekend, made a lovely pork roast and kiwi-cheese pie, and binged. Noting that I am a "coffee maven," she recalled two dreams. In the first dream she was living in a house connected to another house by a giant moving van with detachable parts. As she went through the house she observed scary cats with sharp, brightly colored teeth. In the second dream, as she was driving her car her foot got stuck on the accelerator and the breaks failed. She ended up at the football stadium where there were 50 or 60 working-class men dressed in janitor suits. Her associations were to "raging hormones," wanting to spend more time in therapy with me, and the thought that love is the first step toward separation, the beginning of the end. She felt she needed inspiration to diet and lose weight: "The only inspiration I know is frustration."

For this patient, the meaning of sexuality was intimately related to the death of her mother and later her husband. The fear was that once she let herself go she would not be able to stop. Food for Ms. F. represented gratification, protection from destructive impulses and their imagined consequences, and self-punishment, since it effectively removed her from dating.

CONCLUSION

The focus of this chapter has been on a group of patients with subclinical eating disorders, who demonstrate a particular clinical presentation, character style, form of maternal identification, resistance in treatment, and underlying fantasy structure. They have identified with particular conflictual aspects of the mother's psychopathology as a model of identification, which is reflected in their "false self" presentation, their object relations, and in many aspects of their psychological structures. Their early histories are dominated by a view of a mother deeply involved in her own conflicts in which she was unable to protect the child. This was experienced during infancy as an "impingement," a premature separation in which the mother's conflicted self was globally "taken-in" by the developing child as a core sense of self. This disruption of normal development, in which vitally intimate aspects of the mother–infant relationship are associated with pain, sets the stage for the development and transformation of masochistic impulses. A common feature of this developmental course is the miscarriage of empathy and the repair of communicative mismatches, which result in an "omnipotent self" featuring a system of magical thinking and power that interferes with the normative evolution of the reality principle. All events and happenings are experienced magically, as caused by the omnipotent self, limits and commitments, as well as separations implying loss, are intolerable; and the experience of growing up, in which pleasure is achieved in reality through work and mature relationships, becomes impossible. Development becomes uneven. Disturbances in eating, such as fluctuations in weight, bingeing, and excessive exercising, become futile attempts to achieve omnipotent perfection, reunion with the mother, protection against aggressive destruction and object loss, and gratification.

REFERENCES

Blatt, S. J. (1974). Levels of object representations in anaclitic and introjective depression. *Psychoanalytic Study of the Child, 29,* 107–158.

Boesky, D. (1989). A discussion of evidential criteria for therapeutic change. In A. Rothstein (Ed.), *How does treatment help? Models of therapeutic action of psychoanalytic therapy* (pp. 171–180). Madison, CT: International Universities Press.

Bowlby, J. (1969). *Attachment.* London: Penguin Books.

Brenner, C. (1983). *The mind in conflict.* New York: International Universities Press.

Demos, E. (1985). The elusive infant. *Psychoanalytic Inquiry, 5,* 553–568.

Escalona, S. K. (1968). *The roots of individuality.* London: Tavistock Publications.

Freud, S. (1961). The ego and the id. In J. Strachey (Ed. and Trans.), *The standard edition of the complete works of Sigmund Freud* (Vol. 19, pp. 3–66). London: Hogarth Press. (Original work published 1923)

Freud, S. (1966a). A child is being beaten. In J. Strachey (Ed. and Trans.), *The standard edition of the complete works of Sigmund Freud* (Vol. 17, pp. 175–204). London: Hogarth Press. (Original work published 1919)

Freud, S. (1966b). On narcissism: An introduction. In J. Strachey (Ed. and Trans.), *The standard edition of the complete works of Sigmund Freud* (Vol. 14, pp. 69–102). London: Hogarth Press. (Original work published 1914)

Hartmann, H. (1958). *Ego psychology and the problem of adaptation.* New York: International Universities Press.

Klein, G. J. (1976). *Psychoanalytic theory.* New York: International Universities Press.

Kohut, H. (1971). *The analysis of the self.* New York: International Universities Press.

Kohut, H. (1977). *The restoration of the self.* New York: International Universities Press.

Krohn, S. (1978). *Hysteria: The elusive neurosis.* New York: International Universities Press.

Laufer, M., & Laufer, M. (1984). *Adolescence and developmental breakdown.* New Haven, CT: Yale University Press.

Lerner, H. (1991). Masochism in subclinical eating disorders. In C. Johnson (Ed.), *Psychodynamic treatment of anorexia nervosa and bulimia* (pp. 109–127). New York: Guilford Press.

Mahler, M. (1971). A study of the separation–individuation process and its possible application to borderline phenomena in the psychoanalytic situation. *Psychoanalytic Study of the Child, 26,* 405–424.

Mahler, M., Pine, F., & Bergman, A. (1975). *The psychological birth of the human infant.* New York: Basic Books.

Novick, J., & Novick, K. (1991). Some comments on masochism and the delusion of omnipotence from a developmental perspective. *Journal of the American Psychoanalytic Association, 39,* 307–332.

Novick, K., & Novick, J. (1987). The essence of masochism. *Psychoanalytic Study of the Child, 42,* 353–384.

Papousek, H., & Papousek, M. (1975). Cognitive aspects of preverbal social interaction between human infants and adults. In *parent–infant interactions.* New York: Association of Scientific Publishers.

Piaget, J. (1954). *The construction of reality in the child.* New York: Basic Books.

Pine, F. (1985). *Developmental theory and clinical process.* New Haven, CT: Yale University Press.

Rapaport, D. (1967). *The collected papers of David Rapaport* (M. Gill, Ed.). New York: Basic Books.

Schwartz, H. (1986). Bulimia: Psychoanalytic perspectives. *Journal of the American Psychoanalytic Association, 34,* 439–462.

Shapiro, T., & Perry, R. (1976). Latency revisited: The age 7 plus or minus one. *Psychoanalytic Study of the Child, 31,* 39–106.

Stern, D. (1985). *The interpersonal world of the infant.* New York: Basic Books.

Tronick, E. Z., & Gianino, A. (1986). Interactive mismatch and repair. *Zero to Three, 6,* 1–6.

Werner, H. (1948). *Comparative psychology of mental development.* New York: International Universities Press.

Winnicott, D. (1965). Ego distortion in terms of true and false self. In *The maturational processes and the facilitating environment.* London: Hogarth Press. (Original work published 1960)

Winnicott, D. (1971). *Playing and reality.* New York: Basic Books.

Commentary

KELLY BEMIS VITOUSEK
LINDA S. EWALD
University of Hawaii

WHEN THE FORMAT of this book was first outlined, we cautioned one of the editors that companion psychodynamic and cognitive chapters on self-representation in the eating disorders might make rather dull reading, because it has been our impression that an unusually high degree of correspondence obtains between the perspectives in this topic area. The editor reassured us that rapprochement would be at least as welcome as divergence, and that we were under no obligation to enliven the exchange with artificial controversy. After completing our chapter, and reviewing its counterpart by Howard Lerner, we find that our concerns about the redundancy of side-by-side contributions may have been misplaced. In close proximity, these paradigms—at least as they have been exemplified here—clearly clash more than they harmonize with one another.

Two factors complicate a discussion of the points of similarity and differences between these models. The first is that the chapters may well be addressing different phenomena. We elected to restrict our attention to the "classic," or "primary," type of anorexia nervosa, whereas Lerner chose to focus on what he characterizes as "an intriguing and poorly understood subgroup of eating-disordered patients," those with "subclinical eating disorders" (p. 267).

Lerner notes that these individuals "seldom meet rigorous diagnostic criteria for either anorexia or bulimia" (p. 267); however, he does not indicate which criteria they typically fail to fulfill (body image disturbance, amenorrhea, or amount of weight loss for anorexia nervosa? episode frequency, weight concerns, or use of compensatory behaviors for bulimia nervosa?). He does not specify how they are similar to, or different from, clinical cases in terms of background features, dynamics, symptomatology, course, or response to treatment; he does not speculate about the protective factors that prevent the emergence of a full-blown eating disorder; and he does not propose defining features that could be identified reliably by other investigators. The case examples provided seem quite heterogeneous, including a male compulsive exerciser and binger, a young woman characterized as "exquisitely fragile," whose eating patterns are not described, and a 45-year-old overweight binge-eating widow. It is unclear how much of the causal model, and which elements of the causal model, extend to the eating disorders in general, and which pertain only to the minority of cases that are the particular focus of this report. Except for the emphasis on masochism, most of the personality features and childhood experiences attributed to the subclinical group discussed here are identical to those Lerner has listed elsewhere when characterizing a subgroup of clinical eating disorder cases (Lerner, 1986).

We concur that a substantial number of clients who present with eating- and weight-related symptomatology do not satisfy formal criteria, and we agree that these individuals deserve more clinical and research attention than they have received. We suspect, however, that these clients are even more diverse than their diagnosable fellows, and even less likely to be responding to a uniform set of causal variables. We doubt that Lerner means to suggest that all eating-disordered individuals who fall short of diagnostic criteria form a cohesive group of subjects holding key features in common. If so, a new diagnostic category should be designated to contain them; if not, the subgroup for which Lerner's model is applicable must be identified with greater precision. As emphasized in our own chapter, we also assume that few generalizations about aspects of the self—or any other variables, for that matter—will apply without exception to every member of a recognized subgroup or diagnostic category; however, unless we define the parameters of category membership, we cannot begin to examine the validity and generality of theoretical constructs or compare alternative models of symptom development and maintenance.

A second factor complicating the comparison of psychodynamic and cognitive models is the existence of numerous and highly disparate variants of the former (Goodsitt, 1985; Lerner & Dyer, 1986). Any attempt to contrast *the* psychodynamic theory of the eating disorders with the cognitive account will be misleading, since the psychodynamic label encompasses the oral impregnation theory of Anna Freud, the maternal introject notion of Selvini-Palazzoli, the object relations models of Masterson and Sours, the ego deficit account of Bruch, the developmental perspective of Strober, the biopsychosocial model of Johnson, and the self psychological theory of Goodsitt. There are numerous similarities between our model and the theories of Bruch and Goodsitt, particularly with reference to formulation of treatment. If one of these authors had contributed a chapter to the collection in place of Lerner, our differences might appear to be trivial. In contrast, we would anticipate even more profound disparity if our approach were to be compared to a drive-conflict model of the eating disorders. In the ensuing discussion, then, our comments should be viewed as applying to the specific model delineated by Lerner, rather than to the psychodynamic theories collectively, although we will hazard some generalizations about the themes that seem to recur across most variant forms.

POINTS OF SIMILARITY

Although different subgroups of individuals have been singled out in the two chapters, common elements are readily discernible in the depiction of the modal premorbid personality of those vulnerable to the development of an eating disorder. Aspects of what we termed the "unworthy self" are echoed in Lerner's discussion of his patients' fragile self-esteem, heightened sensitivity, and tendency toward joyless compliance. His descriptions are often apt and evocative: for example, the image of these individuals hunched over an internal radar screen, scanning the environment in search of potential dangers, perfectly captures the wary vigilance with which they feel they must live in the world. Elements of our "perfectible self" are matched in Lerner's "omnipotent self," and the accounts agree that academic or athletic success often serve an organizing function for eating-disordered clients, while giving them "little sense of pleasure." Our "overwhelmed self" is evident in Lerner's observation that these individuals' "self-perception is often one of being fragmented, unreal, and out of control" (p. 273). The cognitive model of primary anorexia nervosa does not incorporate the masochism that dominates the clinical picture Lerner describes in his subgroup of subclinical cases; however, most of the proximal variables that represent aspects of the self appear to be congruent across these two perspectives.

POINTS OF DEPARTURE

Remote Origins of Aspects of the Self

One obvious distinction between the cognitive model and all psychodynamic variants is a differential willingness to speculate about the remote origins of the traits we mutually recognize as predisposing variables. The cognitive model is conspicuously and deliberately silent about the distal sources of the feeling of unworthiness, the drive for perfection, and the sense of confusion that seem to precede the onset of symptomatology. In contrast, Lerner's theory confidently attributes these aspects of the self to the influence of the conflicted and disturbed mother, who warped the emerging personality of her child. She failed to provide empathic mirroring during the symbiotic phase of development, occasioned "chronic frustration of normative childhood needs . . . to be noticed, responded to, and understood by the mother" (p. 272), was experienced as "nonresponsive, distracted, or aloof" (p. 277), and caused her child to feel responsible for her mother's "pain, rage, and helplessness" (p. 279). The product of this "not good enough" mothering is a child who transforms "experiences such as overstimulation, inappropriate physical contact (e.g., frequent administration of enemas, sleeping with the child), and parental neglect" into "fantasies of triumph [and] oedipal victory" (p. 280), and begins to employ "attacks on the self [as] a powerful weapon for attacking the mother" (p. 279).

We do not find this or related models compelling, and recognize a number of problems in Lerner's analysis:

1. *Lack of evidence.* Lerner does not indicate that he has interviewed the parents or siblings of his patients, observed family interactions, or systematically compared the relationships of these individuals and their families with those experienced by other normal or psychiatrically affected subjects, nor does he include citations of supportive studies conducted by researchers who have attempted such investigations. Presumably, his conclusions are based on the retrospective accounts of currently symptomatic individuals who must recall events that transpired during early childhood—the most theoretically crucial of these during a preverbal stage of development. The high probability of distortion introduced by the client's selective memory or the clinician's conceptual framework makes this an extremely perilous enterprise, but we are not informed about the precautions taken to minimize bias or warned about the tentative nature of the data that result. No attempt is made to ascertain whether these mothers really were aloof, neglectful, or overstimulating relative to other mothers, or whether their offspring were in fact subjected to an exceptional number of enemas during their formative years. Evidence of a failure in empathic mirroring in the histories of these clients has not been (and cannot be) provided; rather, it is assumed, because it makes sense theoretically. If something is manifestly wrong during adulthood, it must have gone amiss during childhood, and the particular psychodynamic variant to which the therapist subscribes specifies what "it" is likely to have been. Thus, the same maternal sins of omission and commission turn up with monotonous regularity within—if not always between—psychodynamic schools of thought concerning different disorders.

The risk of confirmatory bias in reconstructions of the familial causes of symptomatology may be particularly great in the case of the eating disorders, since these clients are so eager to fulfill the expectations of their interviewers. The eminent (and psychodynamic) clinician Hilde Bruch (1978) noted that:

> [an] overlooked factor is the enormous compliance with which these youngsters can approach treatment, having lived their whole lives in an overconforming way. They agree with everything that is being said, will elaborate upon it, even fabricate material that they feel the therapist wants to hear. This is one more reason why an interpretive approach is so ineffective in this condition. Anorexics will agree with what has been said, quote it in a different context, but actually feel that it means nothing. While dutifully and compliantly agreeing, anorexics cherish the secret knowledge that things as they are being discussed are not so. (p. 138)

Bruch cautioned that "pseudo-agreeing may manifest itself in every area under discussion" (p. 139), and urged clinicians working with this population to be most skeptical when their interpretations are being confirmed.

2. *Assumption of uniformity.* The homogeneity in family characteristics and interactional patterns assumed by Lerner in his descriptions of the developmental histories of these clients is not supported by preliminary empirical data in this area. Few well-controlled studies have been conducted; however, what is known about the families of eating-disordered individuals suggests considerable diversity in parent–child interaction patterns (Kog & Vandereycken, 1985). The families of anorexics, in particular, appear to be quite heterogeneous in presentation (Grigg, Friesen, & Sheppy, 1989). Although a number of studies have found greater disturbances of various kinds in the family relationships of eating-disordered clients compared to normal controls, there is little evidence that the types of problems exhibited are in any sense unique to the eating disorders (Strober & Humphrey, 1987; Yager, 1982); similar characteristics have been reported in distressed families in general (Stern et al., 1989).

3. *Failure to consider alternative explanations.* Even if some of the predictions of psychodynamic theory were affirmed through more adequate methods of data collection, plausible alternative interpretations would have to be considered. If it could be demonstrated that eating-disordered individuals, before any exposure to therapeutic suggestion, were more likely than controls to characterize their parents as harmful or deficient, we would have to entertain the hypothesis that this difference was a function of distortions in clients' views of their families. Typically, the mother is assumed to be the *cause* of the dominant reaction patterns displayed through the phenomenon of transference; another possibility is that she has been historically—as the therapist is currently—the object of the patient's tendency to overidealize and then feel rejected, unloved, and mistreated by significant figures. If comparative research verified that the

parents of eating-disordered individuals were more depressed or isolative or anxious than the parents of controls, it would of course be necessary to consider genetic as well as environmental determinants of the pathology manifested by their children. If observational studies confirmed that families with an eating-disordered member interacted differently from families of controls, it would be important to examine the possibility that their disordered communication represented a reaction to, rather than an explanation for, symptomatic behavior. Inquiry in this domain presents the same dilemma of disentangling cause from effect that has confounded research into the families of schizophrenic and autistic individuals (Bemis, 1978; Lawrence, 1979); it is hoped that we will avoid committing the same egregious errors and compounding the suffering of those directly affected. Our record of accuracy in identifying the remote causes of psychopathology suggests that when we venture theoretical speculations of this sort, humility is more warranted than confidence.

4. *Lack of specificity*. As noted earlier, psychodynamic theories tend to invoke the same familial characteristics and processes repeatedly in explaining many forms of psychopathology. Etiological models cannot be considered adequate unless they either suggest a link between specific remote variables and specific proximal variables that can account for the subsequent emergence of specific symptomatology, or propose an interaction among general predisposing variables and other specific contributing factors. The kinds of family variables that Lerner implicates may indeed be associated with diverse forms of psychopathology, including the eating disorders, but they cannot be assigned a central position in causal models of any particular disorder because they lack discriminant power (Levine & Smolak, 1989). They can neither explain why an individual deprived of "good enough" mothering would develop an eating disorder, instead of some other syndrome, nor account for the steep increase in incidence of these conditions over the past two decades.

When reviewing an edited collection of psychoanalytic papers on anorexia nervosa, Lerner castigates many of the contributors for their "consistently demeaning attitude toward the anorexic's mother which verges on mother-baiting" (Lerner & Dyer, 1986). He goes on to criticize outdated analytic models for omitting any mention of the role of the father, noting that the papers reviewed made no attempt to relieve the burden of blame from the shoulders of the mother. We endorse Lerner's concerns, but find them puzzling in juxtaposition with his own unqualified indictment of the mothers of subclinical eating-disordered clients in the present chapter—from which fathers are again conspicuously absent. In this account, the words "mother" or "maternal" appear 54 times, often in the context of phrases such as "disturbed mother–child relationship," "maternal impingement," "mother's failings and shortcomings," and "mother's psychopathology." The words "father" or "paternal" appear 4 times: once to identify the occupation of a patient's male parent, and three times in summarizing a paper of Freud's on the topic of sadomasochism.

Linkage between Proximal Variables and Eating Disorder Symptomatology

Although the cognitive model declines to speculate about the relationship between specific distal and proximal variables, it does suggest links between the latter (including aspects of the self, sociocultural influences, and environmental stressors) and the emergence and maintenance of anorexic symptomatology. Indeed, much of the cognitive account is concerned with an explication of why and how eating disorder beliefs and behaviors serve a function for individuals with particular characteristics, operating through the effects of positive and negative reinforcement, automatic information processing, and the starvation syndrome. In contrast, Lerner's model provides minimal information about the connection between proximal variables and symptom formation or persistence. Once again, as with the lack of specificity in linking hypothesized remote origins to particular psychopathological outcomes, the problem is one of accounting in theoretical terms for why *this* individual developed *this* psychiatric disorder.

Lerner does offer a few interpretations of eating disorder symptoms that suggest functional significance. With reference to one overweight client, he notes that food represented gratification, protection from destructive impulses, and self-punishment, "as it effectively removed her from dating." Elsewhere, he observes that these patients rely on the body "as a vehicle for expressing affects and exerting control over the environment," and characterizes starvation and bingeing as "masochistic means." The most extended explanation of the specific symptomatology is contained in the following sentence: "Disturbances in eating, such as fluctuations in weight, bingeing, and excessive exercising, become futile attempts to achieve omnipotent perfection, reunion with the mother, protection against aggressive destruction and object loss, and gratification" (p. 285–286). It seems likely that the first of these proposed functions is consistent with the cognitive model, although the remainder appear inconsistent; in each instance, it would be desirable if they could be defined more precisely so that their validity and generality could be examined.

The Role of Secondary and Automatic Maintaining Variables

Our own chapter strongly emphasized the functional aspects of eating disorder pathology, noting that the egosyntonic nature of symptoms forces the theoretician or clinician to consider issues such as motivation and purposefulness, which are ordinarily ego-alien to the cognitive–behaviorally inclined. The cognitive model, however, also implicates two sets of processes that can act to maintain symptomatology in an automatic, unmotivated fashion: the semistarvation syndrome and schema-driven processing. Both of these include elements that may be positively or negatively reinforcing to some anorexic and bulimic individuals, but both also exert influences that may be capable of perpetuating disordered behavior independently of the subjects' wishes, needs, fears, and gratifications. In some cases, the eating disorders seem to become autonomous, outlasting the relevance of variables that were crucial to their initiation and early development. In all cases, these secondary processes contribute to the maintenance of symptoms, and in all cases, the cognitive approach contends, it is important to address them directly in treatment. Accordingly, cognitive–behavioral therapy for anorexia nervosa and bulimia nervosa prominently features strategies for the normalization of food intake and weight, and for the examination of specific schema-driven distortions in information processing (Fairburn, 1985; Garner & Bemis, 1985). These issues do not appear to be addressed in Lerner's theoretical account or therapeutic program, and are rarely discussed by other psychodynamic writers.

Testability and Falsifiability

As we acknowledged in our own chapter, the validation of variables implicated in the etiology of the eating disorders by both cognitive and psychodynamic theorists poses a formidable challenge to the researcher. Most of these variables are private; many of them are complex, abstract, and difficult to operationalize or test with precision. At present, neither model can claim to rest on firm empirical foundations; consistent with the more general orientation from which each arises, however, clear differences can be discerned in the emphasis on the testability and falsifiability of constructs.

We have already discussed the problems attached to an examination of remote etiological variables in the psychodynamic account; some of the same issues also apply to variables presumed to be present at a time when direct evaluation is possible. Key constructs, such as the highly controversial concept of masochism, are not defined with sufficient exactness so that they can be submitted to disproof. From the information provided in Lerner's report, it seems possible that any repetitive behavior that both causes distress and serves an adaptive function might qualify for this appellation. Before the generality, specificity, and utility of this construct can be examined, we need to be provided with clearer criteria for determining when a pain-inducing behavior that is also valued by the actor does or does not represent an instance of masochism.

The evidence offered in support of Lerner's conceptualization is anecdotal: accounts of what individual clients said or did in the context of therapy, and how he reacted to them. We certainly agree that clinical examples can be instructive and illuminating for both the therapist and the theorist. In our view, however, the value of such excerpts is enhanced when they are closely linked to the specific constructs they are intended to exemplify. It was not clear to us what one anecdote about a client's discovery of an au pair having intercourse with her boyfriend was meant to illustrate. It was not obviously connected to the material that immediately preceded or followed, its dynamic significance to the client was not identified, and it was not apparent whether the incident was intended to represent a common theme for eating-disordered patients that distinguishes them from other distressed individuals. Similarly, the implications of one client's string of associations about football players, car crashes, the therapist's fondness for coffee, cats with multicolored teeth, and men in janitor suits were not evident in the absence of additional commentary. We also tend to find clinical examples more useful when they depend minimally on the interpretations or personal reactions of the observer, since our own idiosyncracies as therapists are otherwise entangled with the individual differences of our clients. In one of the cases described, another clinician might be differentially disposed to interpret missed sessions not as an "[invitation] to engage in a sadomasochistic struggle around who was in charge, who was on top, and who was going to win," but as an expression of anger, hurt, or difficulties in establishing trust.

In general, we think it most desirable for anecdotes to be used as vivid and economical means of summarizing some central and recurrent themes for a particular patient group, and as a generative source of hypotheses that can be examined through more formal investigative techniques. In Lerner's chapter, clinical examples may be serving the former function, but there is no indication that the latter is intended. The chapter does not cite any existing research on the eating disorders or mention the need for assessment or suggest possibilities for the subsequent empirical study of theoretical propositions.

Neither the psychodynamic nor the cognitive model of the eating disorders is sufficiently compelling to remain influential in the persistent absence of evidence; both should be proceeding to formulate and test their postulates with techniques acceptable to the wider community of behavioral scientists. We do not consider it illegitimate to speculate on the remote origins of the eating disorders; indeed, we share with dynamic writers a keen theoretical interest in learning more about how the traits we mutually recognize to be present first began to develop. Yet the need for great caution in this sort of speculation is suggested by the very fact that cross-theoretical agreement (both within psychodynamic schools and across psychodynamic and cognitive models) is so high with reference to proximal variables, such as aspects of the self, and so low with reference to the remote variables alleged to have produced them. Clinical insight is unlikely to be helpful in resolving the theoretical issues that remain in dispute, for the obvious reason that the observations of perceptive and experienced clinicians do not always converge on common interpretations (Vitousek, Daly, & Heiser, 1991). We have little doubt that Lerner is a perceptive and experienced clinician; we look forward to an empirical examination of the ideas he has proposed in this forum.

REFERENCES

Bemis, K. M. (1978). Current approaches to the etiology and treatment of anorexia nervosa. *Psychological Bulletin*, *85*, 593–617.

Bruch, H. (1978). *The golden cage: The enigma of anorexia nervosa*. Cambridge, MA: Harvard University Press.

Fairburn, C. G. (1985). Cognitive–behavioral treatment for bulimia. In D. M. Garner & P. E. Garfinkel (Eds.), *Handbook of psychotherapy for anorexia nervosa and bulimia* (pp. 160–192). New York: Guilford Press.

Garner, D. M., & Bemis, K. M. (1985). Cognitive therapy for anorexia nervosa. In D. M. Garner & P. E. Garfinkel (Eds.), *Handbook of psychotherapy for anorexia nervosa and bulimia* (pp. 107–146). New York: Guilford Press.

Goodsitt, A. (1985). Self psychology and the treatment of anorexia nervosa. In D. M. Garner & P. E. Garfinkel (Eds.), *Handbook of psychotherapy for anorexia nervosa and bulimia* (pp. 55–82). New York: Guilford Press.

Grigg, D. N., Friesen, J. D., & Sheppy, M. I. (1989). Family patterns associated with anorexia nervosa. *Journal of Marital and Family Therapy*, *15*, 29–42.

Kog, E., & Vandereycken, W. (1985). Family characteristics of anorexia nervosa and bulimia: A review of the research literature. *Clinical Psychology Review*, *5*, 159–180.

Lawrence, M. (1979). Anorexia nervosa: The control paradox. *Women's Studies International Quarterly*, 2, 93–101.

Lerner, H. D. (1986). Current developments in the psychoanalytic psychotherapy of anorexia nervosa and bulimia nervosa. *The Clinical Psychologist*, *39*, 39–43.

Lerner, H. D., & Dyer, J. F. P. (1986). [Review of *Fear of being fat*]. *International Journal of Eating Disorders*, *5*, 387–398.

Levine, M. P., & Smolak, L. (1989, November). *Toward a developmental psychopathology of eating disorders: The example of the middle school transition*. Paper presented at the Eighth National Conference of the National Anorexic Aid Society, Columbus, OH.

Stern, S. L., Dixon, K. N., Jones, D., Lake, M., Nemzer, E., & Sansone, R. (1989). Family environment in anorexia nervosa and bulimia. *International Journal of Eating Disorders*, *8*, 25–31.

Strober, M., & Humphrey, L. L. (1987). Familial contributions to the etiology and course of anorexia nervosa and bulimia. *Journal of Consulting and Clinical Psychology*, *55*, 654–659.

Vitousek, K., Daly, J., & Heiser, C. (1991). Reconstructing the internal world of the eating-disordered individual: Denial and distortion of self-report. *International Journal of Eating Disorders, 10*, 647–666.

Yager, J. (1982). Family issues in the pathogenesis of anorexia nervosa. *Psychosomatic Medicine*, *44*, 43–60.

V

Borderline Personality Disorder

9

Problems of Self and Borderline Personality Disorder: A Dialectical Behavioral Analysis

HEIDI L. HEARD
MARSHA M. LINEHAN
University of Washington

ALTHOUGH THE EXISTENCE of a "self" remains a point of philosophical and definitional debate, a sense of self and self-referent thoughts are phenomena experienced by individuals throughout Western culture. Those who are unable to experience this sense of self or whose self-referent thoughts, assumptions, and beliefs are unpredictable, unstable, or chaotic often report these experiences as stressful or disturbing and may present them as an issue for therapy. Such problems are particularly likely when the individual meets clinical criteria for Borderline Personality Disorder (BDP). This chapter explores the relevance of problems related to self and to the disorder within a framework of the dialectical-behavioral theory of BDP recently proposed by Linehan (Linehan, 1987a, 1987b, 1989, in press; Linehan & Koerner, in press).

BORDERLINE PERSONALITY DISORDER AND PROBLEMS OF SELF

Until recently, almost all therapeutic attention to BDP has been from psychodynamic clinicians and biological psychiatrists. This situation is changing rapidly as behaviorists become involved in the treatment of borderline clients. However, although behaviorists have always attended to private experiences, such as the experience or sense of self, and to cognitive activities, such as thinking and processing of information, activities regarding one's own self have been accorded neither special importance nor theoretical significance. The relative absence of theoretical work on topics relevant to self, at least when compared to theoretical writings within the psychoanalytic and humanistic traditions, poses difficulties for the behavioral clinician and theoretician when addressing clinical problems related to experiences and thoughts or assumptions about self. These problems are magnified when treating disorders where problems of self are part of the diagnostic criteria for the disorder, as in BDP.

Description of Borderline Personality Disorder

Individuals meeting criteria for the disorder are flooding mental health centers and individual practitioners. Eleven percent of all psychiatric outpatients and 19% of psychiatric inpatients are estimated to meet criteria for the disorder (Kass, Skodol, Charles, Spitzer, & Williams, 1985; Piersma, 1987). The criteria for Borderline Personality Disorder, as currently defined both within DSM-III-R criteria (American Psychiatric Association, 1987) and the Diagnostic Interview for Borderlines (DIB) (Gunderson & Kolb, 1978; Gunderson, Kolb, & Austin, 1981; Zanarini, Gunderson, Frankenburg, & Chauncey, 1989)—the most commonly used research assessment instrument—reflect a pervasive pattern of behavioral, emotional, and cognitive instability and dysregulation. Indeed, these problems are so widespread that one can consider the borderline disorder a pervasive disorder of both the regulation and experience of self, a notion also proposed by Grotstein, Solomon, and Lang (1987).

The difficulties in self-regulation can be summarized in three categories (Linehan, in press). First, borderline individuals generally experience *emotional dysregulation* and reactivity. Emotional responses are reactive, and the individual generally has difficulties with episodic depression, anxiety, and irritability as well as problems with anger and anger expression. Second, borderline individuals often experience *interpersonal dysregulation*. Their relationships may be chaotic, intense, and marked by difficulties. Even though their relationships are difficult, however, borderline individuals often find it extremely hard to relinquish relationships. Instead, they may engage in intense and frantic efforts to prevent significant others from leaving them. More extreme than most, borderline individuals seem to function well when in stable, positive relationships and do poorly when not in such relationships. Third, borderline individuals have patterns of *behavioral dysregulation*, as evidenced by extreme and problematic impulsive behavior. An important characteristic of these individuals is their tendency to direct apparently destructive behaviors toward themselves. Attempts to injure, mutilate, or kill themselves, as well as actual suicide, occur frequently in this population. Difficulties in the experience of self can be summarized in two additional categories. First, borderline individuals are sometimes *cognitively dysregulated.* Brief, nonpsychotic thought and sensory dysregulation (depersonalization, dissociation, and delusions, including delusions about self) sometimes occur in response to stressful situations, and usually cease when the stress decreases. Second, *dysregulation of the sense of self* is common. Borderline individuals frequently report that they have no sense of a self at all, they feel empty, and they do not "know" who they are.

The diagnostic emphasis on a fundamental disorder related to self, at least as defined by DSM-III-R, reflects the emphasis on a disturbed sense of self and inadequate object representations, including self-representations, postulated in the psychodynamic literature. The critical issues for understanding borderline behavior proposed by these theoreticians include concepts such as difficulties with "cohesiveness" (Adler, 1985; Meissner, 1986), "narcissism" (Adler, 1985; Chatham, 1985), "splitting" (Kernberg, 1975, 1984), "identity diffusion" (Kernberg, 1984), "instability of certain kinds of introjects and identifications" (Adler, 1985), and "fused self-object representations" (Chatham, 1985). In behavioral terms (though not necessarily in behavioral theory), one may summarize the issues formulated by dynamic theorists as the borderline individuals' failure or inability to integrate aspects of their experience and to differentiate between their experience and that of others.

Definitions of Self

Definitions of self, self-representation, and sense of self abound, with each definition attempting to capture the full essence of its referent. Ironically, these constructs, which seem such an integral part of human experience, are difficult to define, so the definitions employed in this chapter are meant to serve operational functions, as opposed to attempts to capture the essence of constructs. The terms *self*, *self-representation*, and *sense of self* have appeared synonymously in much of the literature. Although the overlap is understandable in view of the constructs' complexity, it nonetheless remains confusing. We have attempted to differentiate the referents for these terms as we use them, and to remain consistent throughout the chapter.

Whether it is described as a dynamic system or as an internal structure, and whether it is postulated to develop from internal functions or external relationships, self is generally conceived of as something that "is," not in the physical sense but in a psychological sense. As behaviorists, we remain skeptical of structural constructs such as "the self," preferring to focus on processes or activities of the person, or self-referent behaviors. Many of those who use structural constructs mean them to reflect dynamic processes or activities of the individual rather than static structures within the individual. The shorthand use of "structures" to reflect processes, however, can easily result—and often does—in the reification of the process itself. At times, the reified structure is then used to explain the process that it reflects. Constructs relevant to self appear particularly vulnerable to this misuse.

In this chapter, we are primarily interested in self-referent cognitive-verbal behaviors such as thinking about oneself; imaging oneself; spoken, written, and gestural communication about oneself; and recalling and reviewing information about, or stimuli relevant to, oneself. Collectively, we refer to these behaviors as self-referent cognitive behaviors, or for the purposes of this chapter, self-representing behaviors. In addition, we are interested in the experiencing or sensing that is described as "sensing a self." Thus, we address what the individual experiences or *does* as opposed to what he/she *is*. We employ "representing" to refer to verbal or visual cognitive activities, and "sensing" to refer to nonverbal, sensory activities, although we also view these modes of activity as mutually interactive.

Descriptions of self generally share certain characteristics; self is experienced as permanent and continuous, with a sense of locus, unity, and boundaries. With regard to self-representing, however, two related forms of inquiry appear: self as subject ("I") and self as object ("me"). James (1968) viewed these forms as two components of self, describing them respectively as self as "knower" and self as "known." Skinner (1974) also differentiated between the knowing self and the known. Erikson (1959, 1963) has been both applauded and criticized for his unclear use of the term *identity* (Aranow, 1988), which alternatively refers to subjective and objective functions. Although we concur that these are complementary and integrated constructs for study, most empirical research has focused on self as object (Harter, 1983).

Self as object refers to self as the object of reference and representation. It includes personal identity in terms of self-image, roles, relationships, and values. Research has explored the concepts of possible selves (Markus & Nurius, 1986), the effect of familiarity on differences between self and other representations (Prentice, 1990), and the relationship between self-esteem and clarity of self-concept (Campbell, 1990), among other topics. Self-representation in this context refers to the content, or "what," of individuals depicting and imaging themselves.

Self as subject refers to self as the perceiver or actor. Deikman (1982) discussed four domains in which self as subject can apply: the thinking self that "seems to be in charge" (p. 92), the emotional self that feels and wants, the functional self that is aware of acting, and the observing self, "the transparent center, that which is aware" (p. 94). In the tradition of Piaget, Kegan (1982) defined self or ego, as "the meaning-making dimension of personality" (p. 6). Empirical research of self as subject is developing and includes process constructs such as integrating disparate aspects of self and differentiating self from other (Fast, Marsden, Cohen, Heard, & Kruse, 1991). Self-representation in this context refers to the process, or "how," of individuals imaging and describing themselves.

DIALECTICAL BEHAVIORAL THEORY OF SELF AND SELF BEHAVIORS

Although constructs relevant to self play a major role in cognitive theories of psychopathology, until recently, little theoretical work has aimed at constructing a behavioral approach to phenomena relevant to self per se. This absence of attention is changing, however, at least within the theoretical paradigm of radical, or contextual, behaviorism, a behavioral approach based primarily on operant conditioning. Since much of our theoretical position is drawn from a contextual behavioral framework, we will first briefly summarize the position of contextual behaviorism with respect to the topic of self.

Many behavioral scientists, some behaviorists among them, believe that behaviorism denies self or that self behaviors play any influential role in human experience and behavior. This belief often results from a confusion between methodological behaviorism, which attends to and measures only overt behaviors, and radical behaviorism, which "does not deny the possibility of self-observation or self-knowledge or its possible usefulness" (Skinner, 1974, p. 18). What radical behaviorism rejects is a mentalistic concept of self, a concept that a self "exists" and causes behavior.

Although his followers have examined the construct of self more thoroughly and in greater detail, Skinner (1974) did address issues such as self-knowing and self-managing. Self-knowing (Skinner's equivalent of self-representing) is, from a radical behavioral approach, social in origin in that it requires a complex language, which develops only in a human verbal community. Since self-knowing depends on the verbal community, its process and content will vary according to cultural dictates. The knowing self and the known are "products of genetic and environmental histories . . . of both contingencies of survival and contingencies of reinforcement" (Skinner, 1974, p. 247). Skinner suggests that the experience of an identity crisis occurs when changing contingencies cause disruptive change in behavioral repertoires. The individual experiences these new behaviors as unfamiliar and may explain "uncharacteristic behavior by saying, 'I was not myself.'" (Skinner, 1974, p. 187). Individuals may also experience more than one self if they must act in disparate situations requiring conflicting behaviors. Skinner thus directed researchers to observe the environment—its verbal community and contingencies—in order to understand both the process and the content of self-knowing.

In addition to drawing from Skinner, we have drawn heavily from the work of Hayes (1984) and Kohlenberg and Tsai (1991) in formulating our conceptions of self and self-referent behaviors. We have also adopted Linehan's dialectical perspective. A behavioral view of self and self behaviors is less frequently articulated than other positions, and a dialectical approach is not typically paired with a behavioral framework. Thus, before linking self and Borderline Personality Disorder explicitly in a dialectical behavioral framework, we will first describe the major assumptions of both behavioral and dialectical theory that relate to our discussion of self behaviors in BDP.

Self as a Dialectical Process

Dialectical perspectives on the nature of reality and human behavior share three primary characteristics. First, dialectical perspectives stress the fundamental interrelatedness, or wholeness, of reality, similar to dynamic systems perspectives. Like systemic approaches, dialectical approaches view analysis of individual parts of a system as of limited value per se, unless the analysis clearly relates the part to the whole. In addition, individual identity is possible only in relationship to the whole. The self cannot exist without the other. Second, reality is not seen as static but is composed of internal opposing forces (thesis and antithesis) out of whose synthesis evolves a new set of opposing forces. Thus, the constant transaction between parts of self and between self and other results in an ever-changing identity of each element within the whole. Third, and flowing from the previous points, dialectical approaches view the nature of reality as change rather than structure or content, so both change and interrelatedness are considered as the very essence of experience.

A fundamental dialectical assumption that underlies Linehan's theory of Borderline Personality Disorder and our analyses of self is that the relationship between the individual and the environment is a process of reciprocal influence. Clearly, this transactional-analysis assumption implies a powerful effect of the individual's environment on his/her development. A further implication addressed by behavior genetics is that individuals create their own environments (Scarr & McCartney, 1983). Scarr and McCartney proposed three effects through which genetics influence one's experience: passive, reactive, and active. Primarily influential during infancy, the passive genotypic effect refers to those gene–environment interactions that occur independent of the individual's behaviors. Such gene-environment effects result solely from the individual's genetic structure and the parents' "dispositions", and thus not from the individual, since he/she determines neither the genetic structure nor the initial parental structure. Second, the authors proposed a reactive effect in which the genotype elicits particular responses from the social and physical environment. For example, a wounded child who cries or otherwise asks for help will more likely receive the necessary assistance than a child who does not express his/her pain. Finally, genes influence experience by an active genotypic effect that occurs when the individual seeks environments that support his/her genetic potential. The dexterous child who persues a career as a pianist and the athletic child who trains to become a swimmer demonstrate this effect. From the perspective of a dialectical behavioral theory, much of the pathogenesis of BDP, including problems with sensing self, with identity, and with self-control, illustrate exactly these sorts of genotypic influences on the environment, such that individuals predisposed to dysfunctions of self influence their environments in ways that highlight the full systemic dysfunction.

Smith (1978) argued a similar dialectical position with respect to the development of individual "selfhood." Refering to theories of Marx, Piaget, and Mead, he suggested that selfhood is emergent, both conditioned by sociocultural and genetic factors and self-created. Smith proposed a dialectical development of self:

> In his conception of "dialectical" development, Marx held that people work upon the world, and in shaping their world, by the same token, people are shaped by it. The process is interactive, but it is also cumulative. . . . A radically and cumulatively interactive—that is to say dialectical—approach to development of selfhood . . . seems appropriate to human phenomena. (p. 1059)

This proposal echoes the behaviorists' contextual emphasis on the cultural role in defining self and in shaping self behaviors.

Self as Culturally Defined

All cultures distinguish between a personal region referred to as "self" and a region referred to as "nonself"; however, the position of boundary lines between self and nonself, as well as their rigidity, varies extensively by culture. In turn, the emphasis on self-autonomy as representing internal, personal control versus external, contextual control also varies by culture. Sampson (1988), in summarizing the literature on this topic, suggested that because of the generally close correspondence between the locus of control and the nature of the self-nonself boundary, there are two main clusters of thought about the nature of self and autonomy. The individuated self, represented most strongly by Western culture, is defined by sharp boundaries between self and other and by great emphasis on personal, internal control. Sampson referred to this conception of self as "self-contained individualism," while others called it "egocentric understanding of self" or "the autonomous self." The individuated self can contrast with the relational self. The latter, represented most strongly by non-Western cultures, is defined by more fluid and permeable self–other boundaries and by an emphasis on field or social control (where the field includes, but reaches far beyond, the person). The main unit of identity is the family or community. The family and community also serve as the primary determinants of the individual's behavior. Sampson called this second cluster of thought "ensembled individualism"; others have referred to it as a "sociocentric understanding of self," "social individuality," or "the connected self."

The dominant view of self in Western society and psychology implicitly refers to the individual, or single human organism: Experiences belong to the organism. Persons with this view generally compute the formula of one body equals one self, with the skin symbolically functioning to contain and to divide. The self is represented as a unified organism separate from other organisms; thus, this definition of self explicitly excludes other individuals and the community from the individual self. In cultures with this view, the behavior of mature persons is assumed to be controlled by internal rather than external forces. Self-control, in this context, refers to the person's ability to control his/her own behavior by using internal cues and resources. To define oneself differently or to be field-dependent is labeled as immature or pathological, or at least inimical to good health and smooth societal functioning (Perloff, 1987). Although this conception of the individual self pervades Western culture, it is neither universal cross-culturally nor even within Western culture itself. Notions of the individual, and therefore of self, as unitary and separate have only gradually emerged over the last several hundred years (Baumeister, 1987; Sampson, 1988). Since women receive the diagnosis of Borderline Personality Disorder more frequently than men (American Psychiatric Association, 1987), the influence of gender on notions of self and boundaries is of particular interest in our examination of self and BDP.

An increasing number of research findings and theoretical analyses in recent years have demonstrated that both gender and social class significantly influence how one both defines and experiences self. Women, as well as individuals with less social power, more likely have a relational or social self, a self that includes the group, as opposed to an individuated self, or one that excludes the group (McGuire & McGuire, 1982; Pratt, Pancer, Hunsberger, & Manchester, 1990). The importance of a relational or social self among women has been highlighted by many feminist writers, of whom the best known is Gilligan (1982). Lykes (1985) has perhaps argued the feminist position most cogently when she defined the self as an "ensemble of social relations" (p. 364). In particular, Lykes and others do *not* speak simply of the value of interdependence among autonomous selves but rather of a social or relational self that is itself "a coacting network of relationships embedded in an intricate system of social exchanges and obligations" (Lykes, 1985, p. 362). When self is defined as being in relation to—inclusive of others by its very definition—no fully separate self exists, that is, no self separated from others by the skin of the organism. Such a relational self, or "ensembled individualism" in Sampson's terms, characterizes the majority of societies, both historically and cross-culturally (Sampson, 1988).

Attention to these contextual factors is particularly essential when a cultural construct such as self is employed to explain and describe a culturally influenced construct such as mental health. While the traditional definition of self may generally prove adaptive for some individuals in Western society, one must consider that our definitions and theories are not universal but are products of Western society and thus may prove inappropriate for many individuals. As we will argue later, the problems encountered by the borderline individual may, in part, result from the collision of a relational self with a society that recognizes and rewards only the individuated self. Instead of pathology, a poorness-of-fit model may operate between these individuals and their society. We employ such a model to explain some aspects of the borderline individual's experiences of self traditionally labeled as pathological.

Self as Seeing from a Perspective

Another way to conceptualize self is to view it as synonymous with "perspective," a concept proposed by Hayes (1984), who introduced the concept of "you-as-perspective" through his behavioral analysis of self-awareness. Hayes more fully defined the behavior of self-awareness as "the behavior of seeing seeing from a perspective" (p. 103) and labeled it "you-as-perspective," the "you" generally referred to by the community. "Perspective" refers to the collection of stimuli that controls the experiencing of self and the response of self behaviors. This collection of stimuli consists of public, or external, stimuli and private, or internal, stimuli. For example, when one asserts, "I don't feel like myself," or "I see who I am," there is a stimulus that elicits the behavior of feeling or seeing, just as a mountain would function as the stimulus for seeing the mountain and as one of the necessary stimuli for stating, "I see the mountain."

The key characteristics of the experience of perspective include a nonobject state, a permanent locus in space and continuity across time. Within cultures that support the individuated self, the locus of the perspective is internal to the person. Although not addressed by Hayes, the locus of this experience need not require internality and could as well include some aspect of a social network or group. Internal perspective, in Hayes's framework, is the one aspect of the individual that remains constant, while activities such as feeling and thinking, and objects such as mountain and mother change. This is analogous to the relationship between a theater patron and a play. The cast, scenery, and dialogue change in the play, but the patron remains the observer in the audience. In general, since the public stimuli influencing perspective may vary greatly, the private stimuli may allow the most stable control. In addition to this continuity, most individuals experience perspective as a point within, although a more collective or social perspective might occur in cultures emphasizing the relational self.

Kohlenberg and Tsai (1991), who also attempt to explain the individuated self from a behavioral point of view, suggested that perspective indicates an individual's spatial location relative to others: "It is where the child is, right here, as opposed to where the child is not—over there" (p. 139). Organisms can never experience perspective from any perspective but their own. Nor can an individual observe his/her own perspective without changing perspective. It would be analogous to an individual attempting to physically see him/herself, an objective that can be achieved only from the perspective of a photo or a mirror's reflection. Flowing from the experiences of continuity and internal locus, perspective is not an object. Hayes (1984) indicated that "you-as-perspective, then, is not itself fully experienceable as a thing or object by the person looking from that perspective" (p. 103). One may observe another individual as an object with limits and boundaries, but one cannot objectively observe one's own perspective and thus cannot experience its limits. The set of stimuli controlling perspective need not have physical properties like the mountain, since some stimuli, such as pain, can be "private," that is, accessible to or sensed by only the individual him/herself. Perspective need not exist as an entity; it may simply be experienced.

Whether one identifies self with an internal perspective, independent of the social fabric in which the person develops, or a relational perspective, dependent on a fabric of social relationships even though the actual relationships themselves may change, is determined predominantly by the experiences the individual has interacting with his/her environment. In other words, perspective is learned. The apparently universal influence of gender on a preference for a relational self versus an individuated self, however, suggests that contingencies of survival—that is, genetic factors or cultural factors particular to women—may also play a role. More extensively than men, women may create environments that support a relational self over an individuated self.

BEHAVIORAL THEORY OF BORDERLINE PERSONALITY DISORDER

Linehan (1987a, in press) developed the biosocial-behavioral theory of Borderline Personality Disorder primarily to serve as a scaffolding for the dialectical behavior therapy regimen she developed for the treatment of chronically parasuicidal women meeting criteria for the disorder. Although similar to the diathesis-stress model, the model of BDP retains a dialectical nature in that it assumes that the functioning of individuals and environments are continuously interactive and interdependent. Thus, the development of borderline behavior patterns, including dysfunctions of self and self-referent behaviors, are due to continuous, reciprocal transactions (as opposed to static interactions) between the parts and the whole (e.g., the individual with his/her environment, self-referent cognitive behaviors with other-referent motor behaviors, etc.). Although the theory does not directly address self-referent cognitive behaviors or self-sensing per se, it has implications for both of these self behaviors. Since empirical research in this area remains in the early stages, much of Linehan's theory, as well as the derivations of it presented here, is speculative. The hypotheses are generally derived from clinical experiences and from research in related areas.

Biosocial Etiology

According to Linehan (1987a, in press), Borderline Personality Disorder is an outcome of the developmental transaction between an emotionally invalidating rearing environment and an emotionally vulnerable child. The central characteristic of the environment that contributes to the development of borderline behavioral patterns is its tendency to discredit, disparage, and at times deny the individual's own emotional and emotionally relevant cognitive experiences. In an invalidating environment, significant others negate the individual's experiencing of his/her own affect and disqualify verbal descriptions and interpretations of events not publicly observable and agreed to by all. Emotional reactions that are aversive to others or that are viewed as dysfunctional for the individual are labeled inappropriate and are typically punished. Such an environment can exist either in "chaotic" families (families chronically plagued by conflictual relationships, limited resources, mental health problems, etc.) or "perfect" families (families that appear to have no conflict and deny problems of individual members). The essential component is that these families ignore and/or fail to tolerate or respond appropriately to negative emotional displays and communications. Thus, the experience and communication of negative emotions such as sadness, anger, and fear, as well as their complex emotional derivatives, are responded to with rejection and invalidation rather than by acceptance and soothing. This is especially true when these emotional responses are intense, inconvenient, or dysfunctional for the individual or group. Typically, these families have an exaggerated sense of the individual's ability to control emotional reactions internally, ascribing to the individual personal responsibility for the creation of emotional problems and for their resolution. They expect the troubled person to simply endure or prevail over any challenges. Such an environment radically simplifies the problem-solving process. The individual hears simplistic aphorisms, such as "Where there's a will, there's a way" and "Just smile and you'll be happy." Because of this set of beliefs, the invalidating environment fails to provide adequate training in emotion-regulation skills to the individual and conditions a sense of shame in response to emotions such as sadness and anger. The invalidating environment, in some ways, represents the extreme outcome of a culture that promotes and accepts only the individuated self.

Clearly, however, not all individuals experiencing developmentally invalidating environments develop BDP, thus, the theory further postulates a temperamentally based affective vulnerability as important in the etiology of the disorder. Affective vulnerability refers to the individual's exaggerated responsiveness, in terms of frequency and intensity, to emotionally relevant stimuli. Two other aspects of emotional vulnerability, the inabilities to regulate emotional responses and to return quickly to a baseline, further complicate attempts to cope effectively. Biological factors may contribute to affective reactivity range from genetic characteristics to environmental factors influencing early central nervous system development. Transactionally, the very intensity of the child's emotional reactions further increases the attempts on the part of the environment to stop the emotional responses and communications, leading to escalating attempts on the part of the child to provoke a soothing response. Intermittently, these escalating responses elicit a reinforcing response, with the result that the extreme emotional displays become highly resistant to extinction. Reciprocally, the ability of the child to inhibit and/or dissociate from emotional responses and to become quiet under extreme threat, provides a similar intermittent set of reinforcing contingencies for the invalidating responses of people in the environment.

If the child's emotional expressions and beliefs suffers from constant external invalidation, it follows that the child will learn to doubt what he/she believes or feels, based on internal stimuli, and to not trust internal stimuli. The child may begin to invalidate his/her own perceptions and responses in the direction of congruence with the external environment. Establishing congruence with the environment may often require the inhibition of emotional experiences and expressions. Self-invalidation by the borderline individual includes discounting one's own emotional experiences and seeking from others an accurate perception of internal as well as external events.

SELF-REFERENT BEHAVIORS IN BORDERLINE PERSONALITY DISORDER

In most theoretical formulations of Borderline Personality Disorder, dysregulations in the individual's self or sense of self (Dorr, Gard, Barley, &

Webb, 1983), in self-referent cognitive-affective structures or schemas (Young, 1983), or in the structure of self (Kernberg, 1975, 1984) are afforded priority in attempts to explain the origin and maintenance of the behavioral patterns associated with the diagnosis. In contrast, Linehan has suggested that as a result of temperamental characteristics and severely invalidating developmental environments, borderline individuals fail to develop two crucial abilities: the ability to regulate affect and the ability to trust their own emotional reactions, cognitive interpretations, and behavioral responses to events as appropriate or as valid. Thus, they continuously confront two intense yet contradictory messages: the message conveyed directly by their own emotional and cognitive-emotional responses to events, and the message, learned previously, not to trust their own responses to events as valid informational data. The intense, negative emotional experiences typically encountered by borderline individuals are highly aversive and result in sometimes frantic attempts to obtain relief. However, the ability to self-regulate emotional responses, including aversive negative emotions, requires an ability to trust at least some aspects of one's own responses to situations. At a minimum, the decision of where to place one's trust, with oneself or with others, must be accepted as valid. Furthermore, the invalidation of negative emotions leads to secondary emotional responses of shame, fear, and, at times, intense anger directed toward self. These almost immediate secondary emotional responses further complicate the initial response and reduce the ability of the individual to describe or discern his/her own responses, much less change them. Thus, the inability to trust one's own responses to events is itself aversive.

From this perspective, much of dysfunctional borderline behavior operates both as a means of effective affect regulation (either directly or indirectly by mobilizing persons in the environment) and as self-validation. The role of "self" as an etiological factor and as a factor in maintaining borderline behavioral patterns, therefore, is of interest primarily with respect to the emphasis in the biosocial theory on invalidating environments, and the subsequent difficulties in self-validating. We will develop these points more fully with respect to a number of borderline behavioral characteristics. A more comprehensive discussion with respect to the entire complex of borderline behavior is beyond the scope of this chapter, and we refer the interested reader to Linehan (in press).

Interpersonal Dysregulation

As noted earlier, chaotic interpersonal relationships are characteristic of borderline individuals, typically, a series of relationships that are emotionally intense and marked by conflict and that tend to end abruptly. Often these intense relationships develop with caregivers, notably with psychotherapists. The role of interpersonal dependency in borderline relationships is a common theme in theoretical, diagnostic, empirical, and clinical descriptions of borderline behavior. Although many definitions of dependency exist, the essential characteristics seem to involve two related phenomena: borderline individuals' strong preferences for a close interpersonal relationship, and their attention to interpersonal cues to define their own identity, beliefs, values, and, at times, emotional responses. In terms of our prior discussions of the cultural definitions of self, the borderline individual may typify an extreme relational self, without the ability to interact in a way that consistently maintains the relationships necessary to support such a self. One might say, therefore, that the individual cannot maintain his/her self, since the experience and definition of self depend on relationships that are inconsistent, chaotic, and unreliable.

Whether this relational self results purely from learning or whether genetic or biological factors play a part remains unclear, given the absence of data on this point. Certainly learning theory could account for how an invalidating environment would favor a relational self over an individuated one. The cross-cultural data address this point to some extent. Kohlenberg and Tsai (1991) have made such an argument in their radical behavioral analyses of self and Borderline Personality Disorder. However, Eliasz (1985) reported a relationship between high autonomic reactivity and a self-regulation style that appeals to the environment as a source of personal control, suggesting that borderline individuals may have some biological preference for development of a relational self. The relationship between gender and relational selves further supports this idea.

From our point of view, a relational self requires one of two conditions for positive outcomes: either the social network must support it or individuals with relational selves in unsupportive environments must independently maintain a positive self-image (or at least avoid a negative one) and take care of themselves. They must be able to self-validate and to be self-reliant in a context that socially invalidates the relational self and requires autonomous functioning. We would suggest that neither of these conditions exists with borderline individuals. Not only does the larger Western culture not support the relational self, but even when these individuals do form supportive relationships, they cannot maintain them. From Linehan's biosocial perspective, this inability to maintain relationships is due primarily to the effect of unregulated, aversive emotions in close interpersonal relationships. Intense and labile emotional behaviors, especially when unpredictable, do not promote stable interpersonal relationships. Not only do borderline individuals dysregulate their relationships, but their frequent attempts to engage others in regulating their emotions often proves burdensome to others.

Although a relational self and self-reliance may appear incompatible, the emphasis on field control associated with the relational self does not imply an absence of self-control. Only the form of the control differs. Nor is a relational self necessarily antagonistic to self-reliance or independent problem-solving behaviors. Triandis, McKusker, and Hui (1990) compared cultures high on a collective sense of self (where self is defined in terms of one's relationship to the group) to those high on an individualistic self and found that collectivists valued self-reliance as much or more than individualists. As the authors noted, self-reliance can serve the group—by the individual not burdening the group—as well as the individual. They found, however, that those with a relational self within an individualistic culture valued self-reliance less than did others in their culture. In other words, they placed less value on solving problems alone, independent of the social group. A key characteristic of the invalidating environment, however, is that by not taking the individual's communications of difficulty seriously, the community fails to teach the individual how to be self-reliant. Telling borderline individuals to control their emotions parallels telling the hyperactive child to control attention. Without attention and help, such efforts will often fail.

From our perspective, there are several clear implications of this analysis. First, therapies that invalidate the experiences of borderline clients would harm more than they help. In particular, the therapy should not focus on the invalidity of the relational self or on attempts to create an individuated self, but rather on how the relational person can self-validate within an individualistic society. Second, effective therapies must attend to ferreting out the specific interpersonal and self-control difficulties of each individual and implement a specific training program to improve behavioral skills in areas such as interpersonal effectiveness.

Dysregulation of the Sense of Self

Difficulties with the sense of self typically refers to two phenomena. First, borderline individuals often cannot experience a sense of self, or can only experience "self" episodically, and complain of feeling empty. In this case, the experience of "no self" is painful. Second, they may experience a sense of derealization or depersonalization, feeling themselves to be unreal or unconnected to their experience. They often complain of a feeling of numbness similar to that reported in Post-traumatic Stress Disorder (American Psychiatric Association, 1987). The derealization, depersonalization, and numbness seem to be associated with current stress and with prior histories of traumatic stress, especially sexual abuse. One need only review the post-traumatic literature to explain their etiology and maintenance. This section thus will focus on the problems with the sensing of self, including the sense of emptiness.

Whereas the differences between the individuated and relational selves (discussed above) primarily address differences in "self-as-object," problems with the sense of having or being a self, with self-sensing, seem to concern "self-as-subject." The sense of "I" is episodic or absent. This appears most clearly in the tendency of some borderline individuals to employ the third person when referring to themselves or to their own emotions or thoughts. It is interesting to speculate on the exact referent when people say they "have a self," or can experience their own "self." What they are referring to is some set of private, internal sensory experiencing that they have learned to label "self." In other words, it is not a belief or semantic proposition that one has a self (although such a belief would be included) as much as it is a holistic sense of "knowing" or experiencing that one has a self, a response linked to both sensory/proprioceptive and semantic cues. Within the cognitive literature, the sense of self is analogous to subjective experiences associated with the implicational codes or information described by Barnard and Teasdale (1991). Like Hayes (1984), we suggest that this holistic experience of self is primarily a response associated with perspective. In individuated cultures, the sense of self is related to those private, usually internal stimuli that are stable over time and place. Within more assembled cultures, the sense of self is related to a field perspective that includes the individual person and the family or community. In either case, the development of a sense of self requires the consistency of the perspective in relationship to the semantic "I" or "you" or "self" referred to by the community when referring to the individual person.

Such a consistency, however, would not occur within the invalidating environment, especially for the emotionally reactive child. Particularly within chaotic invalidating environments, the response of caretakers to the child depends on their own mood and "public orienting" as opposed to the child's behavior. This dependency on factors other than the child's experience and behavior when teaching the child how to make associations between self or "I" and experience is the crucial factor in the failure to teach a sense of self. For example, the parent who is too tired to help a child with homework may say to the child, "You can do it," or "You just don't want to do it," while the child experiences, "I can't do it," or "I very much want to finish this homework." In these environments, the child experiences various reactions to the same behavior, and thus a sense of consistent perspective fails to develop. Discrimination training fails to occur; that is, the child does not learn to associate the stimuli consistently present when "I" or self is represented or described, as distinguished from stimuli associated with other referents such as pain.

Feelings of emptiness, frequently reported by borderline clients, are commonly reported by people who are grieving (Rando, 1984). An analysis of the sense of emptiness during normal grief may be instructive for understanding the same sense among borderline individuals. Although most work on grief has been conducted in relationship to bereavement, loss is associated with all forms of change, and particularly with traumatic changes. Thus, the ability to adapt emotionally to change is an important skill that all individuals must master. Investigators (Bowlby, 1980; Engle, 1964; Lindemann, 1944; Rando, 1984) have proposed a variety of stages in the grieving process. At some point, however, they all address what Rando describes as the phases of avoidance, of confrontation, and finally, of reestablishment. Feelings of emptiness seem to occur during the confrontation phase, when the individual experiences the intense, negative emotions associated with loss, including despair and anger. While most individuals tolerate the intense negative emotions experienced during the confrontation phase, borderline individuals appear unable to tolerate these emotions (Linehan, 1987a). Instead, they inhibit the emotions and emotional process, which seem necessary, instead of progressing to the final phase of reestablisment and a return to pre-loss functioning.

More specifically, regarding the loss of a significant other, Rando (1984) discussed Lindemann's formulation of three tasks of grief work: "emancipation from the bondage of the deceased" (p. 18), "readjustment to the environment in which the deceased is missing" (p. 19), and "formation of new relationships" (p. 19). Readjustment to the environment in which the deceased held a significant place requires exposure to both physical and "symbolic" environmental cues. The exposure, in turn, may cause a feeling of emptiness. After the departure of the significant other, the individual encounters many physical examples of emptiness: the empty breakfast chair, an empty side of the bed, an empty house. Symbolically, or in terms of self-referent thinking, grieving individuals must cope with how the loss of the relationship affects their way of describing or imagining their own self. For the individual with a relational self, loss of the other equals a loss of a part of self or a part of the external stimuli controlling the experience of self. In part, the task, as described by Rando, is to redefine one's identity "so it reflects the reality of the loss and its consequences" and "to shift from thinking of as part of a couple, 'we,' to a single individual, 'I'" (p. 19). This task may prove more difficult for the relational self than for the autonomous one.

TREATMENT OF SELF BEHAVIORS

Linehan (1984, 1987b, 1989, in press) developed Dialectical Behavior Therapy within a behavioral tradition, but both draw on dialectics as a philosophical base, integrating into the behavioral approach aspects of Buddhist psychology and meditation practice. In particular, the focus on self-acceptance and the decrease in self-invalidation, as well as the emphasis on tolerance of self and events, is developed from Zen practices. The focus on active self-change through problem solving and skills training is from traditional behavioral and cognitive therapies and theories. The dialectical philosophical orientation, the therapeutic strategies employed by the therapist, and the therapy targets or goals define the treatment. We will present a brief overview of some of the important characteristics of the treatment that concern aspects of self discussed above.

The Role of Validation in Therapy

From a clinical perspective, Dialectical Behavior Therapy was developed following failed attempts to apply standard behavior therapy to chronically parasuicidal clients meeting criteria for Borderline Personality Disorder. Although the failure may have been in the application of the various behavioral therapies, the final conclusion suggested an inherent problem in the fit between cognitive and behavior therapies—at least as conducted in the late 1970s and early 1980s—and borderline clients. From Linehan's perspective, difficulties arose becuase these therapies described the client's behavior as an invalid response to events and in need of change. Thus, the therapies focused on how clients' irrational thoughts contributed to dysfunctional negative emotions, how their inappropriate social behaviors contributed to interpersonal problems, how their emotional overreactivity contributed to their overall problems, and so on. These behavior therapies consisted of a technology of change, with the focus of change on client behavior.

In many respects, this focus recapitulated the invalidating environment. The client was the problem and needed to change. In a sense, the therapist validated clients' worst fears—that they indeed could not trust their own emotional reactions, cognitive interpretations, or behavioral responses. As noted before, however, mistrust and invalidation of one's own behavioral (including emotional and cognitive) responses to events is extremely aversive. Depending on circumstances, invalidation may elicit negative emotional reactions such as fear, anger, shame, or a combination of these, so the entire focus of the therapy was aversive since, by necessity, it contributed to and elicited self-invalidation. In addition, successful behavior therapy with adults usually requires a fair degree of self-regulation skills because it often requires homework assignments and diary keeping. For a person with poor self-regulation skills, this approach leads to failure, subsequent shame, and a continuation of avoidance.

Unfortunately, a therapeutic approach based on unconditional acceptance and validation of the client's behaviors proves equally problematic and, paradoxically, can also invalidate. If the therapist urges the client to accept and self-validate, it can appear that the therapist does not regard the client's problems seriously. Acceptance-based therapies discount the desperation of the borderline individual since they offer little hope of change. The client's personal experience of the current state of affairs as unacceptable and unendurable is thereby invalidated.

To resolve this impasse, a treatment attending to the balance of acceptance and validation strategies with change-based strategies was developed. The dialectical behavior therapist teaches the client both to self-validate and to change. This fundamental relationship between change and acceptance forms the basic paradox and context of treatment. Change can occur only in the context of acceptance, and acceptance is itself change (Linehan, 1987a). Of particular importance, the therapy strives to help the client understand that responses may be both appropriate, or valid, and dysfunctional, or in need of change. This balance point, however, constantly changes and requires a therapist who can react flexibly and quickly in therapy. The recognition of the need for flexibility and synthesis, or balance, which first led to the exploration of dialectics is a foundation for the therapy.

Is an Individuated Self a Proper Goal of Therapy?

As previously discussed, the emphasis on, and valuing of, the individuated self is a cultural artifact of Western society. Particularly relevant here are findings that relational selves develop more frequently among women than among men. No data yet suggest that a relational self is pathological, even in an individualistic culture, and some data suggest a relationship with measures of positive attributes (Pratt et al., 1990). Thus, little evidence exists to indicate that permeable self-boundaries are themselves pathological.

We believe that a therapeutic focus on reducing the relational aspects of self and increasing the individualistic focus may prove iatrogenic. We reason, first, that such a position essentially invalidates and pathologizes the clients' fundamental experience of themselves. Second, it remains unclear whether one can change from a relational to an individuated self. Recent evidence linking genetics to primary personality attributes (Tellegen et al., 1988), suggests that attributes correlated with development of a relational self, such as sociability, may be connected to genetic characteristics and thus prove difficult to change. This finding does not, however, necessarily contradict Triandis et al.'s (1990) cultural approach to a definition and behaviors of self. Research integrating cross-cultural and genetic variables should prove quite enlightening. From our perspective, a more effective approach may be to help the individual either find a different social network, one that would support a relational self, or at least learn to validate his/her own self, living in greater comfort in an unsupportive environment.

The benefits of maintaining a relational self does not, however, negate the necessity of learning to attend to internal, private stimuli, to differentiate private stimuli from public stimuli, and to develop self-reliance. We believe that therapy with borderline clients must enhance awareness of private stimuli (awareness of self that is private from the group) and teach self-reliance. Dialectical Behavior Therapy was designed to accomplish these aims.

Skills Training

Dialectical Behavior Therapy conceptualizes the absence of self-reliance in problem-solving terms, that is, as a problem to solve. Like other problem-solving and behavioral therapies, this therapy focuses on ideographic assessment, with treatment planning linked to the assessment. Thus, the inability to take care of and to care for oneself—to be self-reliant—is analyzed in terms of its relationship to (1) behavioral skills deficits (i.e., deficits in interpersonal skills, emotion regulation skills, distress-tolerance skills); (2) contingencies operating in the environment; (3) faulty cognitive expectancies, beliefs, and assumptions; and (4) emotional inhibition. A complex series of skills-training regimens in each of these areas is implemented, together with treatment strategies designed to modify environmental contingencies (especially those produced by the therapist's own behavior), to analyze and modify cognitive responses, and to reduce the inhibiting effects of fear or other emotions. The fundamental goal is to increase the individual's self-reliant behaviors.

In view of the emotional-dysregulation that characterizes borderline clients, emotional regulation skills play a crucial role in self-reliance training and include identifying emotions, reducing vulnerability to emotions, and changing emotions. Reducing emotional vulnerability and enhancing the ability to change emotions enables the clients to regulate behavior better and thus to rely less on others for this function. Enabling them to soothe themselves in stressful situations also enhances the clients' self-reliance. Distress-tolerance skills useful both in crises and in enduring stressful situations, include self-soothing, breathing techniques, and mindfulness, as described below.

Considering the interpersonal dysregulation that characterizes Borderline Personality Disorder, interpersonal skills play a pivotal role in self-reliance because they help the individual to establish a more supportive, stable environment. Training includes teaching clients how to attend to relationships, to balance priorities versus demands, and wants versus "shoulds," and to build mastery. Attention is paid to the relationship and to the individual. This training helps clients to resolve interpersonal dilemmas, such as conflict between maintaining relationships and maintaining self-respect, by reducing the probability of dilemmas and by teaching processes that will help resolve those that do develop.

Attention to the therapeutic relationship further enhances the development of behaviors designed to establish and maintain a supportive environment. Those behaviors that interfere with the client's maintenance of other relationships are expected to occur within the therapeutic relationship as well. The therapy also anticipates that the therapist will contribute to the relationship problems, as any person does in an intimate relationship. Therapy-interfering behaviors of both the client and the therapist are a major focus of the treatment. In the process of resolving these problems, the client learns more effective interpersonal problem-solving strategies, while the therapist actively attempts to foster generalization of these strategies to the client's other relationships.

Mindfulness Training

Both in general and in view of the culture, there are several benefits for the client who can flexibly attend to and identify private stimuli. In general, such attention is necessary to identify and solve one's most basic needs such as food, warmth, and alleviation of physical harm. Hayes (1984) also suggested that the development of a perspective can enable one to gain psychological distance from dysfunctional thoughts, emotions, and behaviors. In view of Western culture, attention to private stimuli is important not only because the culture reinforces it, but also because the culture seldom allows alternatives. In such a transient society, and particularly in a chaotic family, other people may prove neither reliable nor continuously available.

Mindfulness training provides a method through which a person learns to attend to him/herself. Drawn from meditation and other Eastern spiritual practices, the mindfulness skills include activities of observing, describing, being nonjudgmental, and being one-minded (i.e., engaging in one activity at a time, with focused attention). Observing involves simply sensing one's experiences, neither avoiding nor extending the experience intentionally. Such observing enables one to distance oneself from thoughts, emotions, and behaviors, or what Hayes (1984) referred to as the changeable content of life. Describing refers to acknowledging and verbalizing experience, without analyzing it. Observing and describing encourage clients to attend to their own reactions to either themselves or to the external environment.

SUMMARY

We believe that attention to the experience of self and self behaviors, such as self-regulation and self-referent thinking, is relevant to the theory and to the treatment of Borderline Personality Disorder. Indeed, the disorder may be conceptualized in terms of problems with both self-regulation and experiencing self. Self-regulation problems include emotional dysregulation, interpersonal dysregulation, and behavioral dysregulation; problems with experiencing self include cognitive dysregulation and dysregulation of sensing self. This conceptualization of Borderline Personality Disorder as a disorder of self must not be confused with more traditional conceptualizations. We neither describe nor explain the disorder in terms of self-systems or structures, which have their own causal power. Instead, we simply describe the behaviors of the borderline clients in terms of behaviors pertaining to self.

We review dialectical and behavioral theories of self, discussing self as a dialectical process, as culturally defined, and as a perspective, emphasizing that the construct of self develops from interactions between the environment and the individual and that Western culture expects an individuated self as opposed to a relational self. Borderline individuals may have a more relational self than Western society supports. We present a definition of self as a referent to a collection of stimuli, regardless of whether these stimuli are predominantly private or public, and suggest that to a greater extent than usual, public stimuli appear to control the borderline individual's experience of self.

We explain the etiology of Borderline Personality Disorder with a biosocial theory, which postulates that the interaction between an affectively vulnerable individual and an invalidating environment results in failures to regulate affect and to validate or trust one's own emotions and thoughts. Interpersonal dysregulation and dysregulation of the sense of self are discussed according to this theory.

Finally, we describe two treatment goals of Dialectical Behavior Therapy related to self problems: increasing self-reliant behaviors and enhancing attention to and validation of private stimuli. To attain these goals, we focus on teaching new skills and behaviors in the context of a validating environment. These goals, however, do not attempt to change the relational self into an individuated self.

REFERENCES

Adler, G. (1985). *Borderline psychopathology and its treatment.* New York: Jason Aronson.

American Psychiatric Association. (1987). *Diagnostic and statistical manual of mental disorders* (3rd ed., rev.). Washington DC: Author.

Aranow, P. T. (1988). *Psychoanalytic theories of the self: A review and critique from a Buddhist perspective.* Unpublished doctoral dissertation, Harvard University, Cambridge, MA.

Baumeister, R. F. (1987). How the self became a problem. *Journal of Personality and Social Psychology, 52*, 163–176.

Barnard, P. J., & Teasdale, J. D. (1991). Interacting cognitive subsystems: A systemic approach to cognitive-affective interaction and change. *Cognition and Emotion, 5*, 1–39.

Bowlby, J. (1980). *Attachment and loss: Vol. 3. Loss, separation and depression.* New York: Basic Books.

Campbell, J. D. (1990). Self-esteem and clarity of the self-concept. *Journal of Personality and Social Psychology, 59,*538–549.

Chatham, P. M. (1985). *Treatment of the borderline personality.* New York: Jason Aronson.

Deikman, A. J. (1982). *The observing self: Mysticism and psychotherapy.* Boston: Beacon Press.

Dorr, D., Gard, B., Barley, W., & Webb, C. (1983). Understanding and treating borderline personality organization. *Psychotherapy: Theory, Research and Practice, 20,* 397–404.

Engel, G. (1964). Grief and grieving. *American Journal of Nursing, 64,* 93–98.

Eliasz, A. (1985). Mechanisms of temperament: Basic functions. In J. Strelau, F. H. Farley, & A. Gale (Eds.), *The biological bases of personality and behavior: Theories, measurement techniques, and development* (pp. 45–49). Washington, DC: Hemisphere.

Erikson, E. H. (1959). Identity and the life cycle. *Psychological Issues, 1,* 1–71.

Erikson, E. H. (1963). *Childhood and society* (2nd ed.). New York: W. W. Norton.

Fast, I., Marsden, K. G., Cohen, L., Heard, H., & Kruse, S. (1991). *Self as subject: A formulation and an assessment strategy.* Manuscript submitted for publication.

Gilligan, C. (1982). *In a different voice: Psychological theory and women's development.* Cambridge, MA: Harvard University Press.

Grotstein, J. S., Solomon, M. F., & Lang, J. A. (Eds.). (1987). *The borderline patient: Emerging concepts in diagnosis, psychodynamics, and treatment.* Hillsdale, NJ: Analytic Press.

Gunderson, J. G., & Kolb, JE. (1978). Discriminating features of borderline patients. *American Journal of Psychiatry, 135,* 792–796.

Gunderson, J. G., Kolb, J. E., & Austin, V. (1981). The Diagnostic Interview for Borderlines. *American Journal of Psychiatry, 138,* 896–903.

Harter, S. (1983). Developmental perspectives on the self-system. In P. H. Mussen (Ed.), *Handbook of child psychology* (Vol. 4, pp. 275–385). New York: Wiley.

Hayes, S. C. (1984). Making sense of spirituality. *Behaviorism, 12,* 99–110.

Herman, J. L., Perry, J. C., & van der Kolk, B. A. (1989). Childhood trauma in borderline personality disorder. *American Journal of Psychiatry, 146,* 490–495.

James, W. (1968). The self. In C. Gordon & K. J. Gergen (Eds.), *The self in social interaction* (pp. 41–49). New York: Wiley.

Kass, F., Skodol, A. E., Charles, E., Spitzer, R. L., & Williams, J. B. (1985). Scaled ratings of DSM-III-R personality disorder. *American Journal of Psychiatry, 142,* 627–630.

Kegan, R. (1982). *The evolving self: Problem and process in human development.* Cambridge, MA: Harvard University Press.

Kernberg, O. F. (1975). *Borderline conditions and pathological narcissism.* New York: Jason Aronson.

Kernberg, O. F. (1984). *Severe personality disorders: Psychotherapeutic strategies.* New Haven, CT: Yale University Press.

Kohlenberg, R. J., & Tsai, M. (1991). *Functional Analytic Psychotherapy: Creating intense and curative therapeutic relationships*. New York: Plenum Press.

Lindemann, E. (1944). Symptomatology and management of acute grief. *American Journal of Psychiatry, 101*, 141–148.

Linehan, M. M. (1984). Dialectical behavior therapy for the treatment of parasuicidal women: Treatment manual. Unpublished manuscript, University of Washington, Seattle.

Linehan, M. M. (1987a). Dialectical behavior therapy: A cognitive–behavioral approach to parasuicide. *Journal of Personality Disorders, 1*, 328–333.

Linehan, M. M. (1987b). Dialectical behavior therapy for borderline personality disorder: Theory and method. *Bulletin of the Menninger Clinic, 51*, 261–276.

Linehan, M. M. (1989). Cognitive and behavior therapy for borderline personality disorder. In A Tasman, R. E. Hales & A. J. Frances (Eds.), *Review of Psychiatry* (Vol. 8, pp. 84–102). Washington, DC: American Psychiatric Press.

Linehan, M. M. (in press). *Cognitive–behavioral treatment of borderline personality disorder*. New York: Guilford Press.

Linehan, M. M., & Koerner, K. (in press). Behavioral theory of borderline personality disorder. In M. R. Goldfried & J. C. Norcross (Eds.), *Handbook of psychotherapy integration*. New York: Basic Books.

Lykes, M. B. (1985). Gender and individualistic vs. collectivist bases for notions about the self. *Journal of Personality, 53*, 356–383.

Markus, H., & Nurius, P. (1986). Possible selves. *American Psychologist, 49*, 954–969.

McGuire, W. J., & McGuire, C. V. (1982). Significant others in self-space: Sex differences and developmental trends in the social self. In J. Suls (Ed.), *Psychological perspectives on the self* (Vol. 1, pp. 71–96). Hillsdale, NJ: Lawrence Erlbaum.

Meissner, W. W. (1986). Narcissistic personalities and borderline conditions: A differential diagnosis. In A. P. Morrison (Ed.), *Essential papers on narcissism* (pp. 403–437). New York: New York University Press.

Perloff, R. (1987). Self-interest and personal responsibility redux. *American Psychologist, 42*, 3–11.

Piersma, H. (1987). The MCMI as a measure of DSM-III-R axis II diagnoses: An empirical comparison. *Journal of Clinical Psychology, 43*, 478–483.

Pratt, M. W., Pancer, M., Hunsberger, B. & Manchester, J. (1990). Reasoning about the self and relationships in maturity: An integrative complexity analysis of individual differences. *Journal of Personality and Social Psychology, 59*, 575–581.

Prentice, D. A. (1990). Familiarity and differences in self- and other-representations. *Journal of Personality and Social Psychology, 59*, 369–383.

Rando, T. A. (1984). *Grief, dying, and death: Clinical interventions for caregivers*. Champaign, IL: Research Press.

Sampson, E. E. (1988). The debate on individualism: Indigenous psychologies of the individual and their role in personal and societal functioning. *American Psychologist, 43*, 15–22.

Scarr, S., & McCartney, K. (1983). How people make their own environments: A theory of genotype-environmental effects. *Child Development, 54*, 424–435.

Shearer, S. L., Peters, C. P., Quaytman, M. S., & Ogden R. L. (1990). Frequency and correlates of childhood sexual and physical abuse histories in adult female borderline inpatients. *American Journal of Psychiatry, 147*, 214–216.

Skinner, B. F. (1974). *About behaviorism*. New York: Knopf.

Smith, M. B. (1978). Perspectives on selfhood. *American Psychologist, 33*, 1053–1063.

Tellegen, A., Lykken, D. T., Bouchard, T. J., Wilcox, K. J., Segal, N. L., & Rich, S. (1988). Personality similarity in twins raised apart and together. *Journal of Personality and Social Psychology, 54*, 1031–1039.

Triandis, H. C., McKusker, C., & Hui, C. H. (1990). Multimethod probes of individualism and collectivism. *Journal of Personality and Social Psychology, 59*, 1006–1020.

Tsai, M., & Wagner, N. N. (1978). Therapy groups for women sexually molested as children. *Archives of Sexual Behavior, 7*, 417–427.

Wagner, A. W., Linehan, M. M., & Wasson, E. J. (1989, November). *Parasuicide: Characteristics and relationship to childhood sexual abuse.* Poster presented at the annual meeting of the Association for Advancement of Behavior Therapy, Washington, DC.

Young, J. (1983, August). Borderline personality: Cognitive theory and treatment. Paper presented at the annual meeting of the American Psychological Association, Philadelphia.

Zanarini, M. C., Gunderson, J. G., Frankenburg, F. R., & Chauncey, D. L. (1989). The revised Diagnostic Interview for Borderlines: Discriminating borderline personality disorder from other axis II disorders. *Journal of Personality Disorders, 3*, 10–18.

Commentary

DREW WESTEN
Harvard University and
Cambridge Hospital

ROBERT P. COHEN
Detroit Psychiatric Institute and
Michigan Psychoanalytic Institute

JUXTAPOSING THE CHAPTER by Heard and Linehan with our own makes clear that even in the face of clashing paradigms, some "facts" seem to stand for themselves. Both perspectives on self pathology in Borderline Personality Disorder point to the instability in the way borderline patients represent themselves, derived in part from the real instability of their lives. Both approaches, beginning with James's distinction between self as subject and object, note peculiarities in both the subjective experience of self and the way the self is represented.

What Linehan has brought to the field in her conceptualizations is a compelling focus on affect regulation, which has never been central in psychoanalytic formulations of the disorder, and with it some suggestions about ways to teach what cognitive–behavioral clinicians call "self-regulation" to these patients. An explicit focus on affect regulation and the use of therapeutic procedures tailored to address it is essential in any form of treatment with these patients (see Westen, 1991). Gunderson and Phillips (1991) have made a compelling argument against viewing borderline disorders as affect dysregulation disorders on the order of nonborderline major depression. The affect dysregulation of borderline patients is qualitatively different from the dysregulation of other unipolar depressed patients in that it tends to be less episodic, has a different phenomenology (associated with concerns about loss, loneliness, and emptiness), pertains to all unpleasant affects rather than just depression, is more directly tied to interpersonal issues, and has more kinship with impulse dysregulation in the lack of appropriate procedures for regulating feelings and intentions. Treatment of such affect/impulse dysregulation requires treatment procedures that directly target this form of pathology. We will focus in this response, however, on the ways in which we diverge from the perspective described by Heard and Linehan.

Precisely which domains are encompassed by the "self" is somewhat unclear from their chapter. Regulation of emotion, cognition, views of the self, and behavior is no doubt deficient in borderline patients, but the extent to which this is a problem with "self" is unclear, unless by "self" one means the person, in which case all psychopathology is self pathology. Not all cognition is about the self, so that cognitive dysregulation, by which the authors presumably mean a tendency to make distorted attributions, lapse into psychotic thinking, apply schemas inappropriately, and so forth, is not a self problem. *People* have trouble regulating their affects; selves do not.[1]

The dialectical approach to the self in Borderline Personality Disorder offered by Heard and Linehan provides many theses and antitheses, but not enough syntheses. For example, one finds, throughout, a straining to maintain behaviorist language in dealing with a phenomenon that is simply beyond the scope of the radical behaviorist perspective. While we concur in their concerns about reification, referring to "self behaviors," "learning a self," or "external stimuli controlling the experience of self" seems to move away from a focus on cognitive-affective processes that mediate behavior in a way that neither contemporary psychoanalytic nor cognitive theorists would find compelling. One does not need a homunculus to posit the existence of self-representations. There are many occasions in which the language of conditioning is quite compelling and useful, as in describing the ways different aspects of panic disorder are maintained (see Barlow, 1988), but this is not one of them. Conditioning processes need to be understood within the context of a broader understanding of personality and its disorders.

Precisely what borderline patients should be doing with their emotions and beliefs about the self also remains unclear because the authors seem to offer contradictory views. On the one hand, borderline patients are viewed, we believe accurately, as hyperemotional and unable to regulate intense feeling states. On the other, they are described as "inhibit[ing] the emotions and emotional process" related to grief. Why they can inhibit one set of emotions while being unable to regulate others is unclear.

Similarly, Linehan, like theorists such as Harry Stack Sullivan, focuses on an invalidating environment as a prime etiological variable in the generation of severe character disturbance. The authors point to a paradox involved in trying to promote change in patients who have suffered from invalidating environments—that is, helping them change while not further invalidating their current experience of self—but they do not offer a compelling way out of it, except to assert that "change can occur only in the context of acceptance, and acceptance is itself change" (p. 319). Most borderline patients would probably have trouble understanding this statement, especially in the midst of accusing the therapist of indifference, lack of empathy, or malevolence. The authors' point, however, is well taken.

Heard and Linehan are essentially proposing that a sense of selfhood has not developed appropriately in these patients because their emotional states have not been accepted or validated by their caregivers, who find their intense affects difficult to tolerate; presumably this leads, as Sullivan (1953) would argue, to realms of self-experience being redefined as "not self." Two therapeutic implications could be drawn from this: either that the therapist should help these patients stop experiencing such intense states, which would bring consensual and personal selfhood into congruence, or that the therapist should help them focus on and appreciate their intense affects and often correspondingly idiosyncratic attributions (such as malevolent ones) and let the social environment be damned. The authors seem to advocate both of these strategies at different points. The former clearly involves informing the patient that he/she has a problem and needs to change, whereas the latter seems to ignore the central problems of affect regulation and interpersonal functioning that bring these patients in for treatment.

If borderline patients suffer from intense, poorly regulated affects and idiosyncratic ways of understanding people, which we believe they do, one does not help them by validating their experience, which is, from the perspective of reality and adaptation, invalid. (The therapist, for example, is presumably not *really* trying to destroy the patient by taking a vacation.) To empathize with a person's private experience is one thing; to accept it is another. The essence of good psychodynamic treatment with borderline patients is to empathize with the patient's experience while confronting the parts of it that are inappropriate, unrealistic, or counterproductive. In so doing, the therapist provides the patient with both an experience of attunement, in which the therapist's needs and concerns are not central and distorting the way the parents' may have been, while simultaneously addressing ways of feeling, behaving, and perceiving interpersonal reality that are quite clearly identified as problematic, shown to be tied to aversive consequences, and understood in relation to the person's history.

Perhaps the central paradox of the perspective provided by Heard and Linehan is whether borderline patients have a problem at all, or whether they are simply victims of culture (or of a bad fit with their culture). The authors argue, appropriately, that since the nature of self-experience differs cross-culturally, theories of disorders in which self pathology is prominent should be cognizant of cross-cultural issues. They make a particularly intriguing argument about the difficulty in maintaining a "relational self" in the face of an inability to maintain relationships with significant others; the result is likely to be a sense of emptiness and difficulty synthesizing an identity. The ways in which the poorly bounded self-representations of borderline patients are similar to, and different from, the less bounded self-representations of people in the third world are worthy of considerable study, because most contemporary Western theories assume individuation and boundedness as properties of mature functioning.

The question, however, is whether the problem of borderline self-experience can really be transposed into the problem of a relational self in a nonrelational world. Women in our culture have long been largely relational in their orientation, and only a subset of them become borderline. Research evidence linking borderline disorders to disrupted attachments (see Gunderson & Phillips, 1991; Ludolph et al., 1990) suggests, as does psychoanalytic theory, that these patients may be "hyperrelational" in their orientation because of expectations of abandonment, a failure to internalize functions (such as the ability to self-soothe) that would have likely been internalized under different familial circumstances, and a desperate search to maintain the kind of connection to an attachment figure as an adult which could not easily be attained in childhood. Earlier problems in "validation" or empathy seem more decisive here than cultural issues, as does a later history of abuse, which can, for example, contribute to borderline symptoms such as rage, low self-esteem, and dissociation.

Although it is difficult to know whether borderline disorders are in fact more common now than they once were, two cultural shifts that have occurred with technological development probably have contributed to the incidence of borderline pathology, both of which are, at least indirectly, related to issues of self (see Westen, 1985, 1992). The first is a breakdown in family and community structure. This has left many children in the care of a single, disturbed parent or an intact but dysfunctional marital unit. In most previous historical periods, children had far more buffering from extended family and community when their parents were mentally ill. In adulthood, this factor probably influences the expression of borderline disorder because the object-hungry person has no ready-made objects—and particularly none who have been known over the years—to provide a sense of security and satisfaction of interpersonal needs. The contemporary world is, indeed, in one sense a borderline world, filled with people who could one day abandon, in a way that a social structure built upon family, kin, and geographical proximity was not.

A second influence on the solidification of borderline pathology in adolescence stems ultimately from the rise of ideological pluralism and the breakdown of traditional authority structures and worldview that accompany modernization. The breakdown of cultural mechanisms, such as rites of passage, that provide members with a prefabricated, culturally constructed identity has been part of the process that has made identity a problem in technologically developed societies (see Erikson, 1968). A pluralistic, geographically mobile, anomic society in which bonds between people are ephemeral is probably the worst possible environment for individuals with borderline dynamics, who need interpersonal and ideological stability built into the social structure to compensate for their inability to create such stability for themselves.

Precisely how the cultural argument advanced by Heard and Linehan relates to their etiological theory, which focuses on temperamental hyperaffectivity and invalidating childhood experiences, is unclear. The authors do not make explicit whether having one's experience of self invalidated or having poorly modulated affects would also produce borderline pathology in a less individualistic society. The view of etiology proposed by Heard and Linehan has the same nonspecificity of many psychoanalytic theories, which could equally explain the etiology of a host of different disorders. For many years in psychoanalysis, the culprits were unempathic mothers; for Linehan, they are invalidating environments. Heard and Linehan's comments about the difficulty of forming a cohesive sense of self in the face of being told that one is not or does not feel what one experiences are well taken and do seem likely related to severe character pathology, at least in some cases. To this extent, the psychoanalytic and cognitive–behavioral views agree in their focus on empathic failures. Both perspectives also hypothesize an interaction of constitutional and environmental factors in the etiology of the disorder.

Linehan adds, however, a series of propositions about these families that seem idiosyncratic and do not accord with most clinical or research accounts of borderline families. The stoic "Where there's a will, there's a way" orientation, for example, is something neither of us have ever seen in the family of a borderline; the authors' description of parents who "teach that all problems must have a solution and expect the child to find that solution" similarly seems like a prototypical American parenting style that could lead to achievement orientation or to low feelings of competence but not particularly to Borderline Personality Disorder. Not every child who is frequently told "You can do it" in the face of a difficult task becomes borderline. Research suggests, rather, that borderline disorders tend to emerge in the face of disrupted attachments, maternal pathology, sexual abuse, and family chaos (see, e.g., Ludolph et al., 1990).

The recommendations for treatment that stem from this approach seem problematic as well. The authors make two suggestions that leave a great deal unanswered. One is that the therapy should not try to create an individuated sense of self in the borderline patient but should focus "on how the relational person can self-validate within an individualistic society" (p. 315) or live "in greater comfort in an unsupportive environment" (p. 319). Precisely what this means is hard to know; what comes to mind is assigning anthropological readings on less individuated cultures, or bolstering externalizations in patients who are already too prone to find external instead of internal causes for their difficulties.

Heard and Linehan's second suggestion is that the therapist "help the individual . . . find a different social network, one that would support a relational self" (p. 319). Unfortunately, this is just what borderline patients, with their poor boundaries and uncertain sense of self and values, do for themselves: They join cults, which give them unambiguous values and a sense of total belonging, they form intense unbounded relationships that then sour and drive them to wrist-cutting, and they have children who develop personality disorders because their parents cannot distinguish their own feelings and needs from the child's.

This suggestion points precisely to the reason that a behaviorist perspective, however radical or dialectical, cannot account for character pathology: It locates the problem in the environment, in the stimuli that allegedly control behavior. Changing circumstances may momentarily lower borderline patients' distress, but the reason that they find themselves as adults in the same kind of chaotic relationships in which they found themselves as children is that they *create* those relationships. They do so because of internal cognitive, affective, and motivational processes—which psychoanalysis refers to as object relations—that compel them to do so, and they are far more adept at eliciting chaos, aggression, and problematic behavior from the human "environment" than it is in eliciting anything different from them.

Any understanding of borderline disorder must account for both the affect/impulse dysregulation and the pathological object relations of these patients; the latter includes representations of self and others and the cognitive, motivational, and affective processes brought to bear on those representations. The importance of Linehan's approach is that it calls attention to affective dysregulation in these patients and suggests concrete skills training procedures that should be useful in treating this aspect of their pathology. Dialectical behavior therapy is not likely, however, to have a substantial impact upon the enduring motivational, defensive, and representational processes that generate in these patients experiences of loneliness, emptiness, despair, and interpersonal desperation.

The failure of cognitive and behavioral approaches to develop a sophisticated understanding of object relations remains a tremendous gap in both their understanding and treatment of borderline patients. Cognitive–behavioral theorists are beginning to make considerable strides in that direction, as in the recent work on personality disorders by Beck, Freeman, and Associates (1990), whose approach to schemas about the self and the world has moved cognitive therapy in a decidedly object-relational direction. While admirably clear in exposition (in contrast to most object relations theories), this recent work remains problematic in multiple respects. For example, because of their explicit disinclination to examine unconscious processes, Beck and associates fail to note some of the most salient aspects of the self-representations of patients with personality disorders, such as the unconscious sense of worthlessness that alternates with the manifest grandiosity of narcissistic patients, whom they describe as characterized only by their manifest view of self as special and unique. Their description of passive–aggressive personalities is similarly problematic because it does not distinguish between the conscious "I haven't done anything wrong" self-representation and its vastly different unconscious counterpart. Further, while Beck and colleagues have now extended the schema concept to include motives, impulses, plans for action, and processes that regulate impulses and actions—which essentially makes the term *schema* superfluous because now it simply means "psychological process"; calling a "motive" a "motivational schema" does not really do anything for understanding motivation—their explanations and mode of treatment remain squarely focused on cognitions.

Patients with personality disorders, however, are uniformly people with disorders in the way they attach and navigate the world interpersonally, and this is as much a matter of motivation as of cognition. Borderline patients who were physically and sexually abused in childhood are as likely to experience distortions in the way they *seek* relatedness with others as in the way they *construe* relationships, and reducing one to the other seems both theoretically and therapeutically indefensible. Similarly, the essence of passive–aggressive behavior is a motive to hurt or frustrate, which is typically defensively disavowed; the belief that "people always seem to dump on me unfairly" is a cognitive *precipitate* of a conflict-laden way of dealing with impulses, which itself reflects the interaction of cognitive, affective, and motivational processes (such as rage, beliefs about the acceptability of showing anger, etc.). Moreover, patients with personality disorders (not to mention the rest of us) uniformly have some very nasty fantasies, and one cannot convince them to abandon negative self-schemas (e.g., "I am evil and destructive") until one has explored those fantasies with them in a manner that cognitive therapists are not trained to do and the highly structured process of cognitive therapy tends to circumvent.

Issues of self must be considered in the context of a broader understanding of the psychological processes that mediate interpersonal functioning in close relationships. This demands an approach that examines representations as well as behaviors, conscious as well as unconscious representations, and conscious as well as unconscious mechanisms of coping and affect regulation.

NOTE

1. "Self-regulation" is typically used to refer to processes by which a person regulates feelings, impulses, and the like. These processes cannot easily be viewed as aspects of self, except speaking very loosely: They are typically unconscious, are

seldom experienced consciously as aspects of self, and may not be represented as aspects of self by the person at all (unless he/she is a psychologist).

REFERENCES

Barlow, D. (1988). *Anxiety and its disorders*. New York: Guilford Press.

Beck, A. T., Freeman, A., & Associates. (1990). *Cognitive therapy of personality disorders*. New York: Guilford Press.

Erikson, E. (1968). *Identity: Youth and crisis*. New York: W. W. Norton.

Gunderson, J. G., & Phillips, K. A. (1991). A current view of the interface between borderline personality disorder and depression. *American Journal of Psychiatry, 148*, 967–975.

Ludolph, P., Westen, D., Misle, B., Jackson, A., Wixom, J., & Wiss, F. C. (1990). The borderline diagnosis in adolescents: Symptoms and developmental history. *American Journal of Psychiatry, 147*, 470–476.

Sullivan, H. S. (1953). *The interpersonal theory of psychiatry*. New York: W. W. Norton.

Westen, D. (l985). *Self and society: Narcissism, collectivism, and the development of morals*. New York: Cambridge University Press.

Westen, D. (1991). Cognitive–behavioral interventions in the psychodynamic psychotherapy of borderline personality disorders. *Clinical Psychology Review, 11*, 211–230.

Westen, D. (1992). The cognitive self and the psychoanalytic self: Can we put our selves together? *Psychological Inquiry, 3*, 1–13.

10

The Self in Borderline Personality Disorder: A Psychodynamic Perspective

DREW WESTEN
Harvard University and
Cambridge Hospital

ROBERT P. COHEN
Detroit Psychiatric Institute and
Michigan Psychoanalytic Institute

PSYCHOANALYTIC THEORISTS OF Borderline Personality Disorder (BDP) all assert that a pathology of self and identity is an important aspect of the disorder. Precisely what that pathology entails is a matter of debate. The present chapter begins by reviewing psychoanalytic views of borderline self pathology. It argues that these theories offer an understanding of the complexities of self-representation in borderline patients, particularly in their examination of the self–other relationship paradigms that emerge in clinical work; nevertheless, these theories are limited by conceptual confusion over different dimensions of self and by a corresponding failure to operationalize constructs for testing and theoretical refinement. The paper then distinguishes several aspects of self-structure and briefly describes an evolving methodology for assessing some of these dimensions. Next it applies these distinctions to borderline self-structure. Finally, it addresses issues of etiology, suggesting that different dimensions of self pathology in borderline patients may have interdependent but distinct etiologies.

PSYCHOANALYTIC THEORIES OF THE BORDERLINE "SELF"

The way theorists address the self pathology of borderline patients, both theoretically and clinically, depends on their conceptualizations of both the self and the disorder. Psychoanalysts refer to several different phenomena when they use the term *self* (see Westen, 1992); most typically, they refer to self-representations. With the development of Kohutian self psychology (Kohut, 1971, 1977), an alternative usage considers the self a bipolar structure responsible for maintenance of self-esteem and a sense of self-cohesion, which includes ambitions on one "pole" and ideals on the other. With respect to borderline pathology, some theorists (e.g., Gunderson, 1984) focus on Borderline Personality Disorder as defined in DSM-III-R (American Psychiatric Association, 1987), whereas others, notably Kernberg (1975), use the term *borderline* to refer to a form of personality organization that casts a wider diagnostic net, including patients with severe personality disorders of many different varieties. Numerous theorists have offered accounts of the pathology of self-structure in BDP (see Gunderson, 1984); we will focus here on the work of Kernberg, Adler and Buie, and Masterson, which exemplifies the way many psychoanalytic theorists and clinicians understand borderline pathology.

Kernberg's Approach

Kernberg has written extensively about self pathology in borderline personality organization, a class of disturbance that includes most patients diagnosed with Borderline Personality Disorder in DSM-III-R as well as some severely character-disordered patients who would meet criteria for other DSM-III-R personality disorders (Kernberg, 1975; Kernberg, Selzer, Koenigsberg, Carr, & Appelbaum, 1989). In Kernberg's view, the symptoms of borderline personality derive from an inability to successfully integrate good and bad aspects of self and others. Unlike psychotics, borderlines are able to differentiate themselves from others and can maintain a separate, bounded sense of self; however, either because of a constitutional defect or early environmental frustration, borderlines are flooded with aggression that cannot be properly neutralized. Kernberg believes that the isolation of good and bad representations of the self and others is usual in infancy, but that normal development leads to an integration across affective valence so that complex representations of self and others, containing both loving and hostile elements, evolve. This usually occurs between the 2nd and 3rd year of life, during Mahler's (1971) hypothesized separation–individuation stage of development. Patients who have achieved a neurotic rather than a borderline level of personality organization are able to integrate positive and negative representations of self and others because they have presumably passed through this stage with less difficulty.

For borderline patients, however, excess aggression makes this achievement impossible. For stability, borderlines must hold onto good representations of themselves and others. These "good introjects" are repeatedly threatened with destruction by the predominance of negative, hostile images and impulses. The ubiquity of rage, for instance, can potentially eradicate any internal sense a borderline patient has of a good, loving caretaker. To protect against such a devastating outcome, these patients endeavor defensively to maintain "all good" representations of self and others. The hallmark of the borderline syndrome for Kernberg, then, is splitting, a defense in which an individual unconsciously places an impermeable wall between positive and negative representations of self and others in order to protect the positive representations. The result is a constant shifting of representations of self and others. A previously "good object" whom the patient now finds frustrating may suddenly become a totally bad object, who is seen as malevolent and attacking. Since representations of the self are organized in a parallel fashion with those of others, splitting also leads to "extreme and repetitive oscillation between contradictory self concepts" (Kernberg et al., 1989, p. 28).

A consequence of this way of organizing representations is a chameleonlike sense of identity diffusion in borderline patients. According to Kernberg et al. (1989), "The patient, lacking a stable sense of self or other, continually experiences the self in shifting positions, with potentially sharp discontinuities—as victim or victimizer, as dominant or submissive, and so on" (p. 28). A pervasive sense of emptiness also ensues as a result of the chaotic shifting of self and object representations. Another concomitant of borderline identity diffusion is a tendency toward sometimes representing the self as omnipotent and idealized, as the borderline patient attempts to protect self-representations from integration with bad internal representations that threaten to contaminate them. The opposite pole is a sense of worthlessness or profound evil attributed to the self.

The goal of psychodynamic treatment, from this perspective, is to interpret defenses against uniting good and bad representations of self and others. The therapist must also help the patient observe his/her efforts to keep such representations apart, especially as this tendancy becomes apparent in the relationship with the therapist. This requires the therapist to be vigilant to the constantly shifting sense of self and others that the patient experiences and projects during the therapeutic hour.

The Self-psychological Approach

Kohut offered a theory of the unfolding and integration of the self, but his observations centered for the most part on narcissistic patients. In

Kohut's view (1977), borderline patients suffer from a "permanent or protracted breakup, enfeeblement or serious distortion of the self," which cannot be cured through analysis because such patients cannot form the necessary transference to the analyst (p. 192). Kohut (1984) admitted he did not have much experience with what he called "borderline states" and lumped them together with the psychoses as disorders characterized by an underlying "hollowness" of the self, caused by a lack of early empathic responsiveness that would allow the small child to organize and maintain a coherent sense of self (p. 8).

Other writers who take a self-psychological perspective have, however, addressed the self pathology of borderline patients (Adler, 1981; 1989; Adler & Buie, 1979; Buie & Adler, 1982). This pathology, they argue, has a number of clinical manifestations in borderline patients, including "incoherency, or disjointedness of thinking," "feelings of loss of integration of body parts," "a subjective sense of losing functional control of the self," and "concerns about 'falling apart'" (Buie & Adler, 1982, p. 62). Patients with BPD may also share other, less dramatic manifestations of "self fragmentation" with patients who have narcissistic character disorders, including "not feeling real, feeling emotionally dull, lacking zest and initiative, and feeling depleted and empty" (Adler, 1981, p. 46).

The defects in the borderline self are caused, according to Adler and Buie, by the failure to develop a capacity for evocative memory, in which memories of good objects become available to provide self-soothing in times of distress. This capacity should be achieved in normal development between the ages of 2 and 3, during the rapprochement subphase of separation–individuation (Mahler, Pine, & Bergman, 1975). Without this capacity, borderlines cannot hold onto comforting images of others, which is the first step toward developing an internal, automatic ability to self-soothe.The lack of internal, soothing representations leads borderline patients to feel intense aloneness and emptiness.

The absence of a reliable and soothing other, or an accessible representation of one, precipitates not only separation anxiety but a concomitant "loss of cohesiveness of the self" (Buie & Adler, 1982, p. 62). Adler and Buie never clarified explicitly why the loss of contact with soothing and supporting others and the inability to evoke memories of such figures should lead to a collapse of the borderline self and the confusion of identity concomitant with it. This idea appears to derive from Kohut's (1977) notion that the self is built up and nourished through the "transmuting internalization" of soothing and mirroring functions provided by early caregivers. In other words, a sense of self and self-esteem evolve from repeated experiences of minor parental failures in empathy in the context of children's general experience of their parents as both admiring of them and as suitable objects for admiration with whom they can identify. As these minor empathic failures occur, children take on some of the functions previously carried out by the parents and hence build a capacity for self-esteem regulation.

Psychotherapy in which the patient is able to learn that the therapist exists between sessions, in spite of the patient's occasional or frequent rage, allows the patient to develop an evocative memory for the soothing and comforting qualities of the therapist. The functions served by the therapist are slowly internalized, with a gradual development of a more cohesive sense of self and more realistic and adaptive mechanisms for self-esteem regulation.

Masterson's Approach

Masterson and his colleagues (Masterson, 1985; Masterson & Klein, 1989) focus on distortions of autonomous strivings and self-representations that occur in borderline patients. Developmentally, a "real self" should emerge during the first 3 years of life through the separation–individuation process. This self serves a number of functions including self-soothing and self-assertion, and provides the person with a sense of continuity and aliveness. The growth of the real self is nourished by the encouragment and support of the child's emerging autonomous wishes and self-esteem in early life by caretakers who can tolerate a toddler's rage, clinginess, demandingness, and efforts at separation.

A primary caregiver who has tremendous difficulties with separation herself—and thus desperately needs the child to provide her with a sense of security and love to help her minimize her own abandonment fears—is likely to thwart the child's autonomous strivings and efforts at separation and individuation. Masterson believes that such caretakers produce borderline offspring, who consequently develop a set of "false selves" dictated less by their own needs than by the needs of their early caretakers (for a similar formulation of the origins of severe interpersonal dysfunction, see Sullivan's [1953] description of distortions in the "self-system" directed at alleviating interpersonal anxiety). Because of repeated threats of abandonment by the early caregiver, the borderline patient becomes highly vulnerable to "abandonment depression" and develops a fear that "his very existence is dependent ultimately upon the presence of need-gratifying and life-sustaining others" (Klein, 1989, p. 36). This conviction lies at the heart of two fundamental self-representations common in borderline patients: The self is seen as a needy, helpless, dependent child who is rewarded for this stance by maintaining the love of the caregiver; alternatively, the borderline individual views him/herself as a bad, loathesome person who can drive others away by becoming independent and self-reliant. Thus, in Masterson's view, the clinging, demanding, vulnerable self-presentation of borderline patients is a false veneer that may mask a more competent, independent real self.

The real self emerges in treatment when the therapist subtly indicates approval for the patient's active, assertive efforts, and demonstrates an empathic "communicative matching" with the patient. The therapist also attempts to limit acting out in the hopes of thwarting the enactment of scenaries involving pathological self-representations and object-relational paradigms (such as *self demanding from the other for fear that the other will disappear*). As in Kernberg's system, reconstructive work is also used to help the patient understand his/her recurring object-relational patterns and their origins.

Strengths and Limitations of Psychoanalytic Approaches

Although the preceding theories differ from each other in focus and emphasis, they share a concern with trying to explain the sense of identity confusion characteristic of Borderline Personality Disorder. From a psychoanalytic perspective, the self pathology of these patients must be understood within the context of a more general characterological disturbance and hence cannot be treated apart from their disturbed dynamics, defensive functioning, and object relations more generally. Each of the theories also pinpoints mother–toddler interactions as the crucible in which borderline self disturbances coalesce.

Compared with strictly cognitive approaches, psychoanalytic views of BPD are characterized by their emphasis on the structural complexity and shifting patterns of self-representations in borderline patients. Cognitive approaches generally fail to distinguish the self-schemas of depressed borderline patients (which probably comprise all borderline patients at one point or another) from other depressed patients. Even though the majority of patients with severe depression have personality disorders (see, e.g., Shea, Glass, Pilkonis, Watkins, & Docherty, 1987), at least until very recently cognitive theorists have not addressed the differences in the representational processes of personality-disordered and non-personality-disordered depressed patients. Empirical research supports the psychoanalytic view that the quality of depression does, in fact, differ between borderline and nonborderline depressed patients, with borderline depression more infused with concerns about loss, abandonment, alienation, desperation with respect to attachment figures, and emptiness (Westen et al., 1992; Wixom, 1988). This suggests differences in self-representations, such as greater accessibility or availability of representations of self-as-abandoned (on issues of accessibility and availability, see Segal, 1988). Further, as will be described below, psychoanalytic theories of self-representations emphasize the importance of understanding and altering the structure of unconscious representations, which may be qualitatively different from conscious representations of self.

Psychoanalytic conceptions of borderline self-structure have a number of strengths. Perhaps the most important is the subtle analysis of the flux and flow of representational structures that is made possible by long-term observation of patterns of self-representation and their interaction with wishes, fears, and other motivational and affective processes. Crucial to the development of these theories has been the observation of the way borderline patients interact over time in the therapeutic relationship itself, enacting pathological relationship paradigms, experiencing massively fluctuating views of the self, viewing the self as contaminated or contaminating of the therapist, and so forth.

The theories described above offer powerful conceptual tools for understanding and treating patients who had previously been viewed as untreatable and incomprehensible, providing a way of organizing the data of clinical observation to lend coherence and predictability to the behavior of patients whose behavior otherwise seems singularly incoherent and unpredictable. Nevertheless, recent theory and research has questioned a number of their assumptions and assertions about the development and structure of the self (Eagle, 1984; Stern, 1985; Westen, 1990a, 1992) and of object relations more generally (Peterfreund, 1978; Robbins, 1989; Westen, 1989, 1990b). The critiques of these theories cannot be described in any detail here, but what follows are some key points. The theories all presuppose a direct mapping of psychopathology onto developmental epochs, so that, for example, psychosis is linked to infancy, and borderline disorder to the rapprochement period of separation–individuation. The evidence for either of those linkages is tenuous. A corollary assumption is that certain developmental processes viewed as defective or inadequately mastered in borderline patients, such as the integration of elements of self-structure, are essentially complete by the end of the preoedipal period, that is, by about age 4. Developmental data suggest, however, that self-representations continue to develop throughout childhood and adolescence in both their complexity and integration, and that an adult whose representations resembled the allegedly mature representations of the 5-year-old would be highly pathological.

Perhaps the most significant problem with these theories is a conceptual fuzziness and failure to distinguish subprocesses and developmental lines; the result is that clinical and theoretical discussions are filled with statements, such as "the patient suffered from a lack of self-cohesion" or "patients such as these have a defective self," that lack both definitional clarity and any obvious empirical referents. For example, when a patient is described as having "prominent narcissistic dynamics," one could mean that the patient is egocentric (is cognitively embedded in her/his own point of view), has a need-gratifying or exploitative orientation toward relationships, has a globally grandiose view of her/himself, has unrealistic representations of self in some specific domain, has defensively high self-esteem, has an alternation of extremely high and extremely low self-esteem, has shallow and minimally developed representations of self or significant others, has a particularly salient need to demonstrate her/his sexual attractiveness or competence, has a strong need to be admired, and so forth. The extent to which these different meanings covary is an empirical matter, and it is highly unlikely that the presence of one always implies the presence of the others.

The correlative methodological problem with these theories is a general disinclination to operationalize constructs, which tend to remain murky and fluid as a consequence. Clinical observation is an unequalled database for the generation of theories and hypotheses, but the lack of any way to adjudicate among the claims of competing psychoanalytic theories of borderline pathology provides an irrefutable empirical demonstration of the limits of clinical observation for theoretical refinement and testing of competing hypotheses. Nevertheless, one should remember that the theories described offer an understanding of the dynamics of borderline and other personality disorders that clinicians from other theoretical perspectives (particularly those inspired by narrowly empirical traditions) ignored for several decades.

DIMENSIONS OF SELF-STRUCTURE

To describe the problematic self-structure of borderline patients requires a more careful delineation of different dimensions of self-experience. The brief description of domains of self-structure that follows is both psychoanalytically and cognitively informed (Westen, 1985, 1991a, 1992; for similar dynamically and cognitively informed models, see Epstein, 1990; Horowitz, 1988; Horowitz & Zilberg, 1983; Singer & Salovey, 1990).

Theorists of nearly every persuasion (Kohut, 1971; Markus & Cross, 1990; Rogers, 1959) tend to introduce two confusions into discussions of the self. First, they define the self in a logically inconsistent way to refer to self-representation. For example, Markus and Cross (1990, p. 576) propose that "the self is what one 'takes oneself to be.'" If a self-representation, self-schema, or self-concept is a representation of something, however, it must be a representation of the self, in which case the self cannot be defined as a representation; otherwise, the self-concept becomes a person's concept of his self-concept, which is clearly not what is meant by the term. Having defined the self as a representation, theorists then typically go on to ascribe to it various motivational properties and tendencies, such as goals, plans, and self-esteem motivation (e.g., Epstein, 1973; Kohut, 1971; Markus & Cross, 1990). The self thus comes to denote most, if not all, of personality and hence becomes a superfluous term.

The only logically coherent definition of self is that the *self* is the person—body, mental contents, attributes, and the like. A *self-representation* (Sandler, 1987; Sandler & Rosenblatt, 1962), or *self-schema* (Markus, 1977), is thus a mental model or representation a person has formed of him/herself, much as anyone else might form a representation of that person. Self-representations can be conscious or unconscious. Conscious representations need not be similar to, and can be defensively transformed derivatives of, their unconscious counterparts, as when a narcissistic patient defends against a deflated view of self by waxing grandiosely after perceiving someone's behavior or words as an insult. Unconscious self-representations are frequently disavowed to avoid unpleasant affects, particularly guilt and anxiety.

The distinction between conscious and unconscious representations, and the correlative focus on the role of affective and motivational processes in self-representation, is probably the most important contribution of psychoanalytic thinking to the understanding of self-representations. Conscious self-representations, and to some degree unconscious representations, are compromise formations (Brenner, 1982), that is, compromise structures that reflect several competing psychological processes, including processes directed at veridical information processing and efforts to regulate positive and negative affects (Westen, 1985). In other words, the way people represent themselves depends both on efforts to understand themselves and on efforts to see themselves in ways that have been selected during the course of their development to maximize pleasure and minimize distress.

The self-schema that has been most frequently studied by researchers is the conscious, prototypic, generalized representation of self that people typically offer when asked to describe themselves. This abstract, verbalizable representation is the *self-concept*. (It may be slightly more accurate to say that the conscious prototypic self-concept is the conscious component of a preconsciously constructed prototypic self-concept.)

The self-concept is one of many representations of self in the person's system of self-representations, or *self-system*. Representations of self that are currently activated—that is, through which information is currently being processed consciously or unconsciously—can be called *working self-representations*. An individual's working representations are highly diverse and reflect the interplay of enduring ways of representing the self and current experience. Representations of self are encoded simultaneously in multiple modes, including semantic and sensory modalities (i.e., as propositions as well as in visual, auditory, tactile, or other forms); they are almost always affectively imbued (i.e., associated with feeling-states). Self-representations may be organized a number of ways in long-term memory, including hierarchically (as when a representation of self-as-therapist includes subcategories of self-with-borderline-patients and self-with-nonborderline-patients) and along networks of association. Two particularly important ways in which self-representations are associatively connected (and which have received empirical support) is that they are associatively linked with each other (Segal, 1988), and they are linked with representations of other people or role categories to form *relationship schemas* (Baldwin, in press; Baldwin, Carrell, & Lopez, 1990; Horowitz, 1988) or *self-with-other schemas* (Ogilvie & Ashmore, 1991). These are similar to basic self–other units described by theorists such as Kernberg and Masterson and studied empirically by Luborsky and his colleagues (Luborsky & Crits-Christoph, 1990).

Self-representations are not themselves motivating—I can represent myself as a terrible tennis player but have no inclination to hone my serve because I have no investment in tennis—but can be linked to motivation through affectively charged *wished-for*, *feared*, and *ideal self-representations* (see Higgins, 1990; Markus & Nurius, 1986). The extent to which a person is motivated to act (cognitively or behaviorally) on the basis of such representational processes is a joint function of the degree of discrepancy between cognized self and these evaluative representations, and the strength of the affective "charge" associated with them. Thus, a patient who is strongly invested in a consciously or unconsciously wished-for representation of self-as-victor-over-therapist may feel tremendous shame and anger at therapeutic progress if he/she experiences this as a competitive defeat. This is likely to motivate acting out, a defensively or realistically altered representation of the situation as not involving competition between patient and therapist, or a reevaluation of the wished-for representation presumably based on insight into the dynamic.

Self-esteem refers to the person's affective valuation of the self, which may be momentary or enduring. *Self-presentation* (Jones & Pittman, 1982) refers to ways people present themselves behaviorally in order to influence other people's representations of them. Self-presentation strategies presuppose that people have *representations of others' representations of the self* as well as wished-for and feared representations of the way others view the self.

The distinctions above apply primarily to what William James (1890) called "the self as object," that is, the way one views oneself. The *sense of self*, akin to what James called "the self as subject," includes an experiential sense of self as thinker, feeler, and agent, as well as a sense of continuity in time, based on the relatively uninterrupted flow of consciousness. Perhaps the broadest category of self-experience, *identity*, encompasses a number of features, including this sense of self; a recognition of one's selfhood by the social milieu; a commitment to certain self-representations, ideal self-representations, and role relationships as centrally defining and worthy of investment; and acceptance of, or commitment to, some kind of implicit or explicit worldview that renders life meaningful both cognitively and emotionally (Epstein, 1990; Erikson, 1968).

METHODOLOGIES FOR ASSESSING DIMENSIONS OF SELF-STRUCTURE

The reader who has survived this barrage of definitions and distinctions may no doubt wonder whether the authors would have been better suited as tax accountants, or more personally, whether it has been worth slogging through this chapter. Rather than relying solely on cognitive dissonance to convince the reader that it has, we will shortly present what we believe is a more comprehensive portrait of the pathology of borderline self-structure. Before doing so, however, some words about method are in order.

If self-structure has many components, then there is little reason to believe that a single method is optimal for exploring them all. Clinical observation, and particularly observation of transferential processes in which patients bring their characteristic ways of thinking, feeling, wishing, and behaving into the treatment situation, provide an invaluable source of data about the elements of self-structural pathology of borderline patients. We have noted earlier, however, the limits of clinical observation in deciding among the competing psychoanalytic theories of borderline pathology, let alone among psychoanalytic and other theoretical viewpoints, so we focus here on methods that might allow more definitive hypothesis testing.

Different methods are likely to be optimal for assessing different dimensions of self-structure. Some dimensions are more amenable to self-report. Our experience has been that subjects are usually quite able to report on disruptions in the *sense* of self, such as dissociative episodes or periods of amnesia (see Silk, Lohr, Westen, & Goodrich, 1989). Questionnaire methods can thus be used to ask questions about these or similar experiences, such as whether the person feels like the same person from day to day, whether feelings or perceptions seem to be centered within the self or whether they sometimes seem to be outside the self, and so forth. In conducting pilot interviews, we asked questions that assess issues of sense of continuity through time, which could be readily addressed by questionnaire, such as whether the person has had name changes and under what circumstances, whether he/she felt the same while using different names, whether he/she has ever felt like a totally different person, and the like. Wiss (1991) recently completed a dissertation in which he developed a questionnaire (which he originally called the Wiss Integration of Self Scale—or WISS—demonstrating considerable integration himself) to assess this sense of integration.

For assessing self-representations, in contrast, self-report methods are far more limited despite their widespread use by researchers. The most obvious source of bias in self-reports is defensive—that people are motivated to see themselves in particular ways. With borderline patients this is frequently problematic in the direction opposite to what one finds in most people: Borderline patients often endorse every possible pathological item on any inventory, so that they may look more psychotic on the MMPI (Evans, Ruff, Breff, & Ainsworth, 1984), for example, than even schizophrenics. The potentially invalidating biases of self-report questionnaires have recently been demonstrated in research by Shedler, Mayman, and Manis (in press), who have found that subjects who report that they are mentally healthy and happy on various indices but who are assessed as psychologically unhealthy on the basis of their early memories can be distinguished from subjects who are psychologically healthy in both assessments on a number of dimensions, including cardiac functioning. Weinberger's (1990) research on repressive personality styles similarly documents the tremendous impact of defensive biases of this sort on self-reported data.

Cognitive biases and limitations also render self-reports highly problematic as a way of assessing self-representations. There is little reason to believe that people can gain access to unconscious schematic processes, such as the activation of self-schemas (see Nisbett & Wilson, 1977), so that their self-reports are likely to be post hoc constructions of what they *think* they must think about themselves. Further, many representations of self only become accessible in the context of specific relationship experiences and are not likely to be represented as part of a prototypical conscious self-concept. Many borderline patients, for example, have a view of themselves as evil and contaminating, but they would be unlikely to report that on a standard self-concept inventory except under very particular circumstances. The optimal way to gain access to the representations that are probably the most important—that is, self-with-someone-who-matters—is, of course, to engage the patient in a relationship, as in a therapeutic relationship. An important distinction to bear in mind here is between the working representations that guide information processing at any given time (and that are largely unconscious), and the self-consciously generalized self-concept that people will typically divulge in answering questionnaire items about themselves.

Researchers have begun to think creatively about ways to go beyond assessment of the prototypical self-concepts that are readily available to researchers but are probably functionally far less important than the self-representations that emerge in social interactions. For example, Ogilvie and Ashmore (1991) have developed a procedure for assessing self-with-other schemas by having subjects rate themselves on a set of dimensions across a large number of relationships of their choosing. A hierarchical-classes analysis then reduces the data on each subject to a small set of clusters of prominent self-with-other themes, that is, ways the person describes the self-with-others that seem to cut across a subset of relationships.

Drawing upon Ogilvie and Ashmore's work as well as upon the interview techniques employed in Main and Goldwyn's Adult Attachment Interview (Main, Kaplan, & Cassidy, 1985) and Luborsky and Crits-Christoph's (1990) Relationship Anecdotes Paradigm (RAP) Test, we have been piloting an interview procedure for assessing several dimensions of self-representations across relationships. Initially we asked subjects to describe themselves at different ages and at periods in which they were relatively happy and stable as well as unhappy and unstable; they were then asked to describe what they believed to be continuities and discontinuities. We intended to code their self-descriptions at different periods for similarity, integration, and so forth, as well as to assess the extent to which they could provide a coherent representation of themselves and their history. Although this yielded some interesting data, it did not transcend many of the problems of self-reports adumbrated above because we were largely assessing subjects' conscious ability to synthesize representations (or meta-representations) that cut across many domains and eras. Borderline patients may well differ from others in their inability to do that successfully, but that is only one dimension of self-structure, and not likely to be the most important dimension of their self pathology.

In our latest version of the interview, subjects are first asked to describe a series of important relationships (such as those with mother, father, lover, important friend, disliked other, and child, if applicable). After providing a global characterization of a particular relationship, subjects are then requested to describe three to five specific episodes with that person that were meaningful or problematic in some way. As in Luborsky's RAP Test, administration is similar to that used in eliciting Thematic Apperception Test (TAT) responses. When subjects have completed this part of the interview, which has been used previously for assessing patterns of object relations and social cognition (for a more complete description of this part of the procedure, see Block, 1990), they are instructed to go back and describe themselves in each episode, then more generally within each relationship across episodes, then more generally across relationships. Finally, they are asked to describe themselves more generally at different points in their lives, as described above.

The aim of this procedure is to elicit narrative material that allows assessment of both implicit representations of self, revealed in episode descriptions, and conscious beliefs about the self, abstracted across episodes, relationships, and eras. Episode descriptions, self-in-relationship descriptions, self-across-relationship descriptions, and self-across-time descriptions can be coded for their complexity, integration, and affective quality. In addition, episode descriptions can be compared with one another within and across relationships for recurrent thematic content and degree of overlap in self-representations.

DIMENSIONS OF SELF PATHOLOGY IN BORDERLINE PERSONALITY DISORDER

We are still piloting this procedure and hence cannot yet report any statistically meaningful findings. In what follows, however, we use examples from pilot interviews with borderline patients reliably and validly diagnosed using the Diagnostic Interview for Borderline Patients (Gunderson, Kolb, & Austin, 1981) to flesh out the different dimensions of self pathology that appear to be present in borderline patients from clinical and research experience. We hope that subsequent research will shed light on the extent to which the clinically derived assertions that follow provide an accurate portrait of the pathology of borderline patients in this domain. In what follows, we briefly examine each dimension of self delineated earlier, applying the distinctions of different aspects of self to Borderline Personality Disorder.

Self-representations

Several features characterize the self-representations of borderline patients. The first, acknowledged by all theorists, is that these representations are *split*; that is, the patient has difficulty keeping contradictory representations, particularly representations of differing affective qualities, in consciousness simultaneously. More broadly, contradictory representations seem to come to mind for borderline patients one after another, and the patient often does not see the need to integrate them or to recognize the contradiction. Thus, one might hypothesize two processes involved in the production of split conscious representations: The first is a primary tendency for conscious activation of only one representation at a time; the second is a secondary deactivation of the self-observational or metacognitive processes by which a person typically monitors ongoing thought for coherence and accuracy. These processes could potentially reflect cognitive-structural properties of borderline social cognition, defensive strategies, or both.

The responses of several pilot subjects demonstrate the transitory, split, poorly integrated quality of borderline self-representations. One patient described changes in herself over time in black-and-white terms: "I was always a person who could do anything and now I can't do nothing." The fleeting and contradictory nature of borderline representations is revealed in another subject's depiction of her experience of her mother reading to her as a child: "I loved it. The books were enjoyable to me . . . and being close to my mother. [Interviewer: So there was a feeling of closeness with her?] Well, in a way . . . Um, I never let her know what was really going on with me. I told her everything that was really nothing and nothing that really meant anything." The subject then continued, without noting or commenting on the contradiction between the two ways she had just described experiencing the situation with her mother. The same subject, in describing herself as a child of 6 or 7, stated: "I was a good kid. I can't ever remember causing trouble. I was well liked by teachers and peers. I was very active. [Interviewer: Is that all?] I would say that I was disturbed at that age. [Interviewer: How do you mean?] I can remember being emotionally unstable and sometimes becoming physically ill. I can remember crying a lot and throwing temper tantrums." One should note here not only the lack of awareness of contradictions in the account but also the egocentrism in not imagining the listener's perspective; even if the subject did not see her account as contradictory, she should have recognized that the interviewer might be confused by the seeming discrepancy.

An important point to note is that we really do not know what the difficulties borderline patients have in integrating conscious representations imply about the enduring unconscious organization of representations (in more cognitive terms, their organization in long-term memory or the structure of schemas or networks of association). Associational networks may not be as densely connected as they should be across different affective categories of self, so that activation of "good" representations does not spread activation to, or prime, "bad" representations. Alternatively, the inhibition of recognition of contradictory elements may occur defensively at the time of activation of working representations. In the latter case, splitting would not be a structural property of the organization of the unconscious schemas or representations of self.

A second feature of borderline self-representations is a tendency to differentiate poorly between representations of self and of others, as when a patient who was manifestly hostile to a therapist evaluating her persisted in asserting that the therapist was being hostile. As noted by the theorists described earlier, borderline patients do not manifest the level of disturbance in this regard as do psychotics, who may believe that images or voices in their heads are actually external to them. One does see in borderline patients, however, "soft signs" of poor differentiation, which can sometimes lead to mistaken diagnosis of psychosis by clinicians who are inexperienced or who think less in terms of the phenomenology of the patient than in terms of a standard checklist of psychotic symptoms. For example, borderline patients will sometimes answer "yes" to a question about hearing voices, but upon further questioning one finds that these are generally poorly integrated superego components ("I can always hear in my head my mother telling me how awful I am") and that the patient does not really believe they are external.

A third aspect is the profoundly negative content of self-representations, which theorists such as Kernberg describe as a sense of "primitive badness." One patient, in describing her experience of confession to a priest as a child, noted, "When I was younger, I was always afraid that the devil would be able to reach up between the headboard and the mattress and pull me into hell. [Interviewer: What do you think the priest was feeling and thinking?] He must have felt repulsion. He must have just felt repulsion. [Interviewer: At what?] Me."

One should not lose sight of the fact that these aspects of borderline self-representation are not present at all times. What may distinguish borderline patients is not an all-or-none functioning at a globally lower level of object relations than neurotic patients, but a vulnerability to activation of certain pathological processes under particular situations. In fact, our pilot subjects at several points demonstrated impressive insight into themselves and complexity of self-representation. Studies of the representations of borderline patients in TAT responses have similarly documented the capacity of borderline patients at times to provide very complex, if sometimes highly distorted, representations (Westen, Ludolph, Lerner, Ruffins, & Wiss, 1990).

Self-with-Other Representations

Perhaps the most striking phenomenon observed in our pilot interviews with borderline patients thus far has been the regularity across subjects of three aspects of their self-with-other representations. The first is one of content: In line both with clinical observation and with several studies documenting the malevolent relationship schemas of borderline patients (Bell, Billington, & Cicchetti, 1988; Nigg, Lohr, Gold, & Silk, 1992; Westen, Lohr, Silk, Gold, & Kerber, 1990), the subjects we interviewed repeatedly described interpersonal interactions in which self and others fell into the roles of victim and victimizer. This prominent relationship paradigm probably reflects a number of pathological processes: the social learning of malevolent expectations through disrupted, unempathic, or abusive caretaking; the projection of aggressive impulses onto others; the tendency to experience interpersonal events in an egocentric and need-gratifying way, so that failure to have one's needs met elicits a feeling of having been deliberately abused; and an interpersonal stance designed to elicit both saving responses and abuse and avoidance from others. The second aspect of borderline relationship paradigms, or self-with-other schemas, also in accord with clinical observation and theory, was the interchangeability of self and other in these schemas (see Fast, 1985; Kernberg, 1975): Although the self was generally the victim when victimization themes were prominent, with many relationship paradigms the roles could reverse in an instant. Third was the remarkable fluidity and transitory nature of these relationship schemas, which, like the self-representations described above, would often come into consciousness one after another, with minimal apparent recognition by the subject of their shifting presence or their sometimes contradictory nature.

The interchangeability of self and other along an affective or role axis is illustrated in the description by one subject of an incident in which a friend came to stay with her because the friend "always hated being alone when her husband was gone." When asked what she, herself, was thinking and feeling during the incident, the subject replied, "Just fortunate that I had that person I knew I could depend on, that I knew I could call a friend"; when then asked what was on her friend's mind, she replied, "I think she was enjoying the friendship and the source of someone to be depended on. . . . She knew that she had someone that she could call on in a time of need." In this example, self and other momentarily shift as the subject describes herself as the one doing the depending; the role relationship then shifts back as her friend once again becomes the needy one. One might hypothesize that this is a person for whom dependency and concerns about being safe and nurtured are so intense that she quickly overidentifies with these qualities when observed in another person. She thus experiences many of the same feelings, and activates many of the same self-representations, whether she is in the role of the nurturer or the nurtured. One could see how such a tendency could be highly problematic in parenting, particularly in dealing with a toddler or adolescent struggling for a sense of autonomy and wrestling with conflicts between dependence and strivings for independence.

Wished-for, Feared, and Ideal Self-representations

Several features are characteristic of the evaluative representations of borderline patients, that is, the representations of wished-for, feared, and ideal self that are compared with actual representations. One aspect is their all-or-nothing nature: Borderline patients often seem to represent their wishes, fears, and ideals as states that are either totally achieved or totally not achieved (in statistical language, they seem to represent them as categorical rather than continuous variables). When compared with similarly black-and-white representations of actual self, the discrepancies between, for example, wished-for and cognized self, are consequently enormous and total. These seemingly absolute discrepancies elicit unmodulated and extreme affects, which in turn elicit dysfunctional behavioral and intrapsychic responses, such as wrist cutting or massive reality-distorting defenses. For example, borderline patients sometimes appear to lack a capacity for experiencing guilt because even minor transgressions elicit major discrepancies between representations of self as totally bad and ideal self-representations of self as totally good; the result is that the patient projects her/his own misdeed onto the victim, becomes furious, and/or denies any guilt in order to prevent being overwhelmed by it. This reflects what some analytic observers refer to as a primitive and punitive superego (Kernberg, 1975). One might hypothesize that repeated events of this sort in childhood could lead to the failure to develop certain processes that underlie moral development, such as the capacity to recognize and appropriately respond to graded guilt signals.

A second characteristic of the evaluative representations of borderline patients is that wished-for, feared, and ideal self-representations are frequently highly unrealistic and may at times be confused with, or poorly differentiated from, actual representations. Such patients may thus experience or be motivated by childhood fears of themselves as monstrous, contaminating, or unlovable, which were forged in problematic attachment relationships. Kernberg (1975) similarly described the way patients with severe narcissistic pathology fuse or poorly differentiate self-representations and ideal self-representations.

Third, wished-for and ideal self-representations are often highly transitory in borderline individuals, who have difficulty investing in values, standards, or goal-states involving the self over time. The identity diffusion of borderline patients, to be described below, frequently includes a lack of enduring values and particularly of ideal self-standards. Asked about her goals and values, one patient responded, "Wow! Values. . . . Run the question by me again. . . . Well, my children, they were the most important things to me, they were my goals really, to raise them and see them be happy and productive and healthy. My goals are gone now. I have none. I'm just going one day at a time." When queried about the ways her goals and values had changed over time, she replied, "They are gone. . . . Somewhere, I've got to find something again to just get going for." As will be noted below, part of this reflects the borderline patient's constant need to take action to avoid dysphoric affect or to attain momentary gratification. This leads to abrupt and impulsive activities and precludes adherence to long-term plans.

Self-esteem

The self-esteem of borderline patients is subject to extreme fluctuation, particularly in a negative direction. Self-esteem includes both a normal baseline of self-feeling and momentary fluctuations, as particular representations are activated and constructed and are compared with evaluative representations such as ideal self-representations. The normal baseline of self-esteem in borderline patients is frequently very low, the capacity to regulate and modulate fluctuations in self-esteem is typically highly impaired, and the availability and accessibility of severely devalued representations of self is generally much greater than in nonborderline individuals. As one patient put it, "I have never really felt all that good about myself. I always lacked a sense of belonging in any situation, even in my own family. I used to tell people that they really weren't my brothers and sisters, [that] I was the adopted one."

An important question is the extent to which borderline self-esteem differs from the self-esteem of other patients who can become severely depressed. Although answers to that question will require further research, we would hypothesize the following differences. First, in nonborderline patients vulnerable to major depression, "total badness" representations of the type that are potentially always active in borderline patients are only active and accessible episodically. Second, borderlines have greater fluctuations in self-esteem than unipolar depressives because of nonepisodic, characterological difficulty regulating their affects, as well as difficulty consciously and unconsciously regulating mood-congruent cognitive processes (such as seeing life as totally bleak when upset) and attributional processes. Third, the representations underlying poor self-esteem in borderlines are more transitory in their activation than the representations of other depressed patients and hence can come and go in a matter of minutes or hours.

Self-presentation

Perhaps the major feature of the self-presentation of borderline patients is the extent to which these individuals become overly absorbed in current interactions to the extent that they lose contact with any ongoing sense of who they are, and feel as if they are nothing but their self-presentations. It is as if they adopt a dramatic role that they believe is demanded by the situation and then throw themselves into it totally: They become poor players who strut and fret their hour on the stage and lose their selfhood in the process of playing the part. Deutsch (1942) described this as the "as-if" quality of borderline object relations, the seemingly total adoption of different identities at different times, which sometimes gives these patients a chameleonlike appearance. Numerous theorists, such as Winnicott (1971) and Masterson (1985), have similarly described the "false self" of such patients. Our pilot subjects frequently spoke of the power of the masks they wear and the paradoxical sense of self-definition—but also the alienation—they feel while donning them. For example, when asked how someone who likes her might describe her, one subject replied, "See, it depends, because I put a mask on a lot of times and I pretend to be fine and so they see me as energetic and outgoing, and they envy that I can just go out and get a lot of things done, and you know, just be okay. But I know some of them would know that inside I am not okay." Another patient similarly commented, "People never knew how emotionally disturbed I was. I was able to play my game and pretend and put on that happy face and never let anybody see through me."

Sense of Self

The subjective sense of self is usually disrupted significantly in borderline patients. The sense of continuity of experience and of the self as the subjective center of one's thoughts and feelings is often disrupted by dissociative experiences in which the person feels unreal or experiences thoughts and feelings as outside the self (on dissociative experiences in BPD, see Chopra & Beatson, 1986; Silk et al., 1989; Zanarini, Gunderson, & Frankenburg, 1990). A sense of continuity of self can also be disrupted by the tendency to experience wide oscillations of mood, which leaves the person feeling like several different people, each defined by a particular mood state.

The sense of self as agent of one's actions is disrupted in many borderline patients, in part by their tendency to turn impulses immediately into actions, which leaves them with a subjective sense of not having been the author of the act. The tendency to behave in highly irrational ways that they often cannot themselves explain, such as self-mutilation, also leads to disturbances in the sense of agency.

Identity

More generally, borderline patients experience a diffusion of identity manifest in a number of ways. The lack of consistently invested goals, values, ideals, and relationships over time—or the temporary hyperinvestment in totalistic (Lifton, 1963) value systems that offer black-and-white interpretations of events or in idealized and hypercathected relationships—leads to a sense of emptiness and meaninglessness and to a lack of coherence to the way the person behaves. Gross inconsistencies in behavior over time and across situations contribute to what is, in some respects, an accurate self-perception of incoherence. This sense of the self as incoherent or poorly integrated also reflects the difficulty borderline patients have in pulling together representations of self that integrate multiple aspects of their experience. One patient described her lack of identity this way: "I actually don't know what I am or who I am right now."

An important aspect of the identity confusion or diffusion of borderline patients is the lack of a coherent personal history, life narrative, or sense of self as having a retrievable past. The historical memory of borderline patients is often filled with large gaps or discontinuities, or the self is represented as totally different during different life periods. One subject, who was unable to remember several years of her childhood and could not even recognize herself in pictures from that period, described her sense of radical discontinuity in the self over historical time: "I feel like I am a completely different person than I used to be. I know I am. So basically nothing is the same, except that I am the same height" [subject laughs]."

Another factor that probably contributes to the borderline patient's sense of discontinuity over time is as much interpersonal as intrapsychic. Much of a person's history is interpersonal, including episodic memories of incidents in which one interacted with others. When people end important relationships, they often experience a sense of loss of important memories or pieces of their past because the memory can no longer be shared with the person involved, and no one else can really fully comprehend the experience (e.g., a wonderful Broadway musical seen with another, one person helping the other through a personal tragedy, a wedding ceremony). For borderline patients, who cannot sustain many long-term relationships, life is, in certain respects, a series of disconnected episodes with people who come and go from their lives in an uninterrupted stream. Even fundamental aspects of self, such as meaningful nicknames, are often lost as the relationships in which they emerged dissipate. To the extent that identity is socially constructed, the failure to sustain intimate social relationships with family, friends, and lovers will lead to a tenuous sense of identity.

CONCLUSION: THE ETIOLOGY OF DEFECTIVE SELF-STRUCTURE IN BPD

We have distinguished several dimensions of self-structure and described the pathology of borderline patients along these dimensions. This is not to say, of course, that these dimensions are entirely independent of one another; self-esteem, for example, is obviously dependent in large measure on the content of representations chronically or momentarily activated. Nevertheless, we have tried to show that the self pathology of borderline patients is multifaceted. In concluding, a few words about etiology are in order.

Precisely what leads to borderline psychopathology is a matter of considerable debate (see Gunderson, 1984). Research points to problematic attachment relationships in childhood, chaotic family experience, a history of losses from caretakers who seem less than adequate and empathic, sexual abuse, and family history of psychopathology (Loranger, Oldham, & Tullis, 1982; Ogata et al., 1990; Soloff & Millward, 1983; Ludolph et al., 1990). Whether each of these factors is equally contributory to every dimension of self pathology in borderline patients is debatable but seems unlikely. Dissociative experiences in borderline patients, for example, have been linked empirically to the history of sexual abuse found in many such patients (Ogata et al., 1990), as has the tendency to form poorly bounded representations in which the perspectives of self and others are confused (Westen, Ludolph, Block, Wixom, & Wiss, 1990). Failure to establish long-term goals and ideals, in contrast, may be more likely derived from early failures in identification with parents who are inconsistent, abusive, or poorly attuned in ways described by Kohut, or who are threatened themselves by the child's autonomous strivings as described by Masterson (1976).

Some of the more subtle interpersonal processes involved in pathological attachment relationships in early childhood described by many theorists have not yet been tested empirically by researchers who study Borderline Personality Disorder, but they should not be discarded without careful empirical examination. For example, chronically inconsistent or inaccurate reflected appraisals of the child's needs, feelings, or attributes could lead to distortions in self-representation and sense of self, and could reflect the caretaker's lack of empathy or relative absorption in her own needs rather than in those of the young child. Similarly, having a caretaker who cannot tolerate separation and autonomy from the child seems likely to distort various dimensions of self in ways posited by psychoanalytic theorists. Constitutional factors should also be considered. These include a tendency to experience a flooding of rage that engenders defensive efforts to protect positive representations, as described by Kernberg; a more general deficit in affect regulation, as described by Linehan (1987) and Westen (1991b), which could lead to polarized representations and difficulty integrating representations associated with different affects (because of mood-congruent schematic processes); and subclinical expressions of biologically influenced mood disturbances such as bipolar disorder.

Psychoanalytic theories have offered the most comprehensive and clinically sophisticated understanding of pathological self-structure in borderline patients, and have endeavored to link the disorder as a whole to a small number of relatively nonspecific factors such as poor maternal attunement. The complexity of trying to understand the etiology of pathological self-structure in borderlines is magnified, however, when one acknowledges that "the self" is a many-splendored thing, that different dimensions of self pathology may be influenced to a greater or lesser extent by different etiological variables, and that the same pathology may not reflect the same etiology in all borderline patients. Whether a better understanding of the influence and interaction of various etiologically significant variables will lead to advances in treatment, or whether the primary curative elements will remain less specific factors—the experience of being and identifying with a supportive and empathic therapist, clarification of defenses against more accurate and integrated representations, or the development of skills for affect regulation—remains to be seen.

REFERENCES

Adler, G. (1981). The borderline-narcissistic personality disorder continuum. *American Journal of Psychiatry*, *138*, 46–50.

Adler, G. (1989). Uses and limitations of Kohut's self psychology in the treatment of borderline patients. *Journal of the American Psychoanalytic Association*, *37*, 761–785.

Adler, G., & Buie, D. H. (1979). Aloneness and borderline psychopathology: The possible relevance of child development issues. *International Journal of Psycho-Analysis*, *60*, 83–96.

American Psychiatric Association. (1987). *Diagnostic and statistical manual of mental disorders* (3rd ed., rev.). Washington, DC: Author.

Baldwin, M. W. (in press). Relational schemas and the processing of social information. *Psychological Bulletin.*

Baldwin, M. W., Carrell, S. E., & Lopez, D. F. (in press). Priming relationship-schemas: My advisor and the Pope are watching me from the back of my mind. *Journal of Experimental Social Psychology, 26* 435–454.

Bell, M. B., Billington, R., & Cicchetti, D. (1988). Do object relations deficits distinguish BPD from othr diagnostic groups? *Journal of Clinical Psychology*, *44*, 511–516.

Block, M. J. (1990). *Mothers of female adolescents with borderline personality disorder: Intrapsychic and social funcioning*. Unpublished doctoral dissertation, University of Michigan, Ann Arbor.

Buie, D. H., & Adler, G. (1982). Definitive treatment of the borderline personality. *International Journal of Psychoanalytic Psychotherapy*, *9*, 51–87.

Brenner, C. (1982). *The mind in conflict.* New York: International Universities Press.

Chopra, H. D., & Beatson, J. A. (1986). Psychotic symptoms in borderline personality disorder. *American Journal of Psychiatry*, *143*, 1605–1607.

Deutsch, H. (1942). Some forms of emotional disturbance and their relationship to schizophrenia. *Psychoanalytic Quarterly, 11,* 307–321.

Eagle, M. (1984). *Recent developments in psychoanalysis.* New York: McGraw-Hill.

Epstein, S. (1973). The self-concept resisited, or, a theory of a theory. *American Psychologist, 28,* 404–416.

Epstein, S. (1990). Cognitive–experiential self theory. In L. Pervin (Ed.), *Handbook of personality: Theory and research* (pp. 165–192). New York: Guilford Press.

Erikson, E. (1968). *Identity: Youth and crisis.* New York: Basic Books.

Evans, R., Ruff, R., Breff, D., & Ainsworth, T. (1984). MMPI characteristics of borderline personality inpatients. *Journal of Nervous and Mental Disease*, *172*, 742–748.

Fast, I. (1985). *Event theory*. Hillsdale, NJ: Lawrence Erlbaum.

Gunderson, J. G. (1984). *Borderline personality disorders*. Washington, DC: American Psychiatric Press.

Gunderson, J. G., Kolb, J. E., & Austin, V. (1981). The Diagnostic Interview for Borderline Patients. *American Journal of Psychiatry*, *138*, 896–901.

Higgins, E. T. (1990). Personality, social psychology, and person–situation relations: Standards and knowledge activation as a common language. In L. Pervin (Ed.), *Handbook of personality: Theory and research* (pp. 301–338). New York: Guilford Press.

Horowitz, M. J. (1988). *Introduction to psychodynamics: A synthesis*. New York: Basic Books.

Horowitz, M. J., & Zilberg, N. (1983). Regressive alterations of the self-concept. *American Journal of Psychiatry, 140*, 284–289.

James, W. (1890). *The principles of psychology*. New York: Henry Holt.

Jones, E. E., & Pittman, T. S. (1982). Toward a general theory of strategic self-presentation. In J. Suls (Ed.), *Psychological perspectives on the self*. Hillsdale, NJ: Lawrence Erlbaum.

Kernberg, O. (1975). *Borderline conditions and pathological narcissism*. New York: Jason Aronson.

Kernberg, O. F., Selzer, M. A., Koenigsberg, H. W., Carr, A. C., & Appelbaum, A. H. (1989). *Psychodynamic psychotherapy of borderline patients*. New York: Basic Books.

Klein, R. (1989). Introduction to the disorders of the self. In J. F. Masterson & R. Klein (Eds.), *Psychotherapy of the disorders of the self*. New York: Brunner/Mazel.

Kohut, H. (1971). *The analysis of the self: A systematic appraoch to the treatment of narcissistic personality disorders*. New York: International Universities Press.

Kohut, H. (1977). *The restoration of the self*. New York: International Universities Press.

Kohut, H. (1984). *How does analysis cure?* (A. Goldberg, Ed., with collaboration of P. E. Stepansky). Chicago: University of Chicago Press.

Lifton, R. J. (1963). *Thought reform and the psychology of totalism: A study of "brainwashing" in China*. New York: W. W. Norton.

Linehan, M. (1987). Dialectical behavior therapy and borderline personality disorder: Theory and method. *Bulletin of the Menninger Clinic, 51*, 261–276.

Loranger, A., Oldham, J., & Tullis, E. (1982). Familial transmission of DSM-III borderline personality disorder. *Archives of General Psychiatry, 39*, 795–799.

Luborksy, L., & Crits-Christoph, P. (1990). *Understanding transference: The core conflictual relationship theme method*. New York: Basic Books.

Ludolph, P., Westen, D., Misle, B., Jackson, A., Wixom, J., & Wiss, F. C. (1990). The borderline diagnosis in adolescents: Symptoms and developmental history. *American Journal of Psychiatry, 147*, 470–476.

Mahler, M. S. (1971). A study of the separation–individuation process and its possible application to borderline phenomena in the psychoanalytic situation. *Psychoanalytic Study of the Child, 26*, 403–424.

Mahler, M. S., Pine, F., & Bergman, A. (1975). *The psychological birth of the human infant: Symbiosis and individuation*. New York: Basic Books.

Main, M., Kaplan, N., & Cassidy, J. (1985). Security in infancy, childhood, and adulthood: A move to the level of representation. In I. Bretherton & E. Waters (Eds.), Growing points of attachment theory and research. *Mono-*

graphs of the Society for Research in Child Development, 50(1–2, Serial No. 209), 67–104.

Markus, H. (1977). Self-schemata and processing infromation about the self. *Journal of Personality and Social Psychology, 35*, 63–78.

Markus, H., & Cross, S. (1990). The interpersonal self. In L. Pervin (Ed.), *Handbook of personality: Theory and research* (pp. 576–608). New York: Guilford Press.

Markus, H., & Nurius, P. (1986). Possible selves. *American Psychologist, 41*, 954–969.

Masterson, J. F. (1976). *Psychotherapy of the borderline adult*. New York: Brunner/Mazel.

Masterson, J. F. (1985). *The real self: A developmental, self, and object relations approach*. New York: Brunner/Mazel.

Masterson, J. F., & Klein, R. (Eds.). (1989). *Psychotherapy of the disorders of the self: The Masterson approach*. New York: Brunner/Mazel.

Nigg, J., Lohr, N. E., Westen, D., Gold, L., & Silk, K. R. (1992). Malevolent object representations in borderline personality disorder and major depression. *Journal of Abnormal Psychology, 101*, 61–67.

Nisbett, R. E., & Wilson, T. D. (1977). Telling more than we can know: Verbal reports on mental processes. *Psychological Review, 84*, 231–259.

Ogata, S., Silk, K. R., Goodrich, S., Lohr, N. E., Westen, D., & Hill, E. (1990). Childhood abuse and clinical symptoms in borderline personality disorder. *American Journal of Psychiatry, 147*, 1008–1013.

Ogilvie, D., & Ashmore, R. (1991). Self-with-other representations as a unit of analysis in self-concept research. In R. C. Curtis (Ed.), *The relational self: Theoretical convergences in psychoanalysis and social psychology* (pp. 282–314). New York: Guilford Press.

Peterfreund, E. (1978). Some critical comments on the psychoanalytic conceptualization of infancy. *International Journal of Psycho-Analysis, 59*, 427–441.

Robbins, M. (1989). Primitive personality organization as an interpersonally adaptive modification of cognition and affect. *International Journal of Psycho-Analysis, 70*, 443–459.

Rogers, K. (1959). A theory of therapy, personality, and interpersonal relationships. In S. Koch (Ed.), *Psychology: A study of a science* (Vol. 3.). New York: McGraw-Hill.

Sandler, J. (1987). *From safety to the superego: Selected papers of Joseph Sandler*. New York: Guilford Press.

Sandler, J., & Rosenblatt, B. (1962). The concept of the representational world. *Psychoanalytic Study of the Child, 17*, 128–145.

Segal, Z. (1988). Appraisal of the self-schema construct in cognitive models of depression. *Psychological Bulletin, 103*, 147–162.

Shea, M. T., Glass, D. R., Pilkonis, P. A., Watkins, J., & Docherty, J. P. (1987). Frequency and implications of personality disorders in a sample of depressed outpatients. *Journal of Personality Disorders, 1*, 27–42.

Shedler, J., Mayman, M., & Manis, M. (in press). The illusion of mental health. *American Psychologist*.

Silk, K. R., Lohr, N. E., Westen, D., & Goodrich, S. (1989). Psychosis in borderline patients with depression. *Journal of Personality Disorders, 3*, 92–100.

Singer, J., & Salovey, P. (1991). Organized knowledge structures and personality: Person schemas, self-schemas, prototypes, and scripts. In M. J. Horowitz (Ed.), *Person schemas and recurrent maladaptive interpersonal patterns*. Chicago: University of Chicago Press.

Soloff, P, & Millward, J. (1983). Developmental histories of borderline patients. *Comprehensive Psychiatry, 24*, 574–588.

Stern, D. (1985). *The interpersonal world of the infant: A view from psychoanalysis and developmental psychology*. New York: Basic Books.

Sullivan, H. S. (1953). *The interpersonal theory of psychiatry*. New York: W. W. Norton.

Weinberger, D. A. (1990). The construct validity of the repressive coping style. In J. L. Singer (Ed.), *Repression and dissociation*. Chicago: University of Chicago Press.

Westen, D. (1985). *Self and society: Narcissism, collectivism, and the development of morals*. New York: Cambridge University Press.

Westen, D. (1989). Are "primitive" object relations really preoedipal? *American Journal of Orthopsychiatry, 59*, 331–345.

Westen, D. (1990a). The relations among narcissism, egocentrism, self-concept, and self-esteem. *Psychoanalysis and Contemporary Thought, 13*, 185–241.

Westen, D. (1990b). Toward a revised theory of borderline object relations: Implications of empirical research. *International Journal of Psycho-Analysis, 71*, 661–693.

Westen, D. (1991a). Cultural, emotional, and unconscious aspects of self. In R. Curtis (Ed.), *The relational self: Theoretical convergences in psychoanalysis and social psychology* (pp. 181–210) New York: Guilford Press.

Westen, D. (1991b). Cognitive-behavioral interventions in the psychodynamic psychotherapy of borderline personality disorders. *Clinical Psychology Review, 11*, 211–230.

Westen, D. (1992). The cognitive self and the psychoanalytic self: Can we put our selves together? *Psychological Inquiry, 3*, 1–13.

Westen, D., Lohr, N., Silk, K., Gold, L., & Kerber, K. (1990). Object relations and social cognition in borderlines, major depressives, and normals: A TAT analysis. *Psychological Assessment: A Journal of Consulting and Clinical Psychology, 2*, 355–364.

Westen, D., Ludolph, P., Block, J., Wixom, J., Wiss, F. C. (1990). Developmental history and object relations in psychiatrically disturbed adolescent females. *American Journal of Psychiatry, 147*, 1061–1068.

Westen, D., Ludolph, P., Lerner, H., Ruffins, S., & Wiss, F. C. (1990). Object relations in borderline adolescents. *Journal of the American Academy of Child and Adolescent Psychiatry, 29*, 338–348.

Westen, D., Moses, M. J., Silk, K. R., Lohr, N. E., Cohen, R., & Segal, H. (1992). Quality of depressive experience in borderline personality disorder and major depression: When depression is not just depression. *Journal of Personality Disorders, 6*, 383–392.

Winnicott, D. W. (1971). *Playing and reality*. New York: Basic Books. Wiss, F. C. (1991). *Aspects of the self*. Unpublished doctoral dissertation, University of Michigan, Ann Arbor.

Wixom, J. M. (1988). *The depressive experiences of adolescents with borderline personality disorder*. Unpublished doctoral dissertation, University of Michigan, Ann Arbor.

Zanarini, M. C., Gunderson, J. G., & Frankenburg, F. R. (1990). Cognitive features of borderline personality disorder. *American Journal of Psychiatry*, *147*, 57–63.

Commentary

Marsha M. Linehan
Heidi L. Heard
University of Washington

IN THEIR CHAPTER, Drew Westen and Robert Cohen begin with a review of the three major psychoanalytic theories of Borderline Personality Disorder (BDP). They succinctly highlight the theoreticians' major ideas and then provide an evaluation of these theories. Although we generally concur with their points, we have a few comments, which is to say, we will critique their critique of the psychodynamic theories of BPD. Next, Westen and Cohen review current definitions of self and self-representation, once more examining the "barrage of definitions" that interfere with theoretical and empirical progress. We mostly agree with their arguments here too, but again we have a few remarks to make. Following their review of previous work, Westen and Cohen describe an emerging methodology they are developing to study self-representation among clinical populations. Then, using interview transcripts from several pilot subjects, they construct and describe a number of theoretical positions about self-representation among borderline individuals and the role of such self-representation in the etiology and maintenance of borderline behaviors. Most of our discussion will relate to the authors' methodology and emerging theoretical positions.

Before beginning our discussion, a word about how we will proceed and about the dilemmas that appraising Westen and Cohen has created for us. When one has a clearly defined theoretical position on a topic, critiquing a divergent theoretical position usually elicits a tendency to note all areas of disagreement and to buttress one's own points with the appropriate favorable arguments. The desire to be proved "right" when a competing position is offered usually leads one to assume that the other position must be "wrong" in some important ways. The dialogue between behavioral and psychodynamic therapists is replete with such arguments. The theorist-splitting that has occurred as a result of this resembles the staff-splitting that so often occurs in the treatment of Borderline Personality Disorder. This "if we're right, you're wrong" thinking exemplifies the black-and-white, polarized, nondialectical thinking (or splitting in psychodynamic terms) we ordinarily accuse our borderline clients of doing. We believe that this approach will restrict, not advance, the field of psychology. We will thus attempt to highlight the contradictory positions that we maintain with respect to Westen and Cohen's positions, and then try to find the syntheses and convergences in our ideas.

STRENGTHS AND LIMITATIONS OF PSYCHOANALYTIC APPROACHES

Point 1: Westen and Cohen compare psychoanalytic with cognitive approaches to BDP and suggest that a weakness of cognitive theories is that they fail to distinguish the self-schemas of depressed borderline clients from those of other depressed clients. The authors state that a further advantage of psychodynamic theories is that they emphasize "understanding and altering the structure of unconscious representations." Unfortunately, they do not identify the cognitive theories of borderline disorder to which they allude. Recent theoretical positions of Beck and his colleagues (Beck & Freeman, 1990) seem to clearly propose that cognitive schemas of borderline, depressed (and nondepressed) clients differ in complex ways from nonborderline depressed clients. Whether cognitive schemas, particularly those related to self, prove to be important factors in the development and maintenance of the disorder is, of course, an empirical question still to be tested.

We suspect that Westen and Cohen's critique of cognitive theory is based on their application of standard cognitive theories of depression to the problem of BPD. In other words, the criticism is actually that (until recently) cognitive theorists did not recognize or attend to borderline disorder as a condition that could influence the development, course, and treatment of any other coexisting disorder. Westen and Cohen could have strengthened their argument here if they had included the entire spectrum of cognitive–behavioral and behavioral therapies. From our perspective, this is one of the great strengths of the psychoanalytic school, namely that they recognized, studied, and attempted to understand a class of clients who did not respond to classical applications of their own therapy. As Linehan has noted elsewhere (Linehan, in press), the position that psychoanalysis holds in this regard is most likely a function of its longer history. Psychoanalysts began discussing "borderline" clients in the third decade after Freud first presented psychoanalysis as a method of therapy. Interestingly, as cognitive, behavioral and cognitive–behavioral schools have matured, they too have turned from defending the efficacy of their therapeutic approaches to analyzing their own failures (see Foa & Emmelkamp, 1983)—once again in the third decade or so after their "founding." Thus, in terms of the history of both schools, the focus on developing theories specific to Borderline Personality Disorder have occurred at approximately the same points.

Point 2: Westen and Cohen list two strengths of psychoanalytic conceptions of borderline self-structure. The first is that the theories have been developed by observing how borderline clients interact over time in the therapeutic relationship itself. The second strength, in their view, is that psychoanalytic theories offer powerful conceptual tools for understanding and treating borderline clients. It is simply not clear to us on what basis they claim these two attributes as strengths. We know of no body of data that demonstrates that clinically derived theories are superior to other theories for understanding psychopathology. Behavioral and cognitive theories of psychopathology, derived largely from empirical psychology as opposed to clinical observation, certainly do not suffer when compared to psychoanalytic theories.

We also believe that a claim that psychoanalytic theory aids treatment of borderline clients is an empirical question yet to be addressed. Although experts differ on whether behavioral and cognitive theories and therapies are superior to psychoanalytic theory and therapy overall, no body of scientific research (as opposed to scientific discourse) makes the reverse argument—that psychoanalytic observation, theory, and treatment have led to better understanding or treatment of psychopathology, including that of BPD. Indeed, therapy for the disorder derived from behavioral and cognitive theory and practice, namely dialectical behavior therapy, is currently the only psychosocial treatment that has demonstrated effectiveness within a controlled treatment trial (Linehan, Armstrong, Suarez, Allmen, & Heard, 1991).

The points of synthesis here, as yet unmade but promising, are twofold. First, Linehan's treatment was derived from empirical, psychological research on personality functioning, as well as from a procedure that involved long-term observation of her treatment of several borderline clients. Thus, like psychoanalytic therapy, her behavioral theory and treatment of borderline disorder were based on long-term, clinical observation. Second, there may be considerable overlap between dialectical behavior therapy and the usual psychoanalytic therapies applied to borderline clients. Colleagues of both Kernberg and of Linehan have noted substantial similarities between Kernberg's and Linehan's treatment, in some respects, and between Adler and Buie's and Linehan's, in other respects.

We concur completely with Westen and Cohen's analyses of the weaknesses of psychoanalytic theory. Although in our view the authors have corrected some of the problems, a number of conceptual problems seem still unresolved.

DIMENSIONS OF SELF-STRUCTURE

Westen and Cohen's discussion of problems with self-definitions make some very good points, and we generally concur with these. We remain unclear, however, about what they themselves mean by many of their own terms, especially terms such as *unconsciousness self-representations, mental structures,* and *schemas.* The one operational definition they do present—that of self-concept as the abstract, verbalized representation of oneself that an individual provides when asked for a self-description—is very clear. Equally clear operational definitions of their other constructs are needed as well, however. Such operationalization is especially crucial when defining concepts concerning unconscious representations, since the authors propose this construct as a particularly important psychoanalytic contribution.

We are especially unclear about the rules for inferring "unconscious representations" from observations of verbal statements. How does one know when the context is responsible for the verbal shifts and when hypothetical, internal, and unconscious representations are responsible? We are not as prone as Westen and Cohen to attribute differences between self-report measures and other measures (such as physiological or observational) to biases in self-report. They suggest, for example, that borderline clients view themselves as evil and contaminating but do not report that view on standard inventories except under very particular circumstances. We would suggest that the tendency to represent oneself as evil and contaminating may indeed be linked with very particular circumstances; that is, how, when, and even whether one self-represents may itself be contextually linked, a proposition very different than saying that reports of self-representations are biased in particular contexts.

METHODOLOGIES FOR ASSESSING DIMENSIONS OF SELF-STRUCTURE

The interview procedure Westen and Cohen are piloting appears to be a procedure for eliciting and structuring clinical material from clients such that the material can be systematically observed and coded. Although their method may hold much promise, we are somewhat dismayed that the authors have not attended yet to whether they can *reliably* code the narratives. Without information on reliability, the pilot narratives presented here do not differ in principle from transcripts of clinical interactions used to illustrate theoretical points. We worry that readers may mistake the term *pilot data* to imply more than this.

REPRESENTATIONS

The rest of the chapter, and what we surmise is the substance of their own theoretical position, presents hypotheses and corresponding examples of self-representations that Westen and Cohen believe are important in Borderline Personality Disorder. We have several comments here.

Point 1: The authors state that "psychoanalytic views of BPD are characterized by their emphasis on the structural complexity and shifting patterns of self-representations in borderline patients" (p. 339). The statement implies that this is a strength, rather than a weakness, of psychoanalytic theories. Later, they note that self-representations are not themselves motivating, but then proceed to imply that self-representations can be motivating if there is sufficient affective "charge" associated with them and discrepancies among various self-representations. Just exactly how this motivation works, what determines affective "charge" and how it is measured, what the outcomes of this motivation are, and what the relationship of this motivation to borderline pathology is not at all clear in their presentation. We remain unclear about whether their theory posits that the motive to maintain certain self-respresentations causes or maintains that borderline pathology, borderline pathology causes certain self-representations, or both. In particular, it is not clear whether changing self-representations is viewed as important or not important in therapy. We believe that elucidating these points is essential, since they provide the main substance of the theory.

We agree with Westen and Cohen that psychodynamic theorists often inappropriately ascribe "motivational properties" or other causal explanations to these constructs. But assertions indicating motivation in the opposite direction—that is, statements that certain states or situations motivate individuals to represent themselves in certain ways—do appear. Although motivational factors may sometimes be important to how one self-represents, they do not have exclusive rights as actors in this creation. For example, Adler and Buie suggest a capability deficit model, while Westen and Cohen provide a variety of explanations for the etiology of self problems, including insufficiently dense "associational networks" and social learning. Still, in the review of traditional psychodynamic theories, motivational assertions appear without data to support them or alternative explanations to consider. For example, splitting is said to occur "in order to protect" certain representations. If one operationalizes splitting as a particular type of extreme, dichotomous thinking, we could also hypothesize that splitting is a behavior that normally and naturally occurs in response to stress, and that borderline individuals more frequently and intensely engage in this behavior because they more frequently experience stress. Testing such hypotheses against each other may allow for more effective treatment.

The problem occurs when theoreticians make unidirectional causal statements instead of proposing hypotheses when they lack the experimental data to support their statements. Fortunately, Westen and Cohen appear more sensitive to this issue than their predecessors, who assert that "the lack of internal, soothing representations leads borderline clients to feel intense loneliness and emptiness," (p. 337), and "a pervasive sense of emptiness also ensues as a result of the chaotic shifting of self and object representations" (p. 336).

At the other extreme from psychoanalysis, radical behaviorism asserts that the environment, and only the environment, causes behavior. We suspect that neither perspective—internal or external causality alone—will suffice clinically. Instead, a more balanced view may be necessary, positing that different forms of causal attribution (e.g., environmental, emotional, cognitive) are useful for different purposes and different levels of analyses.

Point 2: Westen and Cohen have a marked tendency to take verbal behavior of borderline clients and to make unquestioning (it seems to us) inferences about internal states and characteristics. For example, they suggest that when a hostile acting client asserts that the therapist is being hostile, this pattern gives evidence of a tendency to differentiate poorly between representations of self and of others. The alternate hypothesis is that the client's representations are influenced by therapist's responses to a hostile client. We would suggest that hostile clients are likely to evoke subtle, hostile responses from therapists, and subtly hostile therapists are likely to evoke overt hostile responses from borderline clients. It seems that one would have to conduct a very thorough behavioral analysis of the entire interaction sequence to rule out these hypotheses. In our experience, clients who describe hostility from the therapist are almost always reacting to subtle cues the therapist unknowingly emits.

The fact that we disagree with many of the authors' interpretations does not make them wrong and us right. Instead, it highlights the absolute necessity of operationally defining all constructs. We suspect that in order to obtain coding reliability, Westen and Cohen will be forced to create these behaviorally anchored definitions. Once accomplished, their work will represent a substantial advance in theoretical work on borderline pathology and offer an opportunity for collaborative research between cognitive, behavioral, and psychodynamic theorists.

Point 3: More generally, the main substance of the paper describes various hypotheses concerning the characteristics of borderline clients' self-representations, self-with-other representations, wished-for and feared self-representations, sense-of-self, and identity. These hypotheses appear to flow from the authors' analyses of pilot interactions with these clients while developing their assessment interview. As such, the hypotheses were derived in exactly the same manner as were the dialectical behavioral hypotheses we propose in our chapter: that is, both sets of hypotheses were generated from clinical contact and observation. Westen and Cohen seem to be a step ahead, however, because if their interview coding proves reliable, then they have a readily available method to test many of their descriptive theories. This represents a considerable advance over all previous psychoanalytic theories of borderline behavior. It is also an advance over our own theoretical positions since, to date, our research has focused more on treatment efficacy than on basic theoretical work.

POINTS NOT CONSIDERED: THE ENVIRONMENT

We find the brevity of focus on environmental influences disappointing. Westen and Cohen fail to discuss the reciprocal influences between the various components affecting self behaviors, such as between individual temperament and familial response to the individual. A transactional approach would suggest a poorness-of-fit model that does not *presuppose* that either the individual's temperament or the family's behavior are necessarily dysfunctional, but that their interaction can result in serious problems. Such a viewpoint provides an explanation that better maintains respect for those concerned and discourages the assignment of blame either to the individual or the family. Even though traditional psychodynamic theories, as summarized by Westen and Cohen, "pinpoint mother–toddler interactions," we cannot ignore the fact that a majority of borderline clients report histories of early sexual abuse, which, although rarely committed by the mother, we expect would have a critical effect on the development of self behaviors.

The second environmental issue concerns the limited scope of environment addressed by Westen and Cohen, which limits the discussion of environmental influences to the borderline individual's family. The culture defines self and expectations for self behaviors as much as psychologists and families do. Theoreticians must, therefore, expand their theorizing to consider the impact of the borderline individual's culture and any relevant subcultures. Not only will considering the cultural context enhance accuracy of theories of self behaviors in borderline personality disorders, it may also challenge traditional assumptions of which behaviors and whose behaviors (the borderline individual's or the community's) should be treated. Living within the culture, we easily forget that the culture subtly shapes our beliefs and attitudes and that what we often accept as facts are only assumptions of the culture. In our chapter we discuss at length the particular problem of idealizing independence and devaluing dependence.

The balance between individual and social influences on psychopathology for any individual case is not only an empirical question, it also concerns where one decides to place the magnifying glass on the interactions between individuals and their social milieu. Perhaps clinical theoreticians can serve the general community as well by correcting extremes on either side and encouraging movement toward a more stable balance.

CONCLUSION

We are impressed by the number of issues discussed by Westen and Cohen that are similar to those we address in our chapter. Many of the same points are made, albeit in different language and with different emphases. We would suggest that psychodynamic theory and research is slowly becoming more behavioral and scientific. We must acknowledge, however, that the theory and therapy described in our chapter expands upon the traditional behavioral theory and technique as well. It may be a credit to our borderline clients that their complexity and our difficulty in developing effective treatments for them has caused theorists to question some basic assumptions in traditional theory, researchers to design more complex scientific research, and clinicians to acknowledge the limitations of traditional therapy techniques. We have all been required to move beyond traditional boundaries and to learn from each other.

REFERENCES

Beck, A. T., & Freeman, A. (1990). *Cognitive therapy of personality disorders*. New York: Guilford Press.

Foa, E. B., & Emmelkamp, P. M. G. (1983). *Failures in behavior therapy*. New York: Wiley.

Linehan, M. M. (in press). *Cognitive–behavioral treatment of borderline personality disorder*. New York: Guilford Press.

Linehan, M. M., Armstrong, H. E., Suarez, A., Allmen, D., & Heard, H. L. (1991). Cognitive-behavioral treatment of chronically parasuicidal borderline patients. *Archives of General Psychiatry, 48*, 1060–1064

VI

Epilogue

11

The Self as a Vantage Point for Understanding Emotional Disorder

ZINDEL V. SEGAL
Clarke Institute of Psychiatry,
Unversity of Toronto

SIDNEY J. BLATT
Yale University

THE CHAPTERS AND commentaries in this book comprise an impressive array of scholarship on the question of self-representation and psychological distress and add to the growing literature on this topic (Curtis, 1991; Westen, 1992). Yet to fully appreciate some of the recurrent themes and assumptions being discussed, it is important to understand the larger context in which this work is situated.

Cognitive–behavior therapy has only recently focused on theorizing about the self and accordingly, has rarely incorporated the self into its models of specific disorders. There are instances where the issue of self-representation is addressed (Guidano, 1991; Mahoney, 1991; Safran & Segal, 1990; Segal & Kendall, 1990), though much of the theorizing remains at a fairly general level. Many cognitive–behavioral therapists would agree that modifying patients' perceptions of self is crucial in bringing about enduring psychological change, yet the field has not fully explored the transformation of this theory into therapeutic technique, partly because the theory is still not fully developed. Instead, cognitive–behavioral clinicians seem more inclined toward developing procedures and methods to evaluate various conceptualizations of the self. Although some of the chapters prepared by the psychodynamic theorists (e.g. Horowitz, Westen, Blatt, and their colleagues) actively consider issues of evaluation and assessment, the primary focus of these chapters are theoretical considerations of what is meant by the self, how it develops, and how, at times, it becomes distorted in particular ways and results in particular forms of psychopathology.

Thus, one of the primary differences between the cognitive–behavioral and psychodynamic chapters is the relative emphasis on measurement, evaluation, and experimental verification versus understanding the development of meaning systems of the self and the impact on personality development. Cognitive–behavioral theorists usually take a "bottom-up" approach and consider systematic, detailed, empirical verification as the starting point of theory building. The approach of the psychodynamic theorists, in contrast, is more usually a "top-down" construction of the details of individuals' lives and their development of meaning systems. Relevance and internal consistency of meaning systems are given priority over behavioral observations and empirical support.

The cognitive–behavioral theorist's requirement for accountability of constructs through empirical testing makes good sense when a domain is at a stage in its development that allows for a clear specification of the variables and procedures to be evaluated. Since the study of self processes has probably not yet reached this stage, some authors suggest that an emphasis on the development of assessment methods may be premature (Guidano, 1991; Mahoney, 1991; Safran, Segal, Hill, & Whiffen, 1990). In the absence of a theoretical foundation from which specific hypotheses connecting representations of the self and psychopathology can be framed, cognitive–behavioral theorists are concerned that testing uncompleted or partially complete formulations may be misleading and render an unnecessarily harsh verdict regarding the explanatory power of selfhood processes.

In contrast to the relative neglect of theoretical formulations about the self in the cognitive–behavioral chapters, the psychodynamic chapters present a rich theoretical base and argue for the centrality of the self in most forms of psychological disorder. This work has benefited from a longer history of inquiry, detailed clinical observations, and a view of the self as a fundamental developmental achievement. Yet even within this grouping of chapters there were differences among the authors about how the self develops and how it is represented later in life. Some of these differences may be resolved by the extensive recent research on developmental processes particularly directed to understanding subtle dimensions of mother–child interaction (Stern, 1985; Tronick, 1989) and attachment patterns (Bowlby, 1969; Main, 1983) throughout the early months and years of life.

Perhaps one way to reconcile the hermeneutic thrust of the psychodynamic chapters with the cognitive–behavioral stance of experimentation is to adopt a common language so that concepts can be better understood in theory and applied with greater fidelity in practice. Representatives of differing therapy constituencies (Goldfried, 1991; Horowitz, 1991), for example, have suggested that translating clinical concepts into information processing terms would serve this purpose. In fact, when we consider the chapters by McNally and Eells et al. there is a good deal of convergence in the processes being discussed, precisely because of their joint reliance on a parlance derived from cognitive psychology. For the opposite extreme, one need only examine the veritable chasm separating the two chapters in the section on eating disorders.

SOME THOUGHTS ON FUTURE DIRECTIONS

If the material presented in this book is to be of some consequence for the treatment of emotional disorder, it would seem incumbent upon us to speak practically about whether and how a clinical orientation informed by the self is advantageous. Pathology of the self is often recognized in patients with an extremely brittle view of themselves, a fragmentation in identity such that there seems be a rivalry among self-views, or a vulnerability to loss of self-esteem (Bednar, Wells, & Peterson, 1989; Kohut, 1977; Masterson, 1985). Responding to this, treatments have sought to "repair" self-distortions through provision of a therapeutic relationship that allows for considering these distortions in a context in which the patient can begin to revise his/her sense of self and form new generalizations about him/herself. What we are describing is a generic context, potentially available in most forms of therapy.

Whether one uses cognitive therapy to explore the consequences of self-referent information processing, or traces the developmental trajectory of repetitive maladaptive behaviors in psychodynamic therapy, the attempt in both cases is to allow for revisions of distortions and/or to bolster or build up a self that is fundamentally lacking in important qualities. The goal of these approaches is to enable the individual to recognize both the antecedents and consequences of self-distortions, with the goal of revising them and preventing further distortions and/or fragmentation and to reverse this destructive process (Blatt & Maroudas, 1992). Cognitive–behavioral therapists seek to facilitate this process through the development of self-based resources previously lacking, whereas psychodynamic therapists seek to provide a context in which the self-distortions are expressed in the transference. Procedures such as monitoring automatic thoughts, skills training, empathic listening, mirroring, and identifying conditions of worth in dysfunctional assumptions, or appreciating developmental antecedents, can be considered as attempts to increase the resources that the self can draw upon in the process of its redefinition in therapy. The important point, however, is that the direction of redefinition is usually toward levels of greater self-complexity, unity, and resilience. Most clinicians would agree that changes of this nature, at post-treatment, would predict a positive therapy outcome.

While we would expect these elements to be valid for a variety of therapeutic approaches, it is also clear to us that our dialogue, up to this point, has been framed within the fairly well defined boundaries of our two respective traditions. Future work on the self may broaden this discussion by moving beyond cognitive–behavioral and psychodynamic perspectives and considering approaches that pursue the *dismantling* of the self as an optimal therapeutic strategy, rather than working at helping patients to develop stronger self-representations. It would seem important to understand the essence of such alternative views, since they advocate precisely the opposite actions, to those outlined above, in order to achieve the common goal of reducing emotional distress. Although a comprehensive analysis of these approaches is beyond the scope of this book, a brief examination of their operative assumptions may be helpful.

Informed by Buddhist and constructivist epistemologies that forcefully reject the notion of the self and, by implication, therapies that focus on the elaboration of adaptive self-representations as being privileged in understanding emotional difficulties, these approaches work to *weaken* a person's sense of self. This is often accomplished by challenges to the individual's model of what a self is and how the idea of a self is defined by the boundaries of the body (inside is me/outside is not me) and by autonomous (rather than relational) dimensions which contribute to a segmentation of ongoing experience into essentially arbitrary categories such as my self, my body, my property (Claxton, 1986; 1987; Cushman, 1990; Varela, Thompson, & Rosch, 1991; Wellwood, 1983). Reliance on these categories of perception limits a person's ability to see new options or ways of thinking and is especially problematic in clinical disorders, since viewing the world through these seemingly rigid perceptual categories may end up contributing to the perpetuation of negative emotional states and thereby feed the very problem one is trying to solve.

> Having identified my self as separate and bounded, as persisting in essence through space and time, and at least partially autonomous in thought and action, I have adopted a stance towards life which make unintended, unanticipated change anathema. By confirming my self within the limits of a body, I have conferred on what lies outside the power to threaten "me." By insisting on consistency, I make a hard shell of a self-image for myself that restricts growth and change. (Claxton, 1987, pp. 32–33)

As illustrated in this quote, interventions that promote the dissolution of self-identity are favored by this perspective, since the process of "self-dismantling" can serve a cleansing function for the patient and allow subsequent perception to fall more in line with the nature of reality. The most common techniques employed to get patients to observe (and ultimately challenge) the model of the self that they hold are simple meditation or contemplation exercises in which they are instructed merely to observe the ebb and flow of their thoughts, and the reactions that stem from trying to do so. Ideally, symptom relief is associated with a view of life that is less fettered by perceptual "mistakes" such as the interpretation of ongoing experience through the essentially arbitrary categories of my self, my body, or my property. As a result, patients are less likely to become emotionally devastated by ever-present change in life, exemplified in such occurrences as loss, death, grief, and suffering (Claxton, 1986, 1987; Varela et al., 1991; Wellwood, 1983).

Whichever of the above-mentioned views one chooses to endorse, it seems clear that the self still occupies center stage in our discussion. In any case, to work toward strengthening or weakening a patient's view of him/herself results in a perturbation of a preexisting cognitive structure. Perhaps this is the overarching point to be made, namely, that procedures are successful only in terms of the degree to which such representations are disrupted and subsequently revised.

CONCLUSIONS

As is apparent from the chapters in this volume, the cognitive–behavioral and psychodynamic clinician and investigator addresses different questions, uses very different observational techniques, and establishes very different data to address questions about the nature, etiology, and treatment of various forms of psychopathology. Each orientation has its advantages and its limitations, and yet each has the potential for making important contributions to understanding adaptive and maladaptive functioning. As cognitive–behavioral investigators become interested in more elusive phenomena such as affects, interpersonal relations, and cognitions not in direct awareness, they may find some of the concepts, techniques, and methodologies developed by psychodynamic investigators extremely valuable. And likewise, psychodynamic investigators and clinicians may find of considerable value the techniques developed by cognitive–behavioral clinicians and investigators for identifying salient activating aspects of current cognitive schemas and how they interact with contemporary life events (Blatt & Madouras, 1992).

Careful evaluation of the wide range of findings within the cognitive–behavioral and psychodynamic orientations may allow us to establish linkages that integrate particular typologies of current modes of adaptation with particular types of early life experiences. The integration of the data from these two orientations may provide the basis for the integration of early life experiences so that we may fully appreciate the continuity and organization of cognitive structures and functional systems—how they develop and are maintained, and how we might develop more effective modes of intervention. It might even be possible to conceptualize a treatment process in which different modes of intervention might be more effective at different points or stages in the treatment process.

By choosing to study self-representation as we have done, we have discovered that simple contrasts are not capable of containing the complexities we seek to describe. In one sense we have carved up the self into these contrasts for purposes of comparison. We hope that future clinicians and clinical investigators will be able to develop a more integrated view of this central psychological process and that this work will continue to grow and develop, and eventually go beyond the understanding achieved by the contributions made to this volume.

REFERENCES

Bednar, R. L., Wells, M. G., & Peterson, S. R. (1989). *Self-esteem: Paradoxes and innovations in clinical theory and practice*. Washington, DC: American Psychological Association Press.

Blatt, S. J., & Maroudas, C. (1992). Convergences of psychodynamic and cognitive-behavioral theories of depression. *Psychoanalytic Psychology, 9,* 157–190.

Bowlby, J. (1969). *Attachment and loss*. New York: Basic Books.

Claxton, G. (1986). *Beyond therapy: The impact of eastern religions on psychological theory and practice*. London: Wisdom Publications.

Claxton, G. (1987). Meditation in Buddhist psychology. In M. A. West (Ed.), *The psychology of meditation*. Oxford: Clarendon Press.

Curtis, R. C. (1991). *The relational self: Theoretical convergences in psychoanalysis and social psychology*. New York: Guilford Press.

Cushman, P. (1990). Why the self is empty? *American Psychologist*, *45*, 599–611.

Goldfried. M. R. (1991). Research issues in psychotherapy integration. *Journal of Psychotherapy Integration*, *1*, 5–25.

Guidano, V. F. (1991). *The self in process*. New York: Guilford Press.

Horowitz, M. J. (1991). *Person schemas and maladaptive interpersonal patterns*. Chicago: University of Chicago Press.

Kohut, H. (1977). *How does analysis cure*? New York: International Universities Press.

Mahoney, M. J. (1991). Representations of self in cognitive psychotherapies. *Cognitive Therapy and Research*, *14*, 229–240.

Main, M. (1983). Exploration, play, and cognitive functioning related to infant-mother attachment. *Infant Behaviour and Development*, *6*, 167–174.

Masterson, J. F. (1985). *The real self: A developmental, self and object relations approach*. New York: Brunner/Mazel.

Safran J. D., & Segal, Z. V. (1990). *Interpersonal process in cognitive therapy*. New York: Basic Books.

Safran, J. D., Segal, Z. V., Hill, C., & Whiffen, V. (1990). Refining strategies for research on self-representations in emotional disorders. *Cognitive Therapy and Research*, *14*, 143–160.

Segal, Z. V., & Kendall, P. C. (1990). Selfhood processes and emotional disorders. *Cognitive Therapy and Research*, *14*, 111–112.

Stern, D. N. (1985). *The interpersonal world of the infant*. New York: Basic Books.

Tronick, E. Z. (1989). Emotions and emotional communication in infants. *American Psychologist*, *44*, 112–119.

Varela, F. J., Thompson, E., & Rosch, E. (1991). *The embodied mind: Cognitive science and human experience*. Boston: MIT Press.

Wellwood, J. (1983). *Awakening the heart: East/west approaches to psychotherapy and the healing relationship*. Boston: New Science Library.

Westen, D. (1992). The cognitive self and the psychoanalytic self: Can we put our selves together? *Psychological Inquiry*, *3*, 1–13.

Index

n. indicates that name will be found in the reference list